YOUR PRIVATE PARTS SHOULDN'T BE PRIVATE TO YOU

Being comfortable with your body is not a matter of modesty—it's a matter of good health. For the first time, women have all the information they need in *The V Book,* ensuring the best possible vulvovaginal health, now and in the future.

Dr. Elizabeth G. Stewart answers these common questions and many more in *The V Book:*

▼ How does a woman's V health change throughout her lifetime?

▼ How do you know when you have a simple infection—or a more serious condition?

▼ Which over-the-counter treatments work or should you always call your doctor?

▼ What really happens during a Pap smear?

▼ Why aren't speculums heated?

▼ If sex hurts, what do I do?

▼ Does cranberry juice really help prevent urinary tract infections?

▼ Can yogurt cure a yeast infection?

▼ Are there simple solutions to embarrassing problems such as odor and itching?

▼ Why is it important to see a gynecologist even after menopause?

▼ What questions should you *always* ask your gynecologist?

▼ And much, much more.

The V Book

A Doctor's Guide to Complete Vulvovaginal Health

Elizabeth Gunther Stewart, M.D.
and Paula Spencer

Illustrations by Dawn Danby and Paul Waggoner

BANTAM BOOKS

New York   Toronto   London   Sydney   Auckland

THE V BOOK

PUBLISHING HISTORY
Bantam trade paperback / July 2002

Grateful acknowledgment is given for permission to reprint from the following:
DILBERT © United Features Syndicate. Reprinted by permission.
Helen Gurley Brown from "Don't Give Up on Sex After 60," *Newsweek,* May 29.
Copyright © 2000 Newsweek, Inc. All rights reserved. Reprinted by permission.
Susie Bright from "Sex Education," which first appeared as a column on
Salon.com on March 19, 1999. Reprinted by permission.
The Period Book, Copyright © 1996, used by permission of Walker & Company,
435 Hudson Street, New York, NY 10014
Photos on pages 280, 284, 291, and 367 are reproduced from:
Kaufman, *Benign Diseases of the Vulva and Vagina,* 3/e, Mosby 1989, figs 6-30,
8-5, 9-2, 9-5. Reprinted by permission.
Figure 34 on page 207 is reproduced from "Allergic Predisposition in
Recurrent Vulvovaginal Candidiasis" by Marjorie Crandall, Ph.D.,
Journal of Advancement in Medicine, 4: 21–38 (1991). Reprinted by permission.
For more information go to www.yeastconsulting.com.

Book design by Ark Design

Library of Congress Cataloging-in-Publication Data
Stewart, Elizabeth Gunther.
The V book : a doctor's guide to complete vulvovaginal health /
by Elizabeth Gunther Stewart and Paula Spencer.
p.   cm.
Includes bibliographical references and index.
ISBN 0-553-38114-8
1. Vagina. 2. Vagina—Diseases. 3. Vagina—Care and hygiene.
4. Generative organs, Female—Examination. 5. Women—
Health and hygiene.   I. Spencer, Paula. II. Title.
RG268 .S74 2002
618.1'5—dc21   2001056611

Published simultaneously in the United States and Canada

PRINTED IN THE UNITED STATES OF AMERICA
RRH   10 9 8 7 6 5 4

Disclaimer

The information in this book is designed to supplement, not substitute for, the advice of a trained medical professional. This book should not be used as a manual for self-diagnosis or self-treatment. Matters regarding vulvovaginal care often require medical supervision. Readers are strongly recommended to consult with a clinician before starting any medical treatment, diet, exercise, or other health program. The authors and publisher disclaim liability arising directly or indirectly from the use or application of this book.

For Donald, with heartfelt thanks.

Your unconditional support for all my projects has helped other women as I became first gynecologist, then V specialist, and now *V Book* author.

—E.G.S.

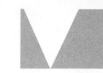

Table of Contents

Acknowledgments   xv

Foreword   xvii

Introduction   xix

PART I   **AN OWNER'S MANUAL**   I

Chapter I   **THE MIND:**
Why V health starts here **3**
     A short history of the Vs ▼ The power of positive thinking

Chapter 2   **THE VULVA:**
A road map to the external genitalia **17**
     Learning what's what ▼ Vulvar self-exam
     PLUS: Labial Enhancement

Chapter 3   **THE VAGINA:**
Demystifying the amazing "secret" organ **41**
     V is for versatile ▼ What's where ▼ A design marvel
     Vaginal secretions ▼ The all-important V bacteria
     So what's "normal" discharge?
     PLUS: Kegels, the Essential Inner Exercise; The G-Spot: Fact
     or Fiction?; Normal Bacteria in a Healthy Vagina

Chapter 4   **AT DIFFERENT AGES:**
V changes throughout the life cycle **61**
     Prenatal and newborn ▼ Childhood ▼ Puberty and
     reproductive years ▼ Pregnancy and postpartum

Perimenopause ▼ Menopause ▼ A controversial rite
of passage
PLUS: Common Questions: Newborn, Childhood, Puberty,
Pregnancy, Perimenopausal Symptoms; Common Questions:
Menopause

Chapter 5   V SMARTS:
Everyday habits that make a difference.................. 81

Tampons ▼ Pads ▼ Panty liners ▼ Alternative protection
Underwear ▼ Douching ▼ Hair removal ▼ Other V styles
PLUS: The Heart of V Health: Ten Rules to Remember;
Tampon Absorbency; More Tampon Dangers to Discount;
Guilty or Not Guilty? The Truth About Common Tampon
Concerns; Does Your Tampon Feel Right?; Instead of Douching

Chapter 6   SEX MATTERS:
V health facts for sexually active women 109

First, desire ▼ Stage 1: excitement (arousal) ▼ Stage 2:
plateau ▼ Stage 3: orgasm ▼ Stage 4: resolution
Masturbation and V health ▼ Passion's pests ▼ Safer sex
Birth control and V health
PLUS: Lubricant Lowdown; Do Women Ejaculate?;
Vibrating with Care; At-a-Glance Guide to STDs;
Contraception and V Considerations

PART II   WHEN YOU NEED HELP 131

Chapter 7   THE MOST BOTHERSOME SYMPTOMS:
Possible causes and cures 133

Odor ▼ Itching ▼ Unusual discharge ▼ Dryness
PLUS: Odors That Talk; Itch Relief Dos and Don'ts; Common
Vulvar Irritants and Allergens

Chapter 8   NOW WHAT?
How to proceed when there's trouble 151

Why you can't tell by looking ▼ Evaluating your symptoms
Why telephone diagnosis doesn't work ▼ Which doctor to see
PLUS: Warning Signs Not to Ignore; Don't Believe These
Medical Myths

Chapter 9   **THE IDEAL V EXAM:**
What to say, what to expect, and a guide to tests 159

Why timing is everything ▼ The vulvovaginal history
The pelvic exam ▼ Three important in-office tests
Other testing methods ▼ Vulvar biopsy ▼ The Pap test
PLUS: How to Talk to Your Gyn; Nagging Little Questions
About Pelvic Exams; The Silent STDs Worth a Routine Test;
Common Questions: Pap tests; All About AGUS;
The First V Exam

PART III   **PROBLEM AND ANSWER GUIDE** 189

Chapter 10   **YEAST INFECTIONS:**
Separating the truths from the popular beliefs 191

What is yeast? ▼ Symptoms of a yeast infection
What causes yeast? ▼ Diagnosing a yeast infection
Self-diagnosing a yeast infection ▼ A yeast infection
action plan ▼ Steps to controlling recurrent yeast
Complicated yeast
PLUS: For Immediate Relief; Are You at Risk?; Common
Questions: Sex and yeast; Can Yogurt Prevent Yeast
Infections?; Common Questions: OTC yeast treatments;
Natural Remedies; Simple Yeast or Complex Yeast?; Is There a
Yeast Hideout?

Chapter 11   **BV:**
The leading cause of vaginal complaints 219

What is Bacterial Vaginosis (BV)? ▼ What causes BV?
Why treatment is important ▼ Diagnosing BV
Treating BV ▼ When BV recurs
PLUS: Is It Yeast or BV?; Treatments for Bacterial Vaginosis

Chapter 12   **TRICH:**
The STD that causes vaginitis 229

What is trich? ▼ Diagnosing trich ▼ Treating trich
Treating resistant cases
PLUS: When a Pap Smear Finds Trich

Chapter 13   VAG ITCH, CONTINUED:
Lesser-known sources of vaginitis 237

> The estrogen-loss vaginitis: atrophic vaginitis
> Strep vaginitis ▼ Mobiluncus vaginitis
> The mystery vaginitis: desquamative inflammatory vaginitis (DIV)
> The discounted problem: lactobacillus overgrowth
> **PLUS:** A Mobiluncus Success Story; A DIV Success Story

Chapter 14   COULD YOU BE ALLERGIC?
Surprising irritants that trigger the body to attack 247

> What is allergy? ▼ Allergy to semen ▼ Other V allergies
> Allergy to latex
> **PLUS:** A Semen Allergy Success Story; The Mystery Allergy:
> Hives

Chapter 15   WHEN SKIN GETS SICK:
The vulva sees these skin conditions too 255

> What to know about cortisone ▼ Eczema/dermatitis/lichen
> simplex chronicus (LSC) ▼ Lichen sclerosus (LS)
> Psoriasis ▼ Lichen planus (LP) ▼ Hidradenitis
> suppurativa (HS)
> **PLUS:** Steroid Safety; The Leading Vulvar Irritants; Handle with
> Care: Hygiene Help for Women with Vulvar Skin Disease;
> LS Success Stories; An LP Success Story; Detecting HS Early

Chapter 16   V BUMPS AND COLOR CHANGES:
Should you be alarmed? Usually not 279

> Common small bumps ▼ Less common small bumps
> Really rare small bumps ▼ Common large bumps
> Uncommon large bumps ▼ Conditions with a red color
> Conditions with a white color ▼ Common dark
> discolorations ▼ Rare dark discolorations ▼ Ulcers

Chapter 17   "IT HURTS":
New insights into the V pain syndrome vulvodynia 297

> Pain theory ▼ Vestibulodynia (VBD) ▼ Vulvodynia (VVD)
> **PLUS:** Ask Yourself: Clues to Vestibulodynia; What to Rule Out
> First; The Q-tip Test; High-Oxalate Foods to Avoid; Tricyclic
> Antidepressants and Their Side Effects; Don't Let Side Effects
> Stop You!; Common Questions: Vestibulectomy; A VBD
> Success Story; A Vulvodynia Success Story

Chapter 18   **SEXUAL HEALING:**
              Help for coping with painful intercourse **329**

              Causes of painful sex ▼ The downward spiral
              The partner's pain ▼ A coping plan ▼ Pregnancy and
              vulvodynia ▼ Vaginismus ▼ A word about Viagra and friends
              PLUS: Common Questions: Vulvodynia and Sex;
              Sex Pain and the Single Woman; The Clitoris's New
              Best Friend?

Chapter 19   **BLADDER PAIN:**
              Feeling the burn that could be UTI or IC **347**

              What is a urinary tract infection (UTI)? ▼ Interstitial
              cystitis (IC)
              PLUS: It's Back! Which Kind of UTI Is It?; Treatment Courses
              for Bladder Infection; What About Cranberry Juice?; Three
              Urinary Problems That Aren't Infections; A Promising New Test;
              Avoid These Foods If You Have IC

Chapter 20   **THE LIFETIME VIRUS:**
              Living with genital herpes **365**

              How herpes works ▼ The big question ▼ What symptoms
              are like ▼ Getting a diagnosis ▼ Treating first infections
              Treating recurrent infections ▼ A special case: herpes
              and pregnancy
              PLUS: A Herpes Success Story; The Bottom Line If You
              Have Herpes; The Bottom Line If You *Don't* Have Herpes

Chapter 21   **THE CRAFTY VIRUS:**
              HPV causes warts, abnormal Paps, cervical cancer—
              and nothing **379**

              Warts from HPV ▼ Diagnosing warts ▼ Treating warts
              HPV and Pap smears ▼ HPV and cervical precancer (CIN)
              Treating CIN
              PLUS: Risk Factors for HPV; Treatments That Destroy or
              Remove Warts; A Genital Warts Success Story; New HPV
              Testing; You're More Likely to Develop CIN If . . . ; An HPV
              Success Story; The Last Word: Be HPV-Savvy

Chapter 22   **V CANCER AND PRECANCER:**
Reassuring facts about uncommon conditions 397

       Vulvar precancer (VIN) ▼ Younger VIN, older VIN
       Diagnosing VIN ▼ Vulvar cancer ▼ Paget's disease
       Vaginal precancer (VAIN) ▼ Vaginal cancer
       PLUS: Pregnancy and VIN; If You've Been Exposed to DES

Chapter 23   **V IS FOR VOICE:**
Some parting thoughts 409

       What I want you to do ▼ Advancing V care

Resources 415

Journal Abbreviations 423

Notes 425

Index 449

Acknowledgments

he V Book **would still be a twinkle in my eye** were it not
for all these people I'd like to thank. Dr. Liz Buechler shared my
vision for a V service at Harvard Vanguard Medical Associates
and has given it her unqualified support. Dr. Marcie Richardson has encouraged me all along the way. Through her suggestions, I found my
agent and ultimately my publisher. She took a weekend out of her life
to read the entire book and offer her suggestions. Dr. Susan Haas has
been a zealot on my behalf, Dr. Robert Barbieri a real friend in camp.
My partner, Diana Parks-Forbes, reinforced my effort to provide this
book for women, has edited chapters and buffed me at every opportunity. My physician colleagues at Vanguard covered for me while I went
for a month of V precepting to start on my way to V specialization in
1990. They, as well as our nurse-practitioners and nurse-midwives, have
enthusiastically supported the V service. The staff and nurses of the
Stewart-Forbes service run the blue-ribbon operation from which I
learned much of what I have written.

Dr. Ray Kaufman and Dr. Stanley Marinoff have my gratitude for sharing their V practices with me as I learned the ropes. The basics they
taught me form a framework on which I built the book. Dr. Lynette
Margesson, vulvar dermatologist par excellence, has generously shared
her expertise regarding V skin issues discussed in the book. I am grateful
also to Dawn Danby, who created the beautiful and anatomically perfect
V illustrations.

Special thanks go to Paula Spencer, whose literary wand transformed my
medical writing rags into a ballgown for public debut. Her imaginative V
notes sequin the pages and her fascinating tidbits of information sparkle
everywhere. Her efforts have truly dressed *The V Book* for the affair.

My entire family has been marvelous in their support of another one of
Elizabeth's Good Ideas. Don—my mentor, manager, consultant, computer
whiz, and cheerleader extraordinaire—is always happy to see women
move forward, and has aided my efforts with unbridled enthusiasm.

The book would not exist without my agent, Loretta Weingel-Fidel,
and my editor at Bantam, Robin Michaelson. It was a pleasure to work
with such experts in their fields. And bouquets to Stacie Fine, who
pulled it all together.

Finally, I thank my patients, who continue to teach and inspire me. They encouraged my writing by declaring that they would crawl if necessary to the bookstore to obtain a copy of such a book as this. They graciously agreed to be included in its pages. Through these women, the twinkle turned into fireworks.

Foreword

F **or centuries a peculiar feature of our society** has been to veil the vulva and vagina in mystery. Women would only speak of the places "down there" with muted voices and eyes lowered. Millions of women suffer from vulvar and vaginal problems, such as constant itching, interminable discharge, and pain with sexual activity. Yet most have been given the worst possible diagnosis: "It's all in your head."

That's why *The V Book* is the right book at the right time, written by the right clinician. Knowledge about and comfort with one's body, including the genitalia, is vital to maintaining good health. This book lifts the veil of secrecy and provides women with an important first step to understanding their bodies and finding relief from their symptoms. Each chapter is thorough, entertaining, accessible, and easy to understand.

Dr. Stewart is the right clinician to help advance our understanding of the health and problems of the vulva and vagina. Having dedicated her professional life to the study of vulvovaginal health, Dr. Stewart's commitment to reducing women's suffering and embarrassment resonates throughout these pages. Her training and experience as a nurse, physician, and gynecologist—hence the term *clinician*—means she has insight into the cultural context and personal meaning of health and disease as well as a deep understanding of the body's biological mechanisms. She is also a wonderful teacher of how to improve our health.

Now is the time to end misguided and dangerous notions about vulvovaginal health. Thanks to Dr. Stewart's expertise and the straightforward information she provides in *The V Book,* she teaches women of all ages to improve their vulvovaginal health. I highly recommend *The V Book* for all women and all clinicians who care for women.

—Robert L. Barbieri, M.D., Chairman,
Department of Obstetrics and Gynecology,
Brigham and Women's Hospital and Harvard
Medical School, and Kate Macy Ladd Professor
of Obstetrics, Gynecology and Reproductive
Biology, Harvard Medical School

Introduction

Ready for a pop quiz like you've never taken before? Here goes:

1. Are you comfortable saying the word *vagina* out loud to your doctor?
2. What's safer in the bikini zone—shaving, waxing, depilatories, or electrolysis?
3. What should you do if a tampon or condom gets "lost" inside you?
4. Why is it normal for sex to hurt sometimes?
5. Do you know where your vestibule is?

Now let's see how you did:

1. The right answer is yes, though it's a rare woman who doesn't feel a little odd about doing so. Funny how we don't feel that way about *elbow* or *toes*.
2. They all have relative pros and cons—be sure you know what they are, and proceed with caution!
3. "Panic" is *not* the right answer. Thanks to its pouchlike shape, nothing's ever gotten lost in the vagina. The key is to be patient and to relax your body as you try to retrieve the AWOL item.
4. That's a trick question. It's *never* normal for sex to hurt. Not when you're in your teens, twenties, thirties, or forties, or in menopause. Yet many women endure vaginal pain that interferes with intercourse and, tragically, are unable to find help for this prevalent problem.
5. I know, I know. You're probably thinking, *I've never even heard of my vestibule!* You've seen it if you've done a vulvar self-exam—but then, who does vulvar self-exams? Even women who religiously do breast exams skip over this useful health basic.

It's surprising how much we women don't know about our own bodies—especially the parts that make us uniquely female. Then again, it's understandable, given that the vulva and vagina are hidden "down there" below layers of pants, panty hose, underwear, and panty liners. The Vs have been kept out of sight metaphorically too, by myths, cultural taboos, and for a long time, a lack of medical interest. Unfortunately, unseen means undiscussed, unappreciated, and ultimately, misunderstood!

The vulva, vestibule, and vagina are body parts, just like the arm or leg or breast. They needn't be unmentionable. Yet we often associate these parts with the realm of the untouchable or dirty. We feel embarrassment over something that should not be embarrassing in the least, particularly in the presence of a doctor. Or we don't think about them at all until a problem crops up, and then we aren't sure what to do about it. Here we are at a time when interest in women's health is soaring, when women have become active participants in their health care, yet the most female parts of our anatomies are still relegated to hushed tones and euphemisms.

I wrote this book because it makes me sad that so many women are unfamiliar with their bodies. I want women everywhere to be informed about—no, to be dazzled by—the parts of our anatomy that represent the beauty of womanhood, the miracle of reproduction, and the joy of sexual function.

I also wrote this book because I desperately want to help the women who make up my typical day as a vulvovaginal specialist, an expert in the care of the vulva and vagina. The following three patients from a recent day are all too typical. There's Susan, who jumps to her feet as I enter the room. (All of the names and identifying details used throughout the book have been changed to protect the confidentiality of my patients.) "Boy, am I glad to see you, Dr. Stewart! This itching is driving me crazy! I keep thinking it will just go away, but it doesn't. I know you aren't supposed to scratch, and I'm good all day. At night, though, the itch wakes me up, and I can't help myself!"

In another room, Ingrid tells me her long story of her inability to have intercourse without pain. "You've got to help me, Dr. Stewart," she sobs. "I'm getting married in a few months!"

Annette's problem—she's certain—is just a bad yeast infection. She's surprised when tests confirm it's something else. She asks, "Is that why the cream I bought at the drugstore didn't work?" (You'd be amazed how often over-the-counter yeast treatments don't work because the woman has a different problem.)

By day's end I will have seen twenty such patients; in a year, thousands. They come with their partners, their mothers, their girlfriends, or just their problems. They bring sheaves of medical records. I learn about itching that persists for weeks, years, even decades. I hear complaints of annoying discharge, dryness, and odor. I see women whose problems make them feel unfeminine or ugly, women who have trouble even talking about what's wrong. Not a day goes by that I don't see someone suffering from perhaps the worst pain of all—being told "It's all in your head."

▼ ▼ ▼

I bring twenty-one years of gynecology, twelve of V specialization, to the exam room and to these pages. That makes me something of a pioneer. Vulvovaginal care is an undeveloped field. It lags behind other aspects of gynecology such as fertility, breast care, or menopause in the amount of medical training and research being done. Clinicians who help women with V problems have a hard time keeping current. Sadly, even good care providers remain stuck on outdated practices that can make conditions worse. And the current era of managed care means that many women first see a generalist, whose vulvovaginal training is even scantier than an ob-gyn's.

If medical professionals don't know this material well, who can blame women for being left in the dark? Reliable information is as scarce as a woman who can say the word *vulva* without a hint of embarrassment. Good luck finding clear anatomical diagrams outside medical textbooks; the cross section of the pelvis on the tampon box insert isn't much help. Mothers may talk to their daughters about their periods or even birth control, but descriptions of what's normal vaginal discharge usually don't come up. Friends don't compare notes about painful intercourse.

So women put up with dryness or itching because they don't think it can be successfully treated, or they write off such symptoms as inevitable aspects of getting older. Postmenopausal women, especially, may be embarrassed about discussing intimate problems with a stranger, particularly when that medical professional is a younger male. Reticence isn't just an American hang-up: Even in Denmark, a country thought of as very open about sexuality, researchers trying to interview women on vaginal matters found them almost too modest to give straight answers. Yet women deserve, and need, the same comfort level about their genitalia, and the same easy access to information, that they have about their reproductive health or any other aspect of their health.

▼ ▼ ▼

My patients are often relieved to discover that someone like me exists: "I didn't know that there was such a thing as a v-v-vul—you know, vagina doctor!" Well, there aren't many. My career started more conventionally. I attended nursing school and then, as the youngest of my three children approached kindergarten, medical school. I specialized in obstetrics and gynecology because I had a strong interest in women's health and because, having been a childbirth educator in the 1970s, I wanted to improve the way women in labor were treated.

But as rewarding as it was to help women give birth to healthy babies, I felt keen empathy for the women who came in with nonobstetric problems. I saw women who had gone from physician to physician for the right diagnosis, only to discover that a few simple tests might have led them to earlier relief. I enjoyed the detective work involved in treating tough cases—tough because the vagina and vulva have been studied far less than other female organs such as the breasts, the ovaries, or the uterus. Soon more and more vulvar cases in my medical group were being referred to me.

I realized I could fill a growing need. In 1990, I started a vulvovaginal service within a large multispecialty medical group after showing the practice's administration that the average woman who came in for a consultation about a vulvovaginal problem had seen more than five other clinicians and had filled ten prescriptions! Nationwide, there are more than ten million office visits a year for vulvovaginal complaints. A suspected vaginal infection is the most common reason a woman visits her gynecologist. Three-quarters of all women get a yeast infection at some point in their lives, for example. Another type of vaginal infection, bacterial vaginosis, is diagnosed more often each year than yeast, although a recent Gallup poll showed that only 34 percent of American women had ever heard of it. Thousands of tubes of cream or antibiotic pills are handed out each year without a clear diagnosis.[1] I decided there was a real need for someone who could handle both routine V problems and the tough cases that left other doctors baffled.

Almost overnight, I was flooded with business.

▼ ▼ ▼

This is not a gynecological sourcebook. That information is plentiful elsewhere. Like my practice, *The V Book* focuses specifically on vulvovaginal matters: the latest research translated into understandable explanations, combined with my experience, the insight of my colleagues, and a framework that aims to make this knowledge both accessible and interesting.

The V Book is divided into three parts: what to know and do when you're well, what to know and do when you develop a problem, and an in-depth guide to specific problems and their treatments.

Part I, "An Owner's Manual," starts far away from the V zone—in your head. In order to feel more comfortable reading about the vulva and vagina, let alone talk about them with your clinician or anyone else, it's useful to understand why this is such a difficult topic for most women in the first place. Chapter 1, "The Mind," walks you through the history of the vulva and vagina, from celebration to confusion to a whole lot of blushing.

Chapter 2, "The Vulva," and Chapter 3, "The Vagina," are perhaps the most important of all, taking you on an eye-opening walk through V anatomy. Because the Vs are anything but static organs, Chapter 4, "At Different Ages," explores how this anatomy changes, from before birth to the menopause. Once you understand what's what, you're ready to learn how to keep everything healthy (Chapter 5, "V Smarts"). That includes everything that comes into contact with the area, from tampons and pads to underclothes, soaps, feminine-hygiene products, even hot wax and razor blades for hair removal. Finally, because sexual function is a primary feature of these organs, I've given it a separate chapter (Chapter 6, "Sex Matters").

Part II, "When You Need Help," is a handy reference for the inevitable times when things don't feel right. (Though it's a good idea to read it over when you're feeling perfectly fine!) Chapter 7, "The Most Bothersome Symptoms," maps out exactly what its title implies: what causes odor, itching, unusual discharge, and dryness, and what you should know about these oh-so-common conditions. Chapter 8, "Now What?," is designed to help you decide how to proceed with self-care or a medical appointment when symptoms develop. I explain why you can't get a good diagnosis over the phone and how to find a good V clinician.

You'll notice throughout the book that I use the word *clinician* instead of doctor. That's because physician's assistants (PAs), certified nurse-practitioners (CNPs), and certified nurse-midwives (CNMs) do an amazing job caring for women. A woman often sees a PA or CNP instead of or in addition to a physician for vulvovaginal care. *Clinician* is therefore a more accurate, all-inclusive term than *doctor*. A complete run-through of what you should expect from your clinician during an office visit appears in Chapter 9, "The Ideal V Exam." Not only do I explain what's happening on the other side of the stirrups, but I'll tell you what tests you want to be sure you get to diagnose a V problem, what your Pap is all about, and how to make pelvic exams less miserable.

Finally, Part III, "Problem and Answer Guide," covers all possible V disorders. You probably don't need to know about all of them in such depth. But if you do develop one of these conditions, I can assure you that you can't possibly read enough on it. I start with all the most common problems, the various sorts of vaginitis (vaginal irritation usually caused by an infection): yeast infections (Chapter 10), bacterial vaginosis (11), trichomonas (12), and then a roundup of other types, such as atrophic vaginitis and strep vaginitis (Chapter 13).

Next come all kinds of skin disorders, many of which are familiar elsewhere in the body but can affect the vulva too. These include allergies to semen, latex, yeast, and other sources (Chapter 14); the diseases eczema, psoriasis, lichen sclerosus, and lichen planus (Chapter 15); and assorted other V bumps and color changes (Chapter 16).

In addition to vaginitis and skin disorders, there's a third major V problem that is of great interest to me—pain. Vulvodynia (vulvar pain) and vestibulodynia (pain in the vestibule) are just beginning to be recognized by doctors, but they have plagued many women for years. Fortunately, there are some exciting advances in their treatment. Chapter 17, " 'It Hurts,' " provides a rundown on V pain never before available to women. Chapter 18, "Sexual Healing," also contains previously unavailable material on maintaining sexuality when intercourse is painful. Though not part of your genitalia, the urinary tract can have two pain problems— bladder infections and interstitial cystitis—that produce V symptoms; they are highlighted in Chapter 19, "Bladder Pain."

Next come two viruses that have become epidemic, with serious impact on V health: genital herpes (Chapter 20, "The Lifetime Virus") and human papillomavirus or HPV (Chapter 21, "The Crafty Virus"). The herpes chapter is so named because it is a permanent infection, which those who have it need to learn to live alongside (which can be done). The HPV chapter uses the word *crafty* because this can cause annoying genital warts, produce worrisome Pap test results, or remain present with no symptoms at all. HPV is what causes cervical cancer. Chapter 22 covers vaginal and vulvar cancers. These are rare, but a book of this sort would not be complete without including them. The final chapter, "V Is for Voice," sums it all up.

I've included medical references so that your clinician can explore the literature on any topic I've covered that you wish to discuss with him or her.

One further note about style: You may have noticed I often shorten the adjective *vulvovaginal* to *V,* as in "V care," "V symptoms," "V area." I also collectively refer to the vulva, vagina, and vestibule as "the Vs." Rest assured, I do so in the interest of brevity and avoiding redundancies, not because I'm being coy. Also, you may notice a lack of information addressed to specific races or to bisexuals and lesbians. This is not from a lack of concern on my part. Rather, V information is scarce at best, and this kind of detail is not readily available. It's much on my mind from future editions.

Finally, let me say that *The V Book* is not out to challenge modesty. Private parts are meant to stay private. But *The V Book* is designed to help you realize that the vulva and vagina should not be private to *you.*

▼

PART I

An Owner's Manual

CHAPTER 1

The Mind
Why V Health Starts Here

Vagina **is hardly a household word.** *Vulva* and *clitoris* might as well belong to another language. They are blushers, vaguely subversive, not ready for prime time. They hide behind pet names and euphemisms ("my privates," "Pookie," "down there") if they're called anything at all. And then there's *vestibule*. That word's easy to say only because 99 out of 100 women have no idea that they have one, let alone where it is or what it does. (Don't worry. I'll show you later.) I feel pretty sure that a man would not allow some important part of his terrain to go uncharted for so long.

Believe it or not, even medical professionals can be uncomfortable about V terms. My own vulvar specialty practice in Boston is called the Stewart-Forbes Specialty Service. It's named after me and my nurse-practitioner partner, Diana Parks-Forbes, because at the time we were deliberating about what to call it, no one in the medical group's administration wanted the word *vulva* or *vagina* in the name. As a result, I surprise many new patients when I first walk into the exam room. "You're a woman!" they'll exclaim. They expected a gentleman named Stewart Forbes. The practice's vague name is hardly helpful to me professionally, either. Whenever I write a business letter or call a colleague, I always have to clarify that I represent the Stewart-Forbes *Vulvovaginal* Specialty Service. (Even so, Dr. Stewart Forbes gets lots of letters!)

I wish everyone could be matter-of-fact about the Vs. How much better my life—and your health—might be.

The first step to being comfortable with your body, after all, is being comfortable thinking about it (if not talking about it). That's why I say that V health starts in your head. As a physician, I'm a big believer in "liberation biology," to use the term coined by Mary Carlson, associate professor of psychiatry and neurobiology at Harvard Medical School. That means using biological information to help you understand your body, shake your hang-ups, and take charge of your full potential as a woman. In V terms, that means recognizing that the vulva and vagina are healthy parts of the body to be protected from disease, explored and treasured in responsible sexual life, esteemed for childbearing. I'd like for every woman to feel free enough to learn her way around her own body, free enough to talk easily to her doctor if a problem crops up.

Why are we so awkward about such commonplace body parts? Reticence about the vulva and vagina is nothing new. I'm no anthropologist or historian, but I do know that a veil has been draped over these parts for not merely a few generations but thousands of years. Knowing this past helps explain where our collective mind-set is today. Moreover, such information points the way to where our thinking ought to go.

So let's start at the beginning.

A short history of the Vs

Once upon a time people did not feel negatively about the vulva and vagina. Tens of thousands of years ago, the beautiful design of the vulva

V NOTE

Hiding behind euphemisms

The British *Cassell Dictionary of Slang* includes hundreds of slang words and phrases for female genitalia. Among them, with their era of origin:

Hey-nonny-no (late 16th century to mid-18th century)

Split mutton (17th century to 19th century)

Honey pot (early 18th century)

Venerable monosyllable (18th century)

Agreeable ruts of life (18th century)

Crinkum-crankum (late 18th century to early 19th century)

Downstairs (19th century)

Fancy bit (19th century)

Botany Bay (i.e., "down under") (19th century)

Cuckoo's nest (19th century)

Upright grin (mid-19th century)

Mole-catcher (late 19th century)

Thingamy (20th century)

Poontang (1920s)

Furburger (1960s)

Joy box (1970s)

was something celebrated, even revered. The *yoni*, a symbol of the female genitalia, took many forms. Flowers, fruits, a triangle, and a double-pointed oval shape were all used to depict the vulva. *Yoni* is a Sanskrit word for "womb, origin, source, sacred place"—honoring the vulva's role as birthplace, bringer of life. Today the word *yoni* enjoys a renaissance as a way to refer to female genitalia, although its use is hardly widespread.

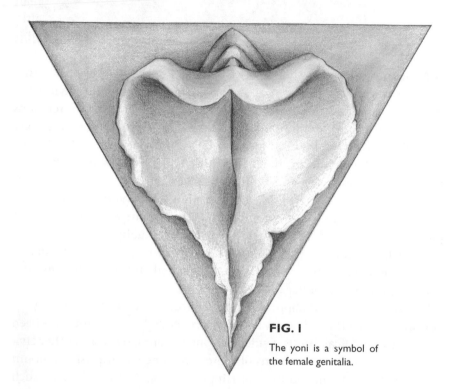

FIG. I

The yoni is a symbol of the female genitalia.

For a time, this symbol was worshiped as more powerful than its male counterpart, the phallus.[1] This was a time when the basic facts of biology that we take for granted today were yet unrecognized. That women were fertile year round, unlike the rest of the animal kingdom, inspired awe. Menstruation—painless bleeding—was a mystery. A woman's periods, not a man's sperm, were linked to the miracle of birth. Women seemed to give birth by their own divine power.

Rock carvings and chiseled figurines of ancient goddesses, their vulvas prominent, have been found dating back as much as thirty thousand years. People are thought to have worn amulets featuring the yoni both to protect them and to bring fertility. They conducted celebratory and fertility rituals at natural rock formations that seemed to echo the shape of the vulva. Some of these sites can still be seen today, in such places as lower Yemen; Tongariro National Park in New Zealand; Koh Samui, Thailand;

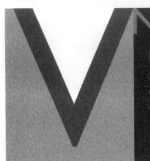

NOTE

Hang a horseshoe over the doorway for luck

It's thought that in ancient times, the horseshoe shape was another symbol of the yoni, perhaps explaining the goodwill associated with them today.

and the southern California desert. Sheila-na-gig statues—stone carvings of a squatting or reclining naked woman prominently displaying her vulva—have been found in old churches or buried in churchyards throughout Ireland and in parts of Scotland, England, and France. Their purpose is unknown. It's been speculated that the Celtic or pre-Celtic statues—many of which were buried or disposed of during the prudish Victorian era—were protectors from evil, bringers of luck, or fertility goddesses.

Many historians suggest that this veneration of the vulva—and in turn of the woman who is able to produce a child from those inner secret places—led to fear of her goddesslike power. Eventually, everything associated with the goddess was denigrated.[2] Goddess worship came to an end around the globe, replaced by the male-oriented cultures, religions, and mythologies we're familiar with today.

We don't know what happened in the centuries after the fall of the yoni culture. Though the vulva was no longer venerated, it may not have been off-limits to medical minds. Evidence from ancient Greece and other civilizations reveals that physicians of these times knew a surprising amount of gynecology.[3] From the time of Hippocrates (c. 460–c. 377 BCE), such things as dilatation of the cervix, uterine infections and prolapse, ovarian cysts, and pelvic infection were accurately described. How much vulvovaginal knowledge existed is unclear. Maybe not a lot, but things such as growths and inflammatory conditions of the vulva were documented.

Methods of examination that women are familiar with today existed long ago too. The Egyptians practiced vaginal examination long before the time of Hippocrates. The position of a woman on her back, knees flexed and legs separated (called lithotomy), for the investigation of gynecological troubles was described by a famous Greek surgeon, Archigenes, who practiced in Rome around 120 CE. We don't have any record of what Greek and Roman women thought of pelvic exams, but I can guess, can't you? Not all cultures were comfortable with genital anatomy and examinations: In ancient China, the diagnostic dolls used for the female patient to discreetly point out the location of her symptoms had no vulva.

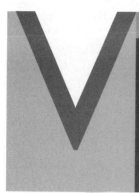

NOTE

And you thought vaginal creams were bad

The commonest form of gyn treatment for practically every kind of vaginal disease from Egyptian times to the 1700s was fumigation. A vessel holding about four gallons of fluid was covered with a tight-fitting lid; a slender reed jutted from the center of the lid. The vessel was placed over a fire until the fluid and herbs inside began to vaporize. Then the reed was placed in the vagina or cervix so the fumes could enter.[4]

Unfortunately, gynecology's early sophistication didn't continue. Thanks to the lack of free communication between various countries, the scanty dissemination of knowledge by means of books, and the overthrow of nations by war, medical knowledge was not transmitted from one generation to another, as it is today. For centuries there was a yawning lack of information; by the beginning of the nineteenth century, Europeans had only a fraction of the gynecological knowledge that had been attained by the Greek and Arabian masters.[5]

Even during the time women's gynecological problems were being treated in ancient Greece, its practitioners were flying a bit blind. No thorough knowledge of anatomy, male or female, existed until the time of Claudius Galen, court physician to Marcus Aurelius, who lived 130–200 CE. A leading medical authority of antiquity, Galen's fame rests solely on his dissections and descriptions of the female genitalia in animals.[6] He never worked on a woman. Along with his successors for the next two thousand years, he thought the human body was basically unisexual and that the two sexes were inside-out versions of each other. The male was primary, and the woman was described based on him.

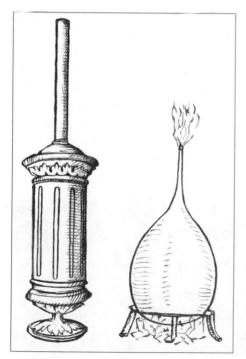

FIG. 2 A 16th-century Italian vaginal irrigation syringe and vaginal fumigator

Source: J. V. Ricci, *The Genealogy of Gynaecology* (Philadelphia: Blakiston, 1943).

Here's how Galen made his point: "Think first, please, of the man's [external genitalia] turned in and extending inward between the rectum and the bladder. If this should happen, the scrotum would necessarily take the place of the uterus with the testes lying outside, next to it on either side.

"Think too, please, of . . . the uterus turned outward and projecting. Would not the testes [ovaries] then necessarily be inside it? Would it not contain them like a scrotum? Would not the neck [the cervix and vagina], hitherto concealed inside the perineum but now pendant, be made into the male member?"

No, it would not, of course. You'd think that by being sexually active themselves, Galen and his contemporaries would have known that women were not inside-out versions of men, but remember that human anatomy wouldn't be perfected for hundreds of years. Galen's faulty logic—of a woman's body being the exact reverse of a man's, like a sock taken off in a hurry—persisted for generations.[7] Following that line of thinking, the uterus was thought to be the female equivalent of the scrotum, the ovaries were like testicles, the vulva was the foreskin, and the vagina was like the penis. The names used for female organs reflect their supposed similarity to the male: Galen called the ovary by the same name he used for the male testes, *orcheis*. Thinking of a woman as merely an inverted man made her automatically secondary and had long-standing repercussions: Why study her very closely if you could derive your basic knowledge by studying men?

Accurate descriptions of female anatomy were a long time in coming. Not until the fifteenth and sixteenth centuries were human dissections systematically done in order to chart the interior of the human body. But they were performed only on male prisoners who had died or had been executed. Andreas Vesalius (1514–1564), a professor of anatomy at the University of Padua, conducted painstaking investigations, resulting in his epochal text *De Corporis Humani Fabrica* (*The Makeup of the Human Body*). To gynecology Vesalius contributed fairly accurate descriptions of much of the genital tract. He perpetuated one very big mistake, though: Women's organs were still represented as versions of man's.

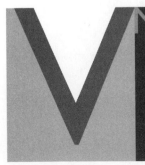

NOTE

Peachy keen

The peach has often represented the female genitals. In Chinese symbolism, a peach blossom meant a virgin, while the ripe fruit represented a mature woman.

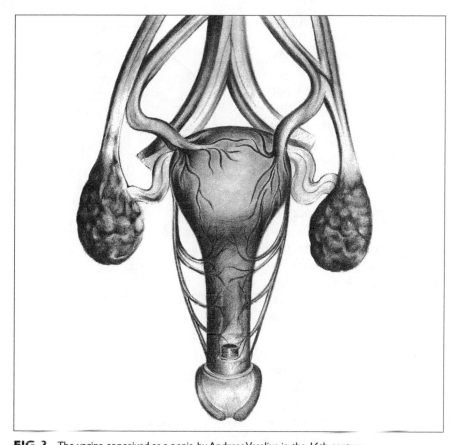

FIG. 3 The vagina conceived as a penis, by Andreas Vesalius in the 16th century

Source: Thomas Laqueur, *Making Sex: Body and Gender from the Greeks to Freud* (Cambridge, MA: Harvard University Press, 1990), 82.

Two of Vesalius's students made progress when they began identifying the distinct parts of female genitalia. Gabriele Fallopio of Modena (1523–1562) named the Fallopian tubes and accurately described the hymen. Matteo Realdo Colombo (1516–1559) was the first to use the term *labia* for structures that he considered essential to protect the uterus from dust, cold, and air. He also introduced the word *vagina*.[8] Not only did Colombo identify the soft inner folds of the vagina and name them *rugae* (the term still used today), but we can also thank him for being the first to describe the clitoris in detail.

The breakthrough in getting the complete landscape of a woman's body right didn't occur until the seventeenth century, when female cadavers were at last dissected along with men's. That's when Regnier de Graaf (1641–1673) mapped all the anatomic structures of the female genitalia, which, with few exceptions, serves well today.[9] His detailed medical text contained separate brief chapters on the external genitalia, the clitoris, the mons, the hymen, the urinary opening, the vagina, and the internal pelvic organs. Hurrah!

Understanding all the V parts and knowing how to help them were two different matters, though. No great advances followed from this new knowledge about the most female parts of the female body. Instead, growing demureness seems to have crept in.

All the way through the nineteenth century, gynecology texts made little mention of the vulva. Dr. Thomas Denman, the leading English practitioner of gynecology in 1805, mentions only clitoral enlargement, hardly a common problem, in his textbook.[10] Bimanual examination at this period was unknown. Vaginal examination was resorted to only on urgent indication, and even then it took place under protective drapes that effectively concealed the patient's genitals from the examiner's eyes. Even once vaginal exams were recognized as useful, toward the end of the 1800s, Victorian discretion often got in the way of effective treatment. Students of Dr. William Goodell (1829–1894) at the University of Pennsylvania, for example, were counseled to keep their eyes fixed on the ceiling while making vaginal evaluations.[11] An upholstered examining chair with concealed stirrups continued the sense of propriety.

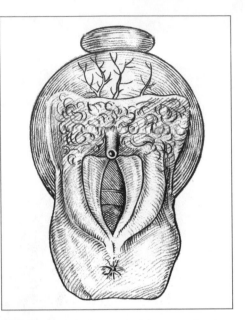

FIG. 4 The earliest picture of the external genitalia, by anatomist Severinus Pineus (1550–1619)

Source: J. V. Ricci, *The Genealogy of Gynaecology* (Philadelphia: Blakiston, 1943), 328–29.

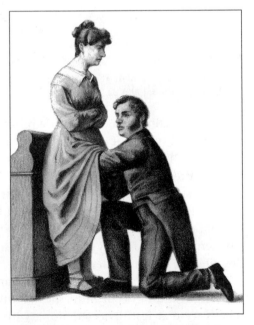

FIG. 5 Pelvic examination in the early 19th century

Source: Maygrier, J. P. *Nouvelles demonstrations d'accouchemens* (Paris, Bechet, 1822).

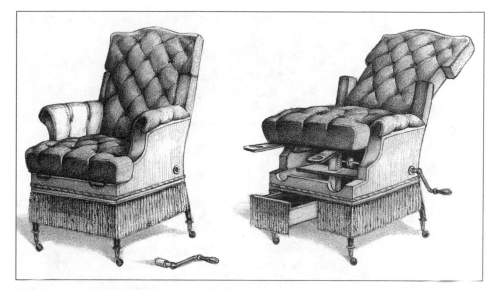

FIG. 6   A plush examining chair of the late 19th century

Source: H. Speert, *Obstetrics and Gynecology: A History and Iconography*
(San Francisco: Norman Publishing, 1994), 488.

Physicians were as clueless about effective therapies as they were about
insightful exams. By the early twentieth century, the treatment for yeast
infection—and, in fact, any of the itching and redness collectively known
as vaginitis—was the same: bed rest. Warm-water vaginal injections med-
icated with opium and belladonna were given every four hours. Opium
rectal suppositories were given at bedtime to bring on sleep. Narcotics and
rest surely eased the pain, but the actual problem was left unaddressed.

It wasn't until 1923 that an American physician, Frederick Taussig, published the first medical book exclusively about the vulva, *Diseases of
the Vulva,* which became the standard medical text in the United States.
In fact, aside from that work and another published in England
nearly twenty years later, there was startlingly little accurate information

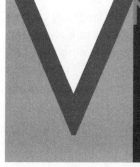

NOTE

No insult

Though now a derogatory obscenity, the word *cunt* has been
traced to Kunthus, the Greek goddess of fertility, and to Cunti
(or Kunti), an Indian earth goddess. In ancient writings, it was a
synonym for "woman." Related words are thought to include
cunabula (cradle), *cunicle* (hole or passage), *cunning* (wiliness or
knowledge), and *conch* (shell).

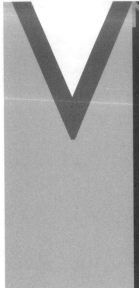

Notorious V moments

1980: Brooke Shields purrs that nothing comes between her and her Calvin Klein jeans.

1990: Comedienne Roseanne Barr grabs her crotch while "singing" the national anthem at a Major League Baseball game.

1992: Sharon Stone flashes her interrogators in *Basic Instinct.*

1998: Monica Lewinsky shows off her thong and plays with a cigar in the Oval Office.

2000: Beaver College in Glenside, Pennsylvania, changes its name to Arcadia University because, according to the school's president, "the word *beaver* too often elicits ridicule in the form of derogatory remarks pertaining to the rodent, the TV show *Leave It to Beaver* and the vulgar reference to the female anatomy."

available to physicians, and in turn their patients, until 1969. That year—well after the birth of such female cultural icons as the tampon, the pill, and Barbie—Americans Herman Gardner and Raymond Kaufman published a groundbreaking book that finally covered all aspects of vulvar and vaginal problems in detail, *Benign Diseases of the Vulva and Vagina.*

Even today, the total number of texts about the vulva and vagina in print wouldn't fill a bookshelf—fewer than a dozen. (Compare that with more than four hundred for the heart.) There is no medical journal devoted to the vulva and vagina. Research is sparse; dozens of papers have been published on the yeast *Candida albicans,* but they deal with the myriad other problems associated with yeast besides vaginitis. Bacterial vaginosis is receiving a lot of attention not because of the miserable discharge and odor it causes but because of its connection with premature labor.

It's not surprising, then, that popular thinking has mirrored the medical community's indifference. For much of the twentieth century, women's genitals remained mired in ignorance and shame, as had been the case for hundreds of years. The vagina was sexual, and you didn't talk about sex. Touching yourself might lead to masturbation; women have had the clitoris removed for that since ancient Egyptian times and are still taught that touching themselves is wrong.[12] The vagina was a birth canal, of concern only to the midwife or doctor attending you. Mothers whispered the facts of Kotex to their daughters at the time of menstruation, and the facts of life on the eve of their weddings—if they told them anything at all. There were no books a woman could consult, only her friends or relatives, should she muster the nerve. Until only recently, women's magazines brought their readers little genital health information alongside the latest fashions and recipes. Into the vacuum of silence fell folklore, misconceptions, and dirty jokes.

Snickers and embarrassed silence are a long way from the primitive celebration of the yoni.

The power of positive thinking

Culturally ingrained habits are hard to change. If, at the dawn of the twenty-first century, you're comfortable with the skin you're in, good for you. It's simply healthy, both mentally and physically, to think about your genitals as yet another intricate part of your human machinery, with important diverse functions, and worthy of considerate care. If you can talk to your doctor about your vulva and vagina without embarrassment, if you can look at your parts and understand what they're for and when something might be amiss, then you're in charge of yourself—and that's a good place to be.

One of my patients, trying to describe her symptoms exactly, said, "Believe me, Dr. Stewart. My fingers have been everywhere. There's nothing that's tender to touch." She was knowledgeable about her body, comfortable with exploring and discussing it, and therefore able to collaborate with me. Compare that to the more common scenario, in which the patient says vaguely, "It itches a lot" or "I have this pain down . . . well, you know, down there."

The fact is that for most of us, unhealthy attitudes have taken root. And revising them is challenging. You may long ago have disconnected that

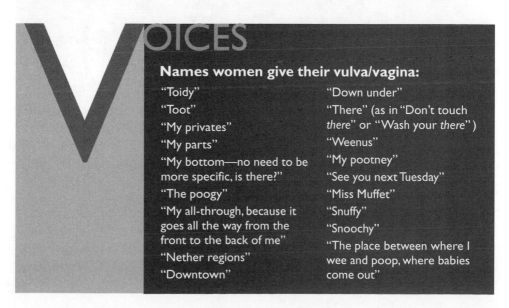

VOICES

Names women give their vulva/vagina:

"Toidy"

"Toot"

"My privates"

"My parts"

"My bottom—no need to be more specific, is there?"

"The poogy"

"My all-through, because it goes all the way from the front to the back of me"

"Nether regions"

"Downtown"

"Down under"

"There" (as in "Don't touch *there*" or "Wash your *there*")

"Weenus"

"My pootney"

"See you next Tuesday"

"Miss Muffet"

"Snuffy"

"Snoochy"

"The place between where I wee and poop, where babies come out"

part of your body from your mind. Or maybe you never connected to begin with because of our do-not-touch society. Hands off, keep away. Don't talk about it, think about it, look at it.

If you feel this way because you have been abused or raped or hurt, my heart is with you. My book will be of little value unless you have done the necessary work to bring closure to what has happened. There are many people who can help you do that. Please see the Resources section.

But if you are separated from your vulva and vagina in your thinking for other reasons, you can work to change. If anatomy is an unmentionable topic in your family, if sex is never discussed, if touching yourself is considered dirty, you may be a long way from feeling comfortable about the vulva and vagina. Reticence is understandable. But it doesn't have to be that way. You can reconnect and move forward.

But how? What can we do to break down all the barriers built up over centuries?

First of all, think about why you feel the way you do about the V area. Think about what topics come to mind when you consider those parts: menstruation, masturbation, what they look like, what they do, what's normal, what's not. Have your impressions been influenced by what your

V NOTE

For art's sake

Women have long found inspiration in their own bodies:

1920s: Georgia O'Keeffe's sensuously magnified renditions of poppies, lilies, and petunias echo the female form.

1965: Performance artist Shigeko Kubota makes waves with her *Vagina Painting*—a piece that involved inserting a brush in her vagina and painting while squatting on the floor.

1960s: Trained artist Betty Dodson begins showing gracefully detailed, anatomically correct erotic drawings well before her later fame as the mother of the masturbation movement.

1966: Niki de Saint Phalle's giantess-sized sculpture *The Figure Hon*, of a woman lying on her back, features a human-scaled doorway at the vulva.

1974: Judy Chicago begins sketches for *The Dinner Party*, her 1979 mixed-media installation celebrating women's history, which draws more fire than praise because of its use of vulval motifs in ceramic plates honoring specific women.

1990s: Dutch artist Christina Camphausen, who paints vulvas almost exclusively (not flowers made to echo vulvas, à la O'Keeffe), offers portraiture online.

mother or grandmother said (or didn't say), or by bad experiences at a clinic or with a partner? Think about where you go for information. Where have you learned information about your genitalia: from pre-adolescent pamphlets about menstruation? Tampon boxes? Your doctor? Your girlfriends? Health magazines? There are no right or wrong answers, of course. But exploring the origins of any embarrassment or reluctance puts it into context.

Then we dump the idea of "dirty." Dirt is dirty. The Vs are not. Yes, they contain bacteria (as do a lot of other places in your body), but I'm going to show you that these bacteria are your friends. Bacteria do not always cause infection and disease, and in the case of the vagina they are essential for health.

Moving on, we need to vanquish the concept of "down there," to get rid of the idea that the vulva is Nowheresville, some mysterious place that you have no right to understand. It's not that far down that you can't check it out. I keep a mirror in the drawer of every exam table, and I pull it out all the time to show women normal anatomy or have them show me an area they've got a question about. Look! The more you look, the better you get. I want you to become comfortable with the correct name of every part and how each part works for you.

Finally, we drop "don't touch." The vulva's not a forbidden garden. There are no serpents lurking about. You have my certified medical guarantee that there's no way that by touching (or enjoying touching) the vulva and vagina, you will cause infection, weaken your character, lower your morals, or spoil your opportunity for normal sexual enjoyment.

Do I expect the vulva and vagina to become cocktail party conversation? That's not my goal. Remember what I said in the introduction—private parts are meant to stay private. But I want you to take ownership. Your vulva belongs to you, not your mother, not your partner, not your doctor. So make my day. Walk into my office and tell me that you have a bump on the labium or pain in the vestibule. That's what I'm waiting for.

▼

CHAPTER 2

The Vulva

A Road Map to the External Genitalia

Vulvar anatomy can be confusing, even for clinicians. So it's not surprising that many women, even those who take an active interest in their health, have a hard time getting it straight. Most of my patients know something about lips and the vaginal opening, and that's about it.

So you might be surprised to discover that this misunderstood hinterland is actually an intricate, magnificent work of design. By understanding this design—the anatomy of the vulva—you'll learn to be comfortable with your body. You already know about your teeth. You worry about your breasts. You think about your bowels. Now on to the vulva! Details about your menstrual cycles and the process of becoming pregnant and having a baby will come into clearer focus. You can also enjoy sex more if you're familiar with your sexual structures and how they

VOICES

"I don't even know what a vulva is—the word makes me think of 'velvet vulvas in Volvos.'"

—Hana, 45, mother of three

work. It's hard to really know what feels good—and harder still to let your partner know—if you've never explored for yourself. Not least, should a problem develop—say, irritation or an allergy, a skin disease, pain, the vulvar challenges that the menopause can bring—you'll pick up on it promptly. And knowing what's where can help you communicate more effectively with your clinician, speeding your path toward answers and relief.

So let's get started toward our mastery.

▼ ▼ ▼

The vulva has three main purposes:

- ▼ It protects the woman's sexual organs, urinary opening, vestibule, and vagina. Obviously, this is a major intersection of bodily functions. So keeping it safe from infection or damage is crucial.

- ▼ It's the center for much of a woman's sexual response. The labia themselves engorge with blood. The sensitive clitoris—yes, it's part of the vulva—is central to orgasm for most women. And the vulva's cushiony, hair-covered outer fat pad makes intercourse more comfortable.

- ▼ The perineum (the area between the vaginal opening and the anus) stretches to accommodate childbirth. The vulva technically stops at the point where the outer lips meet in the back, but the perineum is such an immediate neighbor that it's practically kin.

Learning what's what

You probably do breast self-exams (monthly, I hope). You look in your mouth all the time. Maybe you check between your toes or under your

VOICES

"One of them was talking about the woman painter who was filling the galleries with giant flowers in rainbow colors. 'They're not flowers,' said the pipe smoker, 'they're vulvas. Anyone can see that. It is an obsession with her. She paints a vulva the size of a full-grown woman. At first it looks like petals, the heart of a flower, then one sees the two uneven lips, the fine center line, the wavelike edge of the lips, when they are spread open. What kind of woman can she be, always exhibiting this giant vulva, suggestively vanishing into a tunnel-like repetition, growing from a large one to a smaller shadow of it, as if one were actually entering into it?' "

—Anaïs Nin, *Delta of Venus*

NOTE

Sacred turf

Many historians find feminine symbolism in religious architecture: two sets of doorways, inner and outer (the labia); a central hallway (the vagina) leading to an altar (the uterus). Often there are side paths (the Fallopian tubes) from the altar that lead to small vestries (the ovaries).

arms. Examining one's vulva requires a bit of enterprise, though. A woman's genital anatomy isn't obvious. There is one set of lips tucked inside another, with the vagina hidden up behind both, entirely out of view. Only the tip of the sexual organ, the clitoris, is visible; the rest of this surprisingly extensive organ can't be seen.

So let's start by clarifying the geography. Some of a woman's genitalia is inside the body and some is not. We often use the word *vagina* to refer to anything between the legs. Clinicians, however, know that the vagina is *inside* the body cavity. The vulva is not. The vulva is *outside* the body. In fact, anything between the lips, which are called the labia, is outside the body.

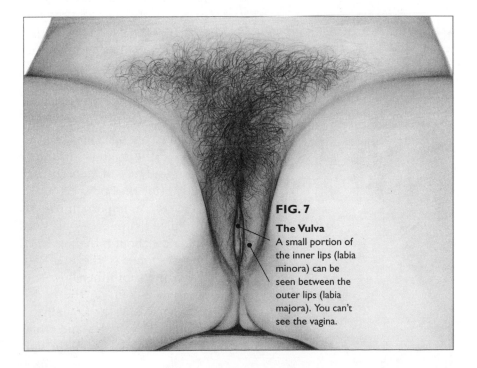

FIG. 7

The Vulva
A small portion of the inner lips (labia minora) can be seen between the outer lips (labia majora). You can't see the vagina.

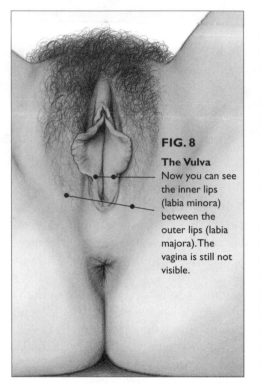

FIG. 8

The Vulva
Now you can see the inner lips (labia minora) between the outer lips (labia majora). The vagina is still not visible.

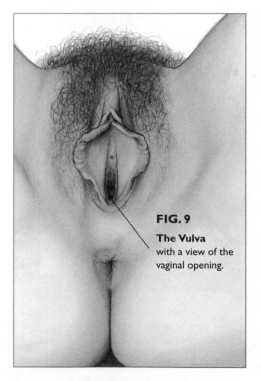

FIG. 9

The Vulva
with a view of the vaginal opening.

Study the following road map to understand all the locations. Then you can interpret the map on your own body.

Before we look at all the interesting details of vulvar parts, let's get the main Vs straight: vulva, vagina, and vestibule.

The vulva includes all the outer genitals you can see between your legs.

FIG. 7 This is the *vulva*. Typically, the outer lips are together, so you can't see any of the other parts beneath. Women vary a great deal in the appearance of the vulva; in some the lips come together completely, while in others the outer lips don't meet and the inner lips are visible.

FIG. 8 This is still the vulva. Now the outer lips are slightly parted so that you can see the inner lips. The inner lips are inside the outer lips, but they are still on the *outside* of the body.

The vagina is internal and separate from the vulva.

FIG. 9 Now the inner lips of the vulva are open so that you can see the vaginal opening. The round tube of the vagina is truly inside the body.

FIG. 10 An important part of the vulva that most women do not know about is the *vestibule*. The vestibule is the area between the thin inner lips. The vestibule is outside the body, although inside the inner lips.

What is the vulva and what does it do? What are all the lips

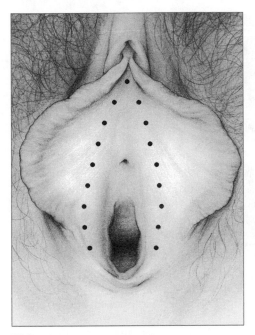

FIG. 10 **The Vestibule** is this hallway between the labia minora. The openings of the urethra, the vagina, and many small glands are in the vestibule.

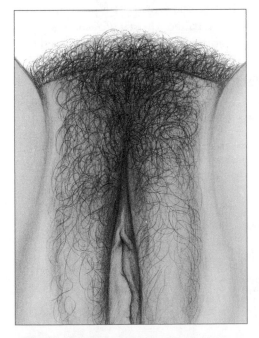

FIG. 11 **The Vulva** with a view of the mons, the padded mountain at the top. You can see most of the labia majora and some of the minora, but no vagina.

about? And what's the big deal about the vestibule?

The word *vulva* means "covering." It's aptly named. It covers the woman's areas of sexual pleasure as well as some passageways. It covers the sexual organs, the clitoris, labia minora, and vestibule. It covers the urinary opening, the urethra. And it covers the organ involved with sexual intercourse, menstruation, and reproduction, the vagina. So the vulva deals with sexual and urinary activity, menstruation, pregnancy and delivery; since the anus is nearby it also deals with bowel activity. All that makes the vulva a real crossroads for several of your body's major transportation routes.

Let's look at all the vulva's parts, one by one.

FIG. 11 The vulva begins at the top with the *mons*. The word means "mountain." On the topography of your body, it's a rounded elevation of skin that lies over the pubic bone. This mountain is made mainly of a fat pad. The skin over the mons is covered with pubic hair. The full Latin name for this area, *mons veneris,* or "mountain of Venus," reveals the function of the mons in lovemaking. The pad of fat, upholstered in hair, forms a cushion so that the hard pubic bone does not cause discomfort during sexual intercourse. The pubic hair also keeps the skin

VOICES

"I think it is a pity that so many women remain who feel uncomfortable and ashamed about their yoni. Some women even think that this most intimate part of them is actually strange, ugly, or even abnormal (size of labia, clitoris, etc.). I, personally, experienced it as a form of inner healing once I learned to look at my yoni as a very beautiful, important, and intimate part of my body. Knowing that other women often struggle with similar misconceptions, I'm very glad to be able to show the flowery beauty of the yoni in a manner that is not pornographic but rather empowering."

—artist Christina Camphausen, who posts
a virtual gallery of her vulvar paintings

surfaces of the two partners from rubbing together and causing irritation. It may also contribute to sexual enjoyment and trap pheromones, natural scents that contribute to desire.

The fat pad of the mons remains even after marked weight loss, one of many cleverly ergonomic aspects of our design.[1] This means that even the skinniest Hollywood actress is as comfortably upholstered for intercourse as her size-12-and-up counterparts in the real world. The pattern of the pubic hair, regulated by hormones, is called the *escutcheon* (say "es-KUTCH-ee-on"). The female escutcheon forms an inverted triangle. A man's escutcheon grows upward onto the abdomen; this pattern can also be seen in normal women, depending on race and heredity. **FIG. 12**

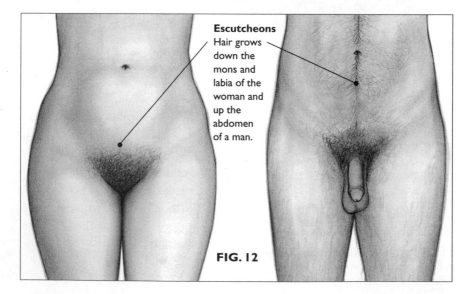

Escutcheons
Hair grows down the mons and labia of the woman and up the abdomen of a man.

FIG. 12

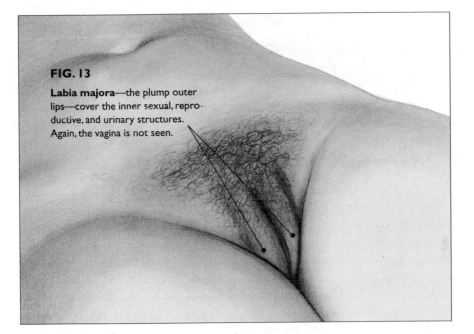

FIG. 13

Labia majora—the plump outer lips—cover the inner sexual, reproductive, and urinary structures. Again, the vagina is not seen.

Pubic hair varies widely among women. Race plays a role: Asian hair is scant and straight, sometimes only a few strands; African American hair is very curly and thick; Caucasian hair tends to be somewhere in between. It's possible to have very little pubic hair (called *hypotrichosis*) or no pubic hair (*atrichia*) because of genetic or hormonal reasons, or from trauma such as burns. Given the social and sexual importance of a hairy mons, there have been many efforts to correct these. But only the relatively drastic measure of surgery—pubic hair grafting—is thought to be effective.[2] (For information on pubic hair removal (clipping, waxing, and shaving), see page 102.)

FIG. 13 The mons leads down on each side to the *labia majora* (large lips), two elongated, rounded folds of skin that are also covered with pubic hair. (Just one is referred to as a *labium*.) In most people, the hair con-

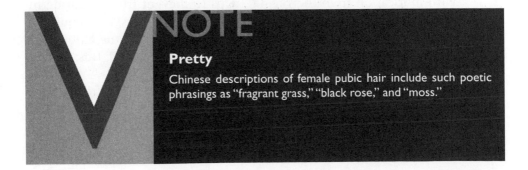

Pretty

Chinese descriptions of female pubic hair include such poetic phrasings as "fragrant grass," "black rose," and "moss."

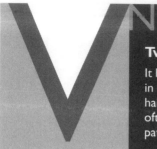

Two-toned?

It happens. The presence of more than one distinct color of hair in the same person is *heterochromia*. (Picture a man whose scalp hair and sideburns are different hues, for example.) Pubic hair is often darker than scalp hair in a fair-haired person. Rarely, a patch of a different color appears.[3]

tinues between the legs and around the *anus,* or opening of the rectum. The labia come together in the front and the back. Where they fuse in the front, the skin is smooth; in the back, the skin may be smooth or form a little ridge like a seam. At this point the vulva ends.

Some supports for the uterus are anchored in the labia. The round ligaments, which are part of the uterine support system, run from the mid-portion of the uterus through the groin and down to the labia. These ligaments become important in pregnancy, since movements that stretch the round ligaments can cause a sharp pain, a "stitch" that runs from the uterus inside the pelvis down into the labia.

The labia, like the mons, contain a fair amount of fat to act as a cushion for sexual intercourse. The labia majora are the same as the scrotum in the male. They not only look like the scrotal sacs, but they are also derived from the same tissue in the embryo before the gender differences form. They contain the same kind of muscle *(dartos)* that tightens up with sexual arousal, although this muscle is less developed in the labia than in the scrotum.

The skin over the labia contains hair follicles, sweat glands, and some special glands that secrete sebum, a blend of oils, waxes, fats, cholesterol, and cellular debris. Sebum serves as waterproofing protection from urine, menstrual blood, and bacteria that might otherwise stick to the surface. Sebum gives the vestibule and the folds between the labia a sleek and slippery feel, a bit like being covered with wax. This, along with lubrication from the vagina, helps to prevent friction during intercourse. Some women make more sebum than others; it can build up on the inside surface of the labia majora and around the clitoris as a yellow-white waxy substance. There's nothing wrong with this; it's similar to earwax.

Any woman who exercises vigorously knows that the wettest parts of her clothing are under the arms and between the legs. This is because there are probably more sweat glands in the vulva than anywhere else in the body. The sweat glands are there because the vulva is such a vascular zone, full of blood vessels that bring blood and therefore heat. Sweat al-

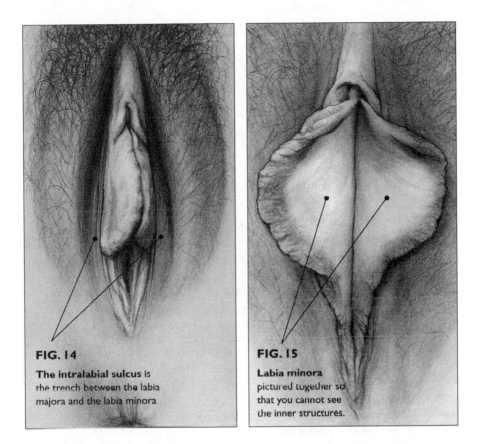

FIG. 14

The intralabial sulcus is
the trench between the labia
majora and the labia minora

FIG. 15

Labia minora
pictured together so
that you cannot see
the inner structures.

lows heat to escape, but it may also be a source of odor that is often erroneously blamed on the vagina. These same skin structures that keep us comfortable can also give rise to assorted bumps and fluid-filled sacs called cysts.

FIG. 14 The areas between the outer lips and the inner lips are called the *intralabial folds*. The fold looks like a little valley between the labium majus and the labium minus. The skin of the intralabial folds can develop lumps and bumps, itching or pain; pinpointing the name and location helps you explain your problem to your clinician.

Together, the mons and the labia majora form a well-padded and sexually responsive covering for the openings below.

FIG. 15 The outer lips (labia majora) surround two smaller, thin flaps of skin without hair, the *labia minora*. They are darker in color than the labia majora, varying by woman from a deep pink to a brownish pink or reddish pink. There's no standard-issue look to the labia minora. Some women have small ruffles, while in others the skin is substantial tissue wide enough to extend past the labia majora. They vary considerably in appearance from thin, small flaps to thick, bumpy bulges. They don't always match either. One can be longer or wider, fatter or thinner, than the other. On average, the labia minora are 1½ to 2 inches (4 to 5 cm) in width when spread open like wings.

The edges of the labia minora (and the labia majora too) often contain tiny glands that make a fine, white, pebbly appearance, almost like tiny pimples. Women often worry that these pebbly bumps are abnormal. Not so—the inner labia minora are smooth and moist from the secretion of the oil glands represented by these bumps. The oil secretions of both the labia majora and the labia minora keep all the skin edges lubricated so that they don't rub against each other and get irritated. The labia minora are part of the protective covering that the vulva provides for the vestibule, urethra, and vagina. Without them, urine would spray. Their main function, though, is sexual. Richly endowed with sensitive nerve endings and blood vessels, the labia minora have a role similar to the corpus spongiosum, the special blood-vessel-rich tissue of the penis. Just as sexual arousal increases blood flow to swell or erect the penis, tissues of the labia minora and the vestibule also swell with sexual stimulation, although not as much as the clitoris (or the penis). Labia minora plumped up with blood

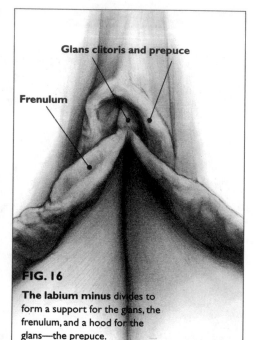

Glans clitoris and prepuce

Frenulum

FIG. 16

The labium minus divides to form a support for the glans, the frenulum, and a hood for the glans—the prepuce.

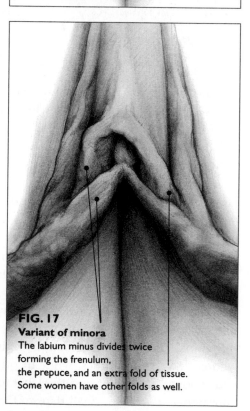

FIG. 17

Variant of minora
The labium minus divides twice forming the frenulum, the prepuce, and an extra fold of tissue. Some women have other folds as well.

increase the pleasurable sensations that go with foreplay.

FIG. 16 At the top, the labia minora split and meet under the clitoris to form the *frenulum,* a small fold of mucous membrane that extends from a fixed part to a movable one. (You have another one under your tongue.) The labia minora also meet above the clitoris to form a hood or prepuce (*prepuce* means foreskin). The clitoris is the most highly sensitive tissue in the body and therefore needs the protective covering of the prepuce.

FIG. 17 Some labia minora split twice, once to form the prepuce and then again to make another fold of tissue next to the prepuce.

In the back the labia minora

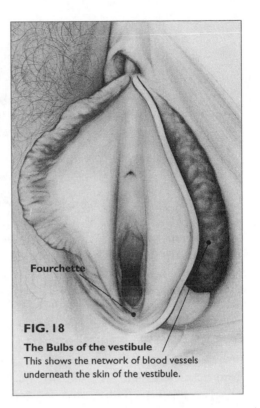

Fourchette

FIG. 18

The Bulbs of the vestibule
This shows the network of blood vessels underneath the skin of the vestibule.

seem to merge into the labia majora, but they actually form a thin fold of skin at the base of the vaginal opening called the *fourchette.* After a woman has a baby, the fourchette may disappear if an episiotomy or tear flattens it out.

FIG. 18 The area between the two sides of the labia minora is the *vestibule.* It's the "other" V part, the one few women are aware of. It's really important to understand that this is a separate part of the body from the labia or the vagina because the tissue of the vestibule functions differently and can have problems of its own. The vestibule is a smooth triangular

V NOTE

Poetic justice

The labia minora are also known as the nymphae, from the Greek nymphs, those graceful maidens of forests and fountains.

area; its sidewalls are the labia minora, with the frenulum of the clitoris at the top and the fourchette at the base, where both sets of labia come together in a slightly raised connecting ridge. The name fits. Like the lobby of a building, the vestibule is the site of several doorways: The upper vestibule contains the urinary opening (urethra), and in the lower vestibule is the vagina. Many openings from vestibular glands enter throughout the vestibule, as described below.

The skin of the vestibule is moist and pinkish; in fact, sometimes it's normally quite red. Its surface contains many small glands. Their secretions keep the lips from rubbing together painfully. Like the labia minora, the vestibule is rich in nerve endings. Bundles of blood vessels—called the bulbs of the vestibule—line the walls and floor of this little hallway. With sexual arousal, blood races into these vessels, making

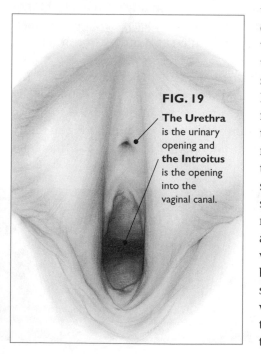

FIG. 19

The Urethra is the urinary opening and **the Introitus** is the opening into the vaginal canal.

them erect and firm like the clitoris. For years, the bulbs were described as being low in the vestibule, limited to each side of the vaginal opening. But recently researchers have found that the erectile tissue in this tangle of blood vessels is much broader than originally thought. The bulbs actually surround the urethra, near the shaft of the clitoris, and can be readily stimulated by a finger against the front wall of the vagina. Perhaps the much-ballyhooed G spot (an area of soft tissue felt within the vagina that's thought by some to be the most sexually sensitive area for certain women;

see Chapters 3 and 6) is actually the bulbs of the vestibule. In normal women there may be spots in the vestibule that are tender to touch with a cotton swab, but if there is no complaint of pain with intercourse, this is not a problem.

The skin here doesn't have the toughness of skin found elsewhere on the body. It more resembles the mucous membrane of the mouth, sensitive and accustomed to moisture.

FIG. 19 In the vestibule just below the clitoris is a small tube that leads to the bladder, the *urethral opening.* This short tube measures about 1½ inches. The *paraurethral glands* open into the vestibule by small ducts on either side of the urethral opening. A pair of these ducts, the *Skene's ducts,* lie just below the urethra on either side. The Skene's ducts and the paraurethral glands are part of the lubrication system of the vestibule. Below the urethra is the larger vaginal opening, the *introitus.* When you note how close the urethra is to the vagina, you can understand how easy it is for the urethra to become irritated, sore, or infected from sexual activity.

Most women are familiar with the clitoris. They know it, however, only as a small raised nubbin between the labia. But the clitoris is far more than the quarter-inch tip (called the *glans clitoris*) that you can see and touch.

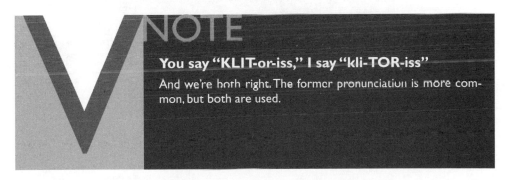

You say "KLIT-or-iss," I say "kli-TOR-iss"
And we're both right. The former pronunciation is more common, but both are used.

Attached to the tip is a firm, rubbery, and movable shaft, about ¾ to 1½ inches (2 to 4 cm) long, connected to the pubic bone. The shaft then divides into two parts that spread out to form the roots *(crura),* two anchoring wishbone-shaped tissues that also attach to the pelvic bones and measure 2 to 3½ inches (5 to 9 cm) across. This is an organ of considerable size! The roots and shaft are covered by overlying muscle so that you cannot see them. Only the glans is exposed.

Part of the misunderstanding about the clitoris is evidenced by its name, which means "shut up" or "concealed." Indeed, the clitoris is well concealed by the labia majora and by the hood (prepuce) that the labia minora form around it.

FIG. 20 The glans of the clitoris is visible under its hood, or if the hood covers the glans, it can be seen by pulling back the hood. (The hood and

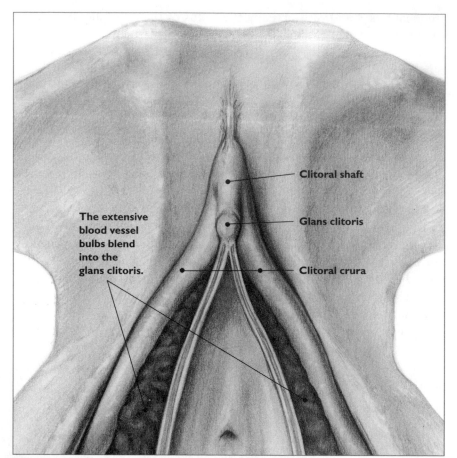

Clitoral shaft

The extensive blood vessel bulbs blend into the glans clitoris.

Glans clitoris

Clitoral crura

FIG. 20

The Clitoris—glans, shaft, and crura. This shows the pubic bones and the clitoris, which is a larger organ than many people think.

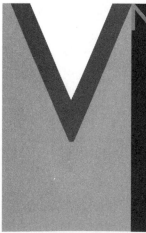

NOTE

Clitistics

▼ The clitoris is fully formed in a fetus by the twenty-seventh week of gestation.

▼ The size of one's clitoris has nothing to do with sexual response.

▼ As many as eight thousand nerve endings sensitive to touch congregate here, more than any other body part (and that's double the number in the penis).

▼ Two pipelines of blood vessels run along either side of the clitoris, with the glans forming a cap at the top.

▼ An aroused clitoral glans swells to twice its usual size.

frenulum are generously supplied with sebaceous glands and mucus-secreting glands so that there's no friction between them and the glans.) It's about the size of a pencil eraser, although this varies among women. Neither your height nor your weight influences the size of your clitoris, but women who have had children tend to have larger measurements.[4] The glans will also enlarge if a woman takes *excessive* amounts of testosterone by mouth, by injection, or by topical application.

Regardless of its size, what's paramount about the glans is its passion potential. Although it's a relatively tiny part of the body, the glans packs in thousands of nerve fibers, which is why few women are strangers to it. In fact, for many women, direct touch is almost painful; they prefer stimulation of the shaft or entire mons.

The shaft of the clitoris, the part you can't see under the skin and muscle of the vestibule, has few nerves; instead, a network of blood vessels within it fill at sexual arousal, pushing the glans forward.

Because of their obvious parallels as the central site for orgasm, the clitoris is often compared with the penis. While it is true that both organs swell with blood upon arousal, there are some big differences between them. The clitoris does not become rigid and erect because there is no venous plexus, the tight-knit network of blood vessels that dam up blood in the penis for an erection.[5] Because blood can flow in and out, the clitoris can swell and relax easily, enabling a woman to have multiple orgasms.

The penis and clitoris also differ in terms of what they're there for. The penis is an organ of pleasure, an organ of reproduction, and part of the urinary system too. For the woman, the clitoris and vestibular bulbs exist solely for sexual sensation. They have no other function.

They are joined in this mission by the entire vulva. From mons to anus, sensation is supplied by thousands of fibers of the pudendal nerve. Branches of the pudendal nerve to the anus explain why anal sex is pleasurable. Researchers have recently proposed that an additional sensory pathway involves the vagus nerve, a long nerve that extends from the cervix to the brain, bypassing the spinal cord.[6] The vagus nerve may

VOICES

"In the clitoris alone we see a sexual organ so pure of purpose that it needn't moonlight as a secretory or excretory device. For this reason, maybe it's best that the clitoris is normally hidden within the vulval cleft: it is, in its way, a private joke, a divine secret, a Pandora's box packed not with sorrow but with laughter."

—Natalie Angier, author of *Woman: An Intimate Geography*

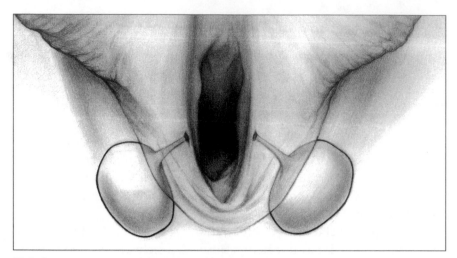

FIG. 21 **The Bartholin's glands** have ducts that empty into the vestibule.

explain why women with spinal cord injuries can have sexual responses.

FIG. 21 *Bartholin's glands* are two small, rounded bodies on either side of the vaginal opening at the base of the labia minora. They are the major vestibular glands. You cannot see the Bartholin's glands, and you cannot feel them unless they are enlarged. Their role is to assist in lubrication; each gland drains its secretion into the vestibule by a small duct. The glands produce only a few drops of fluid that are part of lubrication for sex. Most lubrication for sexual arousal, however, comes from the vagina.

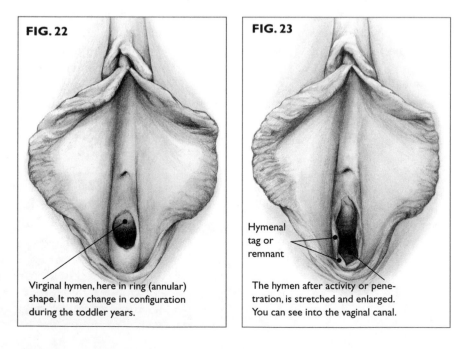

FIG. 22

Virginal hymen, here in ring (annular) shape. It may change in configuration during the toddler years.

FIG. 23

Hymenal tag or remnant

The hymen after activity or penetration, is stretched and enlarged. You can see into the vaginal canal.

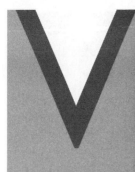

Like a virgin

Hymen was the Greek goddess of marriage—the name means "veil," a logical reference to the membrane of that same name that covers the vagina and has historically been associated with virginity.

FIG. 22 When a female baby is born, a thin membrane with one or more tiny openings in the middle of it surrounds the vaginal entrance. This is the *hymen*. When a young girl reaches sexual maturity, her opening allows menstrual flow to pass out. It's usually a smooth circle of tissue all the way around the vaginal opening (annular) at birth. The hymen may change in shape during the first three years of life (from a ring, say, to a crescent), and these changes may vary by race.[7] Despite the great significance often attached to the presence or absence of the hymen by various cultures, it has no known biological function.

FIG. 23 The elasticity of the hymen varies from woman to woman. Typically, though, with the introduction of a penis, fingers, or sexual devices, the opening stretches and becomes larger. Contrary to popular belief that the hymen can be ruptured by gymnastics, horseback riding, and other vigorous sports, no relation between sports and hymenal changes was found in a study of three hundred females.[8] There is no medical definition of virginity based on the size of the opening in the hymen. The hymen can, as I said earlier, change in various ways, some occurring naturally during the first years of life. With regular sexual intercourse, the small, smooth opening becomes irregular; little petal-like pieces or tags of tissue (myrtiform caruncles, or hymenal tags) remain around the vaginal opening. These are remnants of the hymen.

FIG. 24 After a woman has a baby, the opening becomes larger and more irregular. Women often

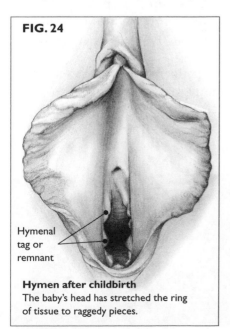

FIG. 24

Hymenal tag or remnant

Hymen after childbirth
The baby's head has stretched the ring of tissue to raggedy pieces.

mistake these hymenal tags for ominous bumps or warts; they are completely normal.

If a hymen has no opening, it is a complete covering over the vagina. This rare variation is called an *imperforate hymen* and needs to be fixed with a simple surgical procedure to make an opening.

Between the vagina and the anus lies a stretch of skin called the *perineum* (Greek for "around evacuation"). Its skin and underlying tissue cover a muscle called the perineal body. Its length, varying from ½ inch to 2¾ inches or more, and its suppleness influence the resistance it offers to the delivery of the baby.

At the time of delivery of a baby, the perineum naturally stretches to make room for the baby's head. For many years, a small incision in the perineum was routinely made to help with delivery. Called an *episiotomy*, this procedure is now a source of controversy in obstetrics. While many doctors stick with the practice, others recognize that epi-

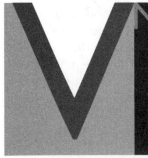

siotomy is associated with an increased risk of damage to the perineum and is not necessary for every birth. Episiotomy is required in some emergency situations where fast delivery at the last minute is essential; it's also often required for assisted delivery with forceps or vacuum suction.

Vulvar self-exam

Now you're ready to go to work becoming acquainted with the details of your own vulvar and vaginal anatomy. You will need time, privacy, and the determination to learn for yourself what you always thought was off-limits, "down there." Some people snicker at the thought of self-exploration. Others merely find the idea uncomfortable; exploring our bodies isn't easy, thanks to generations of taboos against erogenous zones that we've discussed earlier. Also, our culture emphasizes and at the same time forbids sexual arousal. As a result, you may feel very self-conscious when you touch yourself. But it's hard to learn about yourself if you don't look and touch.

The vulva and vagina are body parts, just like hands and feet. I've made the point that there's nothing wrong with exploring them. If

LABIAL ENHANCEMENT

Sometimes labia minora extend past the majora. This is entirely normal and usually of no medical concern. Sometimes, though, large labia minora can extend significantly past the labia majora, a condition called *hypertrophy of the labia minora*. Then women come to me with concerns that are functional, emotional, or purely cosmetic. For example, a woman may complain that when the labia minora stick out past the minora, they look ugly, like "spaniel's ears."[9] This enlargement can be only on one side or on both sides. It can cause irritation, sexual discomfort, hygiene problems during the menstrual period, and discomfort during physical activities such as running or swimming.

Occasionally, if this enlargement is severe, it merits surgical reduction. Such surgery can be done only if it's clear that any irritation and discomfort are not the result of a skin disease or a pain condition called vestibulodynia (see Chapter 17). Reduction surgery should only be done by a plastic surgeon or gynecologist with extensive experience doing this kind of procedure.

Labial reduction shouldn't be thought of like a "nose job," casual cosmetic surgery done to look better. Nor should it be done in the name of fashion, to achieve a certain look (the so-called labial enhancement). It's okay to be uneven. The labia don't have to match exactly. In fact, there's no single standard of what the labia are supposed to look like. Every woman looks a little different. You'll want to consider surgery only if you are troubled by irritation and discomfort from the extra labial size.

in the process of touching you become sexually aroused, fine. That means you're properly wired, which should be reassuring. Give yourself permission to experience the entire range of feelings, both sexual and nonsexual, about the skin in which you live.

To learn about the Vs you need to look at your genital area with a mirror and a bright light as you go through this chapter again; locate each illustrated area on your own body. You'll need good-sized aids. A large hand-held mirror and a gooseneck lamp will enable you to see well; you can't find anything with a compact mirror and a flashlight. Ideally, you'll also want to have both hands free.

The best way to do this is to straddle a mirror. But it has to be close to the vulva or you can't see well. Try this: Put the lid of the toilet down and place a couple of large, thick books on it, in order to raise the height of the mirror. Then lay the mirror on top of the books. Stand over the mirror, with your feet on either side of the toilet. (Adjust the number or size of the books you stack to suit your height.) Now place the lamp on the floor just a few inches away so that it can be aimed at your vulva while you're straddling the mirror on the books on the toilet seat. Prop this book on the toilet tank or anywhere you can see it well. Now both your hands are free to separate the labia so that you can view all the V parts. You may wish to pursue this interesting bathroom research during a private time at your house. On the other hand, learning about your body is no cause for shame.

If you are a woman of size, you will probably do better with a floor-to-ceiling mirror on the wall. You'll need to sit on the floor facing the mirror, as close as you can get, with your legs apart. Prop your head and shoulders with pillows or a backrest against a tipped-over chair in order to see over your abdomen. Adjust the light to shine on the vulva. You may be able to see well straddling a handheld mirror tilted slightly toward the wall mirror. You'll see the vulvar image in the wall mirror.

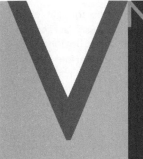

NOTE

For the woman who has everything

Dr. Arnold Kegel once made plaster casts of vaginas to prove the effects of his Kegel exercises. Now an entrepreneur has developed kits that enable a user to "make an exact copy of your lovely labia." Though casting your vulva in wax is billed as "a great way to get in touch with your anatomy without holding a mirror," a mirror is really much simpler and more educational.

You may have to look at one small area at a time. Even if you can't see your entire vulva at once, you can still do this tour if you make up your mind to do it. If you are comfortable with the idea, a friend or your partner can help.

Going step by step will make the job easier. Look, touch, and feel. It's okay. You are doing this because you want to understand how you are designed. You want to turn "down there" into "my vulva." This is not hands-off knowledge. Once you know every nook and cranny, you will *know* your own body.

With the mirror you will first see an overview of your outer genitals or *vulva,* everything between your legs. *Pubic hair* is the first obvious feature; it covers your *mons* over the pubic bone and grows down over your *labia majora* and around your *anus.* Under the hair, you can feel the plump thickness of the mons and the outer lips (labia majora). The outer lips surround the inner lips *(labia minora),* but your inner lips may extend beyond the outer lips. The area in the back between the lips and the anus is your *perineum.*

Take a close look at your inner lips. At their upper portion the thin inner lips divide; their uppermost divisions form a soft fold of skin, the hood or *prepuce* of the *clitoris.* The lower part of the division forms the *frenulum* to support the *glans clitoris.* In some women the inner lips have another division extending along the sides of the clitoral hood. You can gently pull back on the hood so that you see the little pink nub of the glans clitoris. Very gentle touching of this area is stimulating and feels wonderful. Now if you gently feel in and up on the clitoris toward the pubic bone, you will feel a firm, rubbery cordlike structure, the *shaft of the clitoris.* You will not be able to feel the rest of the clitoris, the crura. At the meeting point of the shaft and the crura, the vestibular bulbs await sexual stimulation to fill with blood. You cannot feel the bulbs under the labia.

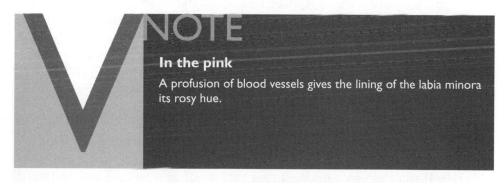

NOTE

In the pink
A profusion of blood vessels gives the lining of the labia minora its rosy hue.

As you spread your inner lips apart you see your vestibule, the tissue around the vaginal opening.

The vulvar self-exam should be comfortable or even exciting. If while you are doing this self-exam you experience pain—for example, if merely touching the vulva or the vestibule hurts or produces a stabbing sensation—you will want to find a clinician who can help you figure out what's going on.

At the base of your outer lips are the *Bartholin's glands.* You cannot see them, and are usually unable to feel a normal gland.

Back between your inner lips and just below your clitoris you will see the *urinary opening (urethra).* It looks like a small dimple or slit. Below this is the *vaginal opening (introitus);* if you have never had intercourse, this is

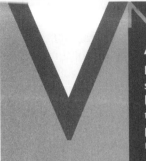

A matter of interpretation

In his classic book *The Perfumed Garden*, a sixteenth-century sheik cataloged forty-two different types of vulvas. Cheikh Nefzaoui's list included the Long One (extending to the anus), the Starling (that of a young brunette), the Humpbacked (with a prominent mons), and the Crested One (with frilled edges that redden upon excitement).

probably smooth and round, but there are many variations. If you have had intercourse, the smooth marginal ring around the opening divides into *hymenal remnants,* small tags of pink tissue all around the vaginal opening. If you have had a baby, your vaginal entrance may look open and the tissue tags may be prominent.

At the vaginal opening, insert your fingers into your *vagina.* As you go in slowly, you can appreciate that the front and back walls touch each other and spread as your fingers advance. The walls feel bumpy from the *rugae,* the interior folds that allow the vagina to expand with intercourse and childbirth. If everything feels dry and tight, you can use a little water or Vaseline to make your self-exam go smoothly. Push down toward the back; you'll feel some rectal pressure. Push up in the front; you'll feel it in your bladder. The vagina may feel a little sensitive everywhere.

With your fingers in the vagina, try to tighten the muscles around your fingers and grip. You are using the *muscles of the pelvic floor.* These muscles hold pelvic organs in place; sometimes they can be tight and cause spasms that make sexual intercourse painful.

A thin layer of tissue separates the vagina from the *rectum* in the back. You may be able to feel lumps of stool in the rectum through the vaginal wall.

If you slide your middle finger back as far as it will go, you will touch your *cervix.* This will feel like the tip of your nose, firm yet wobbly. The po-

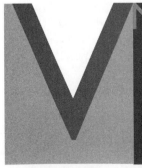

Further interpretations

Five centuries after Cheikh Nefzaoui's categorizations of the vulva, sex educator Betty Dodson came up with her own descriptions, based on architecture. Her list includes the Gothic Vulva (with cathedral-shaped arches), the Baroque (elaborate drapery), the simplistic Modern, and the Art Deco (characterized by graceful fluted lines).

sition of the cervix varies with the menstrual cycle and with sexual excitement, so that it may be easy or difficult to feel, depending on the situation. Note how your finger does not go straight in: The course of the vagina naturally causes your finger to go down and back at an angle toward the small of your back. All around the cervix—front, back, and sides—the vagina ends as a pouch, called the *vaginal fornix*.

There is no way that your finger, a tampon, or a penis can go through the cervix. (The only exception would be if violent force were used.) And because of its pouchlike shape, nothing can get lost in the vagina.

Now you're an expert. You know the names for everything; you know where everything goes and what it does. The vulva and vagina are not secret places; they are part of you. I hope you feel wonderful about your ownership.

▼

CHAPTER 3

The Vagina
Demystifying the Amazing "Secret" Organ

n the simplest terms, the vagina is a passageway. It starts with the opening (the introitus) and ends as a blind pouch around the neck of the womb (the cervix). But that basic architecture conjures up visions of a dull, empty hall rather than the happening, high-tech hostelry that the vagina more closely resembles. How many mere passageways do you know with expanding walls? How many passageways have ten trillion friendly inhabitants? How many passageways have the ability to constantly change their climate according to the varying needs of the surrounding structure?

The vagina is a uniquely specialized thoroughfare. It performs more widely varying functions than most organs of the body. Penises, tampons, and doctors' speculums go in. Babies and menstrual flow pass out. Yet for all this traffic, the vagina is as delicate as it is hardy. To remain healthy, it requires a precarious biological balance among the many bacteria that dwell naturally within it. It's the disruption of this balance that often leads to vaginitis, the collective term for the itching, redness, and swelling that send more adult women to their gynecologist than any other complaint. Understanding vaginal anatomy, the normal condition of the vagina, and what's not normal is the best first step to preventing and diagnosing problems.

V is for versatile

For a body part that is so often taken for granted, the vagina plays a starring role in many different aspects of life. It performs a variety of functions:

▼ *It serves as the passage for menstrual flow.* Rusty color on toilet paper or underpants for the first time marks the passage to womanhood, an event almost every girl grows up anticipating. Monthly egress fuels a billion-dollar industry for menstrual protection, tampons and pads.

▼ *It accommodates the penis during sexual intercourse.* In fact, the word *vagina* means "sheath." Encompassing the penis as a sheath covers a sword, the vagina brings pleasure to both men and women.

▼ *It serves as the birth canal for the delivery of a baby.* In one of the most awe-inspiring acts in creation, the vagina expands easily and naturally during childbirth. Cesarean sections (delivery of the baby surgically from the uterus through an incision in the abdomen) are done for many reasons—but never because the vagina doesn't work.

▼ *It allows access to the cervix for Pap smears and permits examination of the uterus and ovaries.* The vagina acts as a window to other, more internal organs. The Pap smear is one of the few truly effective medical tests, saving countless women from cervical cancer before the disease begins.

▼ *It prevents certain bacteria from entering the body.* The vagina is home to ten trillion lactobacilli, a type of "good" bacteria that produce an acidic environment, which in turn prevents the development of harmful bacteria that can cause infections.

What's where

Women tend to use the word *vaginal* vaguely, to refer to anything between the legs. For example, many patients tell me, "I'm having vaginal itching." Or they say, "It hurts inside." But they often mean that they itch or hurt between the labia, which is *outside* the vagina. Remember that to clinicians, "inside" means inside the vagina. The vagina is internal and completely separate from the vulva. Using a precise vocabulary is the first step to better care.

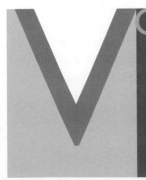

" 'Vagina.' There, I've said it. 'Vagina'—said it again. I say it because I believe that what we don't say, we don't see, acknowledge, or remember. What we don't say becomes a secret, and secrets often create shame and fear and myths. I say it because I want to someday feel comfortable saying it, and not ashamed and guilty."

—Playwright Eve Ensler, author of *The Vagina Monologues*

Why make a point about the difference? Because the vagina is made of a different kind of tissue from the vestibule and often develops different kinds of problems. Precise terminology can affect treatment. For example, if you have vaginitis, a cream medication needs to go *inside* the vagina. If you have a vulvar problem, however, the cream will not help inside the vagina. The medication would likely need to be applied inside the vestibule.

The vagina is an expandable muscular tube that runs from the vestibule to the cervix, which is the lowermost part of the uterus. If you are standing up, the vagina is tipped back 30 degrees. The angle is the same if you are lying down—sloping back 30 degrees. (If you remember your geometry, if you stand straight upright, your body is at 0 degrees. If you lie down flat, your body is at 90 degrees.) This means that the penis entering the vagina (if you are on your back) slides back away from your pleasure points, the clitoris and/or anterior vaginal wall (which may contain the G spot). That's why women usually tip up their hips during intercourse in the missionary position—in order for these areas to be stimulated by the penis on its way south.

The 30-degree angle also means that if you are inserting a tampon, you need to aim down and back (toward your lower back) whether you are standing or lying down. Your cervix also has something to say about where a tampon stays during its tour of duty. A longer tampon (say, Tampax compared to o.b.) often goes to the right or left of the cervix, meaning that when you pull the tampon out it is curved to the right or the left.

Along its front wall (under the bladder and the pubic bone) the vagina measures about 2½ to 2¾ inches (6 to 7 cm) from the opening back to the cervix; it's slightly longer along the back wall (above the rectum), 3 to 3⅜ inches (7.5 to 8.5 cm). That's basically a 2½-to-3-inch-long tube.

Around the entrance to the vagina (the introitus) are other muscles, those of the pelvic floor. These muscles hold the pelvic organs in place; strengthening these muscles through Kegel exercises can help with the enjoyment of sex and with giving birth, and can prevent problems controlling urine flow (urinary incontinence) and dropping (prolapse) of the uterus. Only a thin layer of tissue separates the vagina from the bladder in front and from the rectum behind; if you have some stool in the rectum, you may be able to feel a bump on one side of the vagina. If the wall between the rectum and vagina is really thin, stool in the rectum can raise enough of a bump in the vagina that a partner may feel somewhat of an obstacle on entry. The vagina ends in a blind pouch (the fornix) on each side of the cervix. **FIG. 25**

A design marvel

When not in use, the vagina is collapsed. Its walls touch each other. But they are easily pried apart by the fingers, a tampon, a penis, or a 10-pound

KEGELS, THE ESSENTIAL INNER EXERCISE

Childbirth educators preach them. Sex therapists swear by them. Gynecologists and other physicians recommend them, especially for patients with incontinence and prolapse. Women, however, are often left confused. What exactly is a Kegel exercise, and why is it so important?

Basically, Kegels (which get their name from Dr. Arnold Kegel, and are also called pelvic floor squeezes, perineal exercises, or tightening exercises) strengthen the pubococcygeus (PC) muscle. It's the main muscle of the pelvic floor, which surrounds the vaginal, urethral, and rectal openings. Strong muscles lend good support and improve bladder control.

To locate the PC muscle, imagine that you're urinating and then stop the flow. Or you can locate the muscle while you're actually urinating, although it's not recommended to actually do Kegels then because it can promote urinary tract infections. Hold the squeeze for ten seconds and release. Do this ten times in a row, and build up to about twenty times in a row.

To be effective, Kegels must be done properly and regularly for three months before results can be expected. Just as with sit-ups, these exercises work only when the right muscles are used, when the squeeze is held long enough, and when sufficient repetitions are done.

To make Kegels a regular health habit, try doing them:

▼ While you watch TV

▼ While you're commuting or waiting at red lights

▼ Before or after your usual workout

▼ In the bathroom

▼ During meetings at work (no one can tell!)

▼ As you drift off to sleep

Should everyone do them? Most health professionals agree that Kegels are beneficial to women who have relaxation of their pelvic floor muscles—for example, after pregnancy. Kegels can't change the effect of a weighty pregnant uterus, but women who learn the exercise during the last part of pregnancy and are instructed in the hospital after delivery have better results, including less incontinence, during the postpartum period. (Kegels are also recommended for men after prostate surgery.) Kegels cannot improve a dropped uterus (uterine prolapse).

Kegels can also help strengthen the pelvic floor in women who:

▼ Are born with congenital defects of the pelvic floor

▼ Have a Caucasian background and a family history of dropped uterus or bladder

▼ Had traumatic childhood injuries in the area

▼ Have had vaginal surgery

▼ Have jobs involving heavy lifting and climbing

▼ Often get constipated and strain at bowel movements

▼ Participate heavily in such sports as jumping, hurdling, gymnastics, basketball, volleyball, karate, judo, bodybuilding, and daily horseback riding featuring dressage and jumping

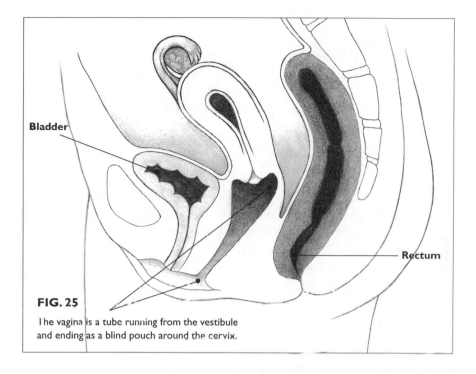

Bladder

Rectum

FIG. 25

The vagina is a tube running from the vestibule and ending as a blind pouch around the cervix.

baby during childbirth. How is this possible? I used to spend a lot of time wondering about this in junior high. I couldn't imagine how a penis could fit, let alone a baby! But Mother Nature is pretty clever. The width and length of the vagina vary from one woman to another, but, as I will say again, the size of the vagina is not a cause for painful intercourse or failure of the baby to come through because of the elastic nature of the surrounding muscles. There is a circular layer and a layer running up and down longitudinally. These muscles are not under your control, unlike the muscles of the pelvic floor that you tighten and release to do Kegels.

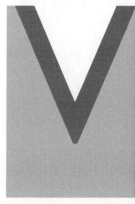

NOTE

Size *doesn't* matter

Vaginal size, anyway. Thanks to the accordion-style folds of skin in its walls, any woman's vagina can accommodate any size penis, no matter how large. Vaginas can also accommodate a baby of any size during childbirth. (Narrow pelvic bones, or a pelvic structure that is too small for the baby, are the reasons some women have trouble giving birth vaginally—not a too-small vagina.) Nor has vaginal size been found to be a cause of painful intercourse.

The elastic muscles of the vaginal wall are covered with *rugae,* soft folds of connective tissue. Other muscular cavities of the body also have a capacity for expansion, like the stomach or bladder. But the vagina's rugae allow even more. They look and function like broomstick pleats in fabric, allowing the muscle to expand to proportions otherwise unimaginable. (Babies are further aided at birth by the fact that the bones of the skull can overlap slightly so that the diameter of the head is compressed to make the trip.) Remember that you can feel these yourself. If you run your finger inside the vagina, you feel little ridges rather than smooth walls.

The vaginal lining *(squamous epithelium)* is key to the clever construction that accommodates the diverse activities that take place in this passageway. The vagina is lined by the same moist, sturdy covering found in the mouth. In the vagina, the cells that form this lining multiply and thicken in response to fluctuating estrogen levels. (This is different from the mouth, where the lining remains at a constant thickness because there are no estrogen receptors there.) Squamous epithelium is designed to be rugged; in the mouth it accommodates chewing as well as food particles and the enzymes in saliva. In the vagina, squamous epithelium is tough enough to deal with all the traffic through the vagina: menstruation, sexual activity, and childbirth. It's also remarkably resilient. When injured (scraped by vigorous sex or scratched by a tampon applicator, for instance), the vagina can heal in forty-eight hours.

Physicians have always been taught that the vagina doesn't have many nerve endings and has very little sensation. The pain of labor was supposed to come from the opening of the cervix. I always wondered how sexual enjoyment could work without any nerves around, but the focus of sexual research at the time was on the clitoris. It was believed that if a sample of tissue (biopsy) was necessary from the vagina, no local anesthetic was needed. Repair of lacerations of the vulva or perineum at delivery were thought to require local anesthesia, but

THE G SPOT: FACT OR FICTION?

The G spot is the name given to an area of sensitive tissue in the front wall of the vagina, just under the urethra. Its name comes from Dr. Ernst Grafenberg, a German ob-gyn who first wrote about it in 1950. While traditional sexual researchers suggest that the clitoris is the main source of female sexual pleasure, Grafenberg (and later others) reported that the G spot is also a significant contributor to stimulation through another nerve source.

Is it really there? Some women insist they've never felt it, while others assert that it's not only there but an erogenous zone worth seeking out. Or is the G spot actually part of the clitoris rather than the vagina? For all of its publicity and ready acceptance into modern sexual beliefs, there's no professional consensus about the existence of the G spot. But couples can have great fun trying to locate it.

For more information, see Chapter 2, "The Vulva," and Chapter 6, "Sex Matters."

not stitching up in the vagina. It turns out that the nerve supply has been there all along—we just didn't have the technology to find it. During the last decade, special staining techniques on tissue from the human vagina show that all its regions have a rich nerve supply. Areas closer to the vaginal opening (the introitus) are richer in nerve fibers than the distant vagina up by the cervix, and the front wall has more than the back.[1]

Vaginal secretions

Most women wonder at one time or another about vaginal discharge. If there is a yellowish stain on your underwear, does it indicate a problem? Is it okay if slippery mucus always seems present? Is discharge something that's supposed to be there or not?

It certainly is normal to have vaginal discharge during the reproductive years. In fact, I'm amazed that women don't have more than they do, given the variety of substances that lurk within the vaginal walls. Actually, the vagina itself doesn't make many secretions. There are no glands in the vagina. What is called "vaginal discharge" is composed of a number of secretions from several sources. Discharge may include:

- ▼ Oil and sweat from oil and sweat glands in the vulva
- ▼ Secretions from specialized vulvar glands called Bartholin's and Skene's glands
- ▼ Moisture that comes through the vaginal walls (called *transudate*)
- ▼ Cells shed from the vaginal walls
- ▼ Mucus from the cervix
- ▼ Fluid from the Fallopian tubes and uterus
- ▼ Products from bacteria that live in the vagina
- ▼ Salt water (the physiologic saline that makes up most bodily fluids and mucus)

As you can see from this list, vaginal discharge is made up of things already in your body—salt water, minerals, cells. It's not waste matter or dirt

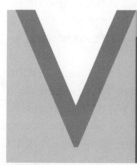

NOTE

How dry I'm *not*

It's a myth that stained underwear is a sign of a problem. Depending on the time of your menstrual cycle, perfectly ordinary secretions may cause stains or wetness.

in the sense of urine or feces. Under ordinary circumstances, then, some discharge is perfectly natural.

Exactly how much vaginal discharge does a woman normally produce? It's not clear. For something that is such a basic aspect of every woman's life, relatively few scientific measurements have been made. Gynecology texts seldom describe how much is normal; older books sometimes included a general statement such as "There is a constant small amount of vaginal discharge present" or an indication that the vagina when examined with a speculum is "no more than moist."[2] How these conclusions were reached is unclear.

A few studies have attempted to measure the exact amount of vaginal secretions by weighing tampons that have been worn by subjects throughout their menstrual cycles. The amount of fluid is estimated by comparing the weight of the tampon before the experiment to its increased weight afterward. In one such study, the average amount of vaginal secretion produced by twenty-two women of reproductive age was 1.55 g per eight hours over all cycle days. (A gram, abbreviated *g*, is about ¼ teaspoon.) Secretion was greatest on day 14, ovulation (1.96 g). The least amount was on day 7 (1.38 g) and day 26 (1.37 g).[3] Women taking the birth control pill showed less variation because oral contraceptives involve less fluctuation of hormones. Another study looked at women fitted with cervical caps. By placing a rubber cap over the cervix, the researchers could measure the amount of fluid from the vagina only. The measured amount of vaginal secretions in twenty-four hours was similar: 1.89 g.[4]

This research has involved only small numbers of women, though. Physicians who work with women constantly know that moisture and wetness are common and normal. We also know that the phase of the menstrual cycle is extremely important. The amount of discharge varies with hormone levels (estrogen generally increases secretions) and with the nature of the cervix (some cervices make more mucus than others).

HOW HORMONES INFLUENCE VAGINAL SECRETIONS

Another important thing to know about normal vaginal discharge is that it is acidic. Acid? The stuff that burns holes in things? What is acid doing in the vagina? Actually, the vagina is only mildly acidic, not enough to be corrosive. But for optimal vaginal health, a certain level of acidity needs to be maintained.

The measure of acidity is called pH, an indication of the concentration of hydrogen in a solution. The lower the pH—which is measured on a scale from 1 to 14—the more acidic a solution is. A pH of 7.0 is neutral. High-pH solutions are alkaline, like lye, which has a pH of 14 and is very corrosive. Low-pH solutions are acidic, such as sulfuric acid (which has a pH of 1), and can burn a hole in nearly anything it touches. The human vagina has a pH of 3.5 to 4.5—on the acidic side, though not as much as lemon juice or soda pop. (My dentist loves to show that cola will erode the enamel of a tooth soaked in it for several hours.)

The vagina, of course, is not acidic enough to be corrosive. But why does it need to be acidic at all? For your protection. Because the vagina opens to the outside world, bacteria can get it. The vagina's acid environment controls bacteria and prevents the harmful types that like a high pH from overgrowing. (One common reason for vaginal discharge, bacterial vaginosis, or BV, occurs when the pH is out of balance; see Chapter 11.)

How does the vagina make and keep its low pH? That's where hormones and bacteria come in. The amount and type of secretions are influenced by the amount of estrogen and progesterone circulating through the body. You always have these hormones, but their quantity rises and falls over the course of the menstrual cycle. The vaginal lining and its purpose also change during the cycle. Discharge is minimal at the beginning of a cycle, becomes most noticeable at ovulation and just afterward, then diminishes. Here's why.

During the first week of the cycle, menstruation, estrogen is low. As estrogen picks up, the cells of the vaginal lining multiply under its influence. Secretions begin to increase. At midcycle, just after ovulation, estrogen levels suddenly plummet and progesterone rises.[5] The buildup of the vaginal lining stops. By now, the lining has become thick and rich in a special kind of starch called glycogen. Glycogen is broken down by the normal bacteria that live in the vagina into glucose, which is their energy source. After the bacteria have used the glucose, the end product is lactic acid. This process is thought to contribute to the acid environment of the vagina, which encourages the survival and growth of such acid-loving organisms as the lactobacilli, one of the major groups of "good" bacteria

HOW DISCHARGE CHANGES		This table shows the relationship between the menstrual cycle hormones and secretions.	
Cycle Day	**Estrogen**	**Progesterone**	**Secretions**
1–7	Low	Very low	Menstrual flow begins and ends Few secretions Dryness
8–13	Rises and peaks	Very low	Secretions increase
14–16	Drops sharply	Starts to rise	Ovulation; maximum clear mucus
17–25	Second small rise	Peaks	Secretions thicken and turn yellowish
26–1	Drops slowly	Drops rapidly	Secretions diminish to low point

living in the vagina. When the vagina is acidic, the lactobacilli can stick to vaginal epithelial cells and stay in the vagina.

So an acidic vagina is a healthy vagina. The acid balance is kept there by your friends the lactobacilli. Nothing you can eat, drink, or douche with is going to change that balance on an ongoing basis.

The uppermost or top layers of the vaginal wall that thickened during the first half of the menstrual cycle are shed during the latter part of the cycle, resulting in a much thinner lining, but a thicker discharge containing all the cells from the vaginal wall. A thin vaginal wall is less elastic, less comfortable during sex, and more vulnerable to injury.

Those extra secretions at midcycle come mostly from the cervix, the uterus, and the Fallopian tubes. At ovulation, the cervix changes to favor the passage of sperm through it on their way to fertilize an egg. The cervical mucus thins and becomes more watery and more plentiful. The mucus is stretchy and will form long strands between two surfaces. Because thin, stretchy mucus is more porous, it is all the better for allowing sperm to swim through. (Thick mucus is hostile to sperm penetration.) This altered mucus is the main component of increased vaginal discharge in midcycle.

After ovulation, levels of progesterone are high in order to support the early stage of pregnancy if fertilization occurs. Progesterone makes vaginal secretions thicker and yellowish. As the cycle winds down toward the time the menstrual period is due, there are fewer secretions. After the period, discharge continues to be scanty for the first week. Then, as estrogen rises, so do secretions, and the cycle begins again.

Oral contraceptives introduce a steady level of estrogen and progesterone daily so that all the normal variations of the cycle are overridden and there are no cyclical variations in the cervical mucus.[6]

HOW THE CERVIX INFLUENCES VAGINAL SECRETIONS

Clearly the cervix is a major player in determining how much vaginal discharge is experienced on any given day. Although the cervix is the neck of the uterus, it's technically not part of the uterus because it's made of different tissue. In fact, it's so different that doctors consider it a separate organ. At the upper end of the cervix, the uterine cavity narrows to an opening called the *internal os* (*os* means "opening" or "mouth"). The internal os connects to a canal (the *endocervical canal*) through the cervix to the vagina. The opening of the cervix into the vagina is called the *external os*. Like the vagina, the cervix has a rugged covering *(squamous epithelium)* designed to be tough enough to withstand sexual intercourse. The mucus that's so noticeable around ovulation originates from a more delicate layer of cells (the *columnar epithelium*) that line the cervical canal. They manufacture the mucus in order to protect the cervix from disease and to help with fertility. Good clear mucus provides a good traveling medium for sperm.

The delicate columnar epithelium is usually buried within the endocervical canal and is not visible. Under the influence of estrogen, though, this layer of cells can spread out of the canal and onto the cervix. When these mucus-producing cells grow out onto the surface of the cervix, they cause a red appearance because they form a single cell layer and their capillaries filled with blood are easily seen. In the past, doctors thought this red appearance represented inflammation or an infection called cervicitis, and treated the cervix with heat (cauterization) to destroy these cells. If you are over fifty, you may have had your cervix cauterized. It's now known, however, that the presence of mucus-producing cells on the outside of the cervix is a variation of what is normal. This condition typically occurs during puberty, during pregnancy, and under the influence of the birth control pill—all circumstances that are associated with raised estrogen levels. Some women who are not pregnant or on the pill have this condition too, just because their bodies make plenty of estrogen. With time, the columnar epithelium can change into squamous epithelium; with age and declining estrogen levels, the mucus-producing cells can retreat back to the cervical canal. None of these situations requires treatment.

Some women complain of having too much vaginal discharge all the time, so heavy that they feel they need to wear sanitary pads or tampons throughout their cycle. First of all, it's unwise to wear such protection continually, so please don't. (See Chapter 5, "V Smarts," to learn why.) Seemingly excessive discharge can happen when there are mucus-producing cells from the endocervical canal on the surface of the cervix; more mucus is produced, which in turn contributes to increased discharge. Unfortunately, we do not have a good way to improve this annoying situation. If cultures for herpes, chlamydia, and gonorrhea—organisms that can infect the columnal epithelial cells of the cervical canal—are negative, if other parts of the evaluation show no abnormal findings, and if a future pregnancy is desired, destroying the cells with heat or by freezing may eliminate the excess mucus, which can impair fertility. But if testing has shown that the mucus or discharge is normal,

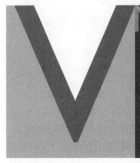

An important distinction

Menstrual flow is entirely different from vaginal discharge. Menstruation comes from the uterine lining and represents cyclical bleeding that is unrelated to the vagina or the cervix.

women of childbearing age who experience this problem are best advised to put up with the wetness.

The all-important V bacteria

Bacteria that dwell in the vagina also influence discharge. All open body cavities—the mouth, the intestines, and the rectum, as well as the vagina—are home to high levels of bacteria. Why don't all these bacteria cause disease? Most of them are harmless. Some (called pathogens) are capable of causing disease. But a major benefit of the "friendly" bacteria normally living in these areas is that they keep potentially harmful bacteria from setting up housekeeping (a process called colonization). Defenses in the vagina such as vaginal secretions, cervical mucus, and the "police patrol" of the white blood cells of the immune system also keep bacteria from invading further and causing disease.

The exact array of bacteria in each area of the body is unique, dependent on different conditions present in that particular site. The vagina and its particular bacteria form a finely balanced ecosystem that favors certain bacteria, which in turn influence the vaginal environment. This

NORMAL BACTERIA IN A HEALTHY VAGINA

Organism	% of Women Harboring the Bacterium
Lactobacillus	68
Corynebacterium	31
Streptococcus	37
Enterococcus	26
Staphylococcus epidermidis	53
Staphylococcus aureus	8
Escherichia coli	20
Gardnerella vaginalis	25
Clostridium	12
Peptostreptococcus tetradius	26
Bacteroides	52
Fusobacterium	21

Source: S. Faro, Bacterial vaginitis, *Clin Obstet & Gynecol* 1977:128:777.

ecosystem changes as hormone levels vary, for example, but cycles back again month after month. Thus the bacterial population is not a fixed and unchanging population but is constantly fluctuating.

It's important to understand the makeup of the normal vaginal bacteria for two reasons: (1) some of the bacteria have key jobs in the vagina, and altering them may result in disease, and (2) although most of the bacteria in the vagina are not ordinarily capable of causing disease there, they can produce disease when normal conditions in the vagina change drastically. In other words, if either the environment of the vagina is changed or the bacteria that live there are altered, vaginal symptoms may result.

Complicating this delicate balance is the sheer number of bacteria. The total number of bacteria in the vagina is over ten trillion per quarter teaspoon of vaginal secretion![7] The most widespread group belong to a family called lactobacilli. *Lactobacillus acidophilus,* the familiar variety you see listed on yogurt cartons, is only one example of this large group. In 1892, when the first extensive study of human vaginal bacteria was done, it was thought that there was only one group of bacteria present, called Doderlein's bacilli, which are now known to be members of the lactobacillus family. When other vaginal bacteria were discovered, they were perceived as unhealthy. Another eighty years passed before science recognized that

VOICES

"I'm fine with the word *vulva* but not entirely comfortable with *vagina,* which is odd since no coy substitute words were used at home when I was young. On the other hand, my mother is Irish Catholic and didn't exactly go out of her way to have long gynecological chats with us. We got bare-bones facts and that was it—not inaccurate, but not delivered in any way that put you at ease.

"I think *vagina* just *sounds* weird. I feel when I say it that it's likely to have the same effect in a room that the words 'E. F. Hutton' did in that old ad—a total hush falls over the room. Which makes one . . . cautious."

—Flora, 47

the normal vagina has a wide variety of bacteria, including some that do not require oxygen for growth (anaerobes) and others that do require oxygen (aerobes).

There are other bacteria that may also be found in the normal vagina. As you look at this list you may recognize names of bacteria such as *E. coli* that are known to cause disease; but, as I mentioned earlier, we're kept safe from dangerous invasion by an intact vaginal lining, the vaginal mucus barrier, and cells of the vaginal immune system. It's very important to realize that any culture done of the vagina will grow a wide variety of bacteria. That's why gynecologists who specialize in vulvovaginal work do not recommend vaginal cultures of bacteria—they can be misleading. A culture positive for *E. coli* or strep or *Gardnerella* merely identifies bacteria that one would expect to find. These bacteria are unlikely to be the cause of symptoms. On the other hand, there are some bacteria that are never normal inhabitants of the vagina. They include those that cause gonorrhea *(Neisseria gonorrheae),* the organism causing chlamydial infection, and the virus causing herpes. These cause sexually transmitted disease in the cervix and are detected with special cultures of the cervix, not the vagina.

THE GOOD GUYS: VAGINAL LACTOBACILLI

Vaginal lactobacilli are worth a closer look because of their crucial role in protecting us from disease. More than any of the many other types of vaginal bacteria, the right amount of lactobacilli seems to help ensure V health. It's not certain how this protection happens, but several ways have been suggested:

1. Lactic acid from lactobacilli may contribute to keeping the vagina acidic.

2. Lactobacilli may keep other bacteria from sticking, or adhering, to the vagina.

3. Production of hydrogen peroxide by lactobacilli keeps other bacteria under control.

VOICES

"I never thought about what my vagina was, or what it looked like. I didn't even really understand whether my urine came through the vagina or where the menstrual flow came from. I don't think girls grow up with a picture of their insides in their heads—and I sure didn't look.

"Even now that I have a baby, I don't feel like I know everything I should. For instance, when I was pregnant, I read about 'the birth canal' but at first I didn't even realize that it was the same thing as the vagina. That might sound dumb, especially coming from someone who has given birth, but there are a lot of euphemisms out there. Even in books about pregnancy. I mean, why do they call it a birth canal when they really mean vagina?"

—Jessica, 30

4. Lactobacilli produce a number of substances that inhibit other bacteria.

5. Lactobacilli may stimulate the vaginal immune system.

One of the keys to diagnosing vaginitis is the absence of lactobacilli under the microscope, in a test called a wet prep. A small amount of vaginal secretion is mixed with a few drops of salt water on a slide. In the healthy vagina, many lactobacilli are present; they predominate on the slide. So if a clinician sees lactobacilli prevailing on the slide, infection is not present. The only exception is a yeast infection, because yeast can grow with the lactobacilli around. In these cases clinicians believe that although there are adequate numbers of lactobacilli, they are not functioning the way they should.

The importance of the lactobacilli is demonstrated by the most common vaginal problem in the United States, bacterial vaginosis. BV, as it's more commonly known, is not an infection but a lack of lactobacilli with a corresponding overgrowth of other normal bacterial inhabitants of the vagina, that leads to discharge and odor. The pH level also becomes elevated from all the bacteria, so the vagina is no longer acidic. What causes the lactobacilli to vanish is not known at this time, and though BV can be improved with antibiotics, it often returns. (A complete picture of BV is in Chapter 11.)

TOURING THE V ECOSYSTEM

The type and number of bacteria that live in the vagina are governed by many different factors. These range from the presence of sperm or antibiotics to such things as douching, immunosuppression caused by drugs to treat diseases, or surgery. Diseases such as HIV, diabetes, and cancer may also influence vaginal bacteria.

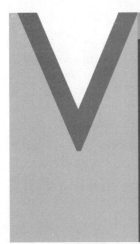

V NOTE

Shakespeare's vagina

While many modern euphemisms for female genitalia sound crude, those used by the Bard have a certain poetic ring:

- ▼ Maidenhead (*Twelfth Night*)
- ▼ The Netherlands (*The Comedy of Errors*)
- ▼ Glass of her virginity (hymen; *Pericles*)
- ▼ Virgin-knot (hymen; *The Tempest*)
- ▼ Tail (*The Taming of the Shrew*)
- ▼ Treasure (*Cymbeline*)
- ▼ Sweet bottom grass (*Venus and Adonis*)

Probably the most important factor, however, is hormonal. Hormonal levels change throughout your life cycle (see Chapter 1) as well as during each menstrual cycle. As I previously mentioned, the vaginal lining also varies considerably during the menstrual cycle. Cells lining the vagina multiply under the influence of estrogen but then become inactive at midcycle, when estrogen levels fall and progesterone dominates. At midcycle the lining is thick and rich in glycogen content; the top layers are shed during the second half of the cycle, resulting in a much thinner lining. Then the cycle begins again.

Vaginal pH varies a lot during the cycle too. At the start of menstrual flow, the pH is already increased, peaking at around 7.0. The pH then drops sharply to between 4.0 and 4.5 over the next three days and remains constant until day 21, although it may rise slightly with ovulation. Bacterial populations show great variations during the menstrual cycle; as would be expected, they are highest in the menstrual flow, possibly because menstrual blood acts as a source of nutrition, or because of the rising pH associated with menstrual blood.[8]

During pregnancy, the carbohydrate content and lactic acid concentration of the vaginal lining increase so that conditions become even more favorable to the acid-loving vaginal bacteria. The changes probably protect the fetus from passing through a birth canal populated with many kinds of bacteria. Immediately postpartum, the vaginal flora change dramatically. Low estrogen levels have a marked influence on the vagina of a breast-feeding mother; the cells are low in glycogen, so the walls are thin and dry, and lubrication may be necessary for comfortable sex.

Sexual intercourse may have an effect on the composition of the bacteria in the vagina. Ejaculate, as well as the lubricating mucus generated by sexual arousal, are strongly alkaline, raising the vaginal pH. It can take up to eight hours after intercourse for the pH to return to normal; women

	Pregnancy and Newborn	Premenarchal	Menarchal or Reproductive	Postmenopausal
Estrogen level	High	Low	Medium	Low
pH	Acid	Neutral	Acid	Neutral
Glycogen content	High	Low	Medium	Low
Number and variety of bacteria	Increased	Decreased	Increased	Decreased

who are very sexually active rarely possess a vaginal bacterial population characteristic of low (4.5) pH.

Not everything affects vaginal bacteria. Sanitary methods and contraceptive techniques have little effect, for example. Nor do tampons have an effect. It's been proven that insertion of a tampon, or the string itself, is not likely to carry fecal bacteria into the vagina from the vulva and skin around the anus.[9]

The table on page 56 summarizes the conditions of the vagina during the life of the normal female.

So what's "normal" discharge?

What all this tells us is that, far from being a static, empty vessel, the vagina is a dynamic organ with its own constantly changing ecosystem. The normal vaginal microflora prevent potentially disease-causing organisms from moving in. Lactobacilli predominate in part because estrogen keeps vaginal cells rich in glycogen to feed them; in turn, they release lactic acid, which contributes to keeping the vagina acidic. Menstruation, intercourse, disease, douching, and antibiotics all change the acid-base and bacterial balances—and this, in turn, affects the discharge you notice when you wipe yourself in the bathroom or change your underwear.

Depending on the time of the menstrual cycle, secretions make a clear, milky white, or faintly yellow discharge. Sometimes there is stringy mucus. The discharge may be somewhat slippery or clumpy. Most women have small white or yellow stains on their underwear, varying with their menstrual cycles. Normal secretions will also form small dry yellow-white flakes or clumps in the pubic hair surrounding the vaginal opening. Some women have enough normal secretions to make them feel wet all the time. What if you never notice any discharge? That's normal too. Your secretions probably remain in the vagina without appearing on the outside.

The important thing is that normal secretions do not itch, burn, or irritate. Normal secretions do not have a bad odor, although secretions that stay on the underwear may develop a slightly sour smell. (For more on odor, see Chapter 7, "The Most Bothersome Symptoms.") Normal secretions do not contain any blood, even in microscopic amounts. Women with normal discharge will have a normal gynecological exam, showing no skin problems on the outside or problems with the uterus, ovary, or tubes on the inside that suggest a contribution to wetness. Women with normal discharge also have a low (acid) pH, normal findings under the microscope, and negative cultures for yeast, chlamydia, and gonorrhea. A culture for bacteria will always grow all kinds of bacteria because all kinds of bacteria live in the vagina. A complete assessment of these factors is needed to properly diagnose and treat vaginal problems. Do not be reassured by a clinician who tells you things are fine based on just looking.

CHARACTERISTICS OF NORMAL VAGINAL DISCHARGE IN REPRODUCTIVE-AGE WOMEN

Amount	Variable depending on menstrual cycle and individual woman
Color	White, mucoid; yellowish during second half of the cycle
Consistency	Floccular (tiny particles mixed in white liquid); clear stringy mucus at midcycle; stringy mucus if cervix is active
pH	Less than 4.5
Microscopic	Some white cells, many lactobacilli, vaginal epithelial cells with sharp borders; small round yeast spores may be seen
Culture for bacteria	Positive for many different kinds, such as *E. coli*, strep, staph
Cervical culture	Negative for herpes, chlamydia, gonorrhea

(For more information on how to be sure to get a proper exam, see Chapter 9.)

The table above summarizes normal secretions.

IF YOU'RE POSTMENOPAUSAL

The preceding information relates to women who are in their reproductive years. With menopause and the loss of estrogen and progesterone, all the cyclical variations cease. The amount of cervical mucus diminishes and the lactobacilli disappear from the vagina. Discharge is minimal to absent.

There are some exceptions to this:

V NOTE

Discharge as birth control?

Predicting ovulation by vaginal discharge is part of natural family planning, a type of contraception in which women observe and touch their cervical secretions on a daily basis and record changes on a chart. Ovulation is signaled by an increase in secretions that are clear, stretchy, and slippery in character. *Perfect* use of this method results in a 3 percent pregnancy rate during the first year of use (that is, three women per hundred who use the method perfectly will become pregnant). One big however: Because it's more difficult than, say, popping a pill or inserting a diaphragm, typical use results in a higher pregnancy rate, around 20 percent.

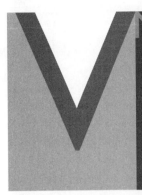

NOTE

Everybody gets it wrong

New York's *Village Voice* newspaper reported that a Halloween parade float was halted before it reached TV cameras, presumably because "one float performer was dressed as a giant vagina for the nationally televised event." Never mind whether or not the costume—which featured a curly-haired mons and anatomically correct labia—was suitable for a national audience. It was technically a vulva, not a vagina.

▼ If you are taking hormone replacement therapy, you may continue to have white or yellow-white discharge.

▼ If you are not on hormone replacement, you may develop such low levels of estrogen that there is a sticky yellow discharge made up of white blood cells, bacteria, and cells from the vaginal wall. This or any unusual discharge in a postmenopausal woman needs to be evaluated by a doctor.

▼ If you are a large woman, you may have significant levels of estrogen in your body after menopause. Although the ovaries cease production, body fat can convert adrenal hormones into estrogen. It is possible to have some of the whitish discharge seen in the reproductive years.

▼ If you are on tamoxifen as treatment for breast cancer, it may act as an estrogen on the vagina of the postmenopausal woman. It's possible to have slightly increased discharge. Since yeast needs estrogen in order to flourish, women on tamoxifen may develop yeast infections.

▼

CHAPTER 4

At Different Ages

V Changes Throughout the Life Cycle

The body you had while surfing in your mother's womb and the body you have when you reach menopause are one and the same—and yet they're different in many ways. You grow. The structures change physically. Your habits, lifestyle, and priorities vary over time. You're vulnerable to different health conditions at different stages of life as well.

All of these life changes bring about vulvovaginal changes. In fact, the vagina is amazingly different throughout a woman's life. While I'll walk you through specific problems later in the book, it's both interesting and helpful to have a grounding in what you can generally expect across your life span. After all, your vagina plays a prominent role in many of the key passages of being female—beginning menstruation, first intercourse, pregnancy, motherhood, and menopause.

So here are snapshots of what happens to your V zone as you age.

Prenatal and newborn

It all starts at conception. In order to be born a female, four important steps must take place: (1) First, as a baby is conceived, an X chromosome from the mother and an X chromosome from the father come together, making a female. The sex of the baby has been determined by the master controls, the genes. (The father determines the gender; if he contributes a Y chromosome, the baby is born male, as the mother always contributes an X.) (2) Under the control of the X chromosome, the ovaries develop in

Q How do I keep the genitals clean during diapering and bathing?

A Wiping carefully from front to back with a damp washcloth or baby wipe is all that's required. Baby lotions or powders aren't recommended. If you do use a powder, choose cornstarch rather than talc because talc has been linked with cancer. A drawback of powders (unrelated to Vs) is that they can be inhaled and gag a baby should they spill.

Q What's that white gunky stuff that seems to collect between an older baby's labia?

A It's normal lubricating secretions (sebum) from the glands of the vestibule. It's seen in adult women as well. Without it, the labia would rub against each other and become irritated.

Q What if my baby's clitoris or labia looks large? How big is too big?

A The labia minora and clitoris always appear prominent in a little girl since the mons and labia majora are diminished. There's a wide variation in size and shape of the normal clitoris and labia minora. If you are concerned, ask your pediatrician.

the female baby. (3) During the development of the baby in the womb, the ovary makes hormones that direct the development of the internal genitalia (uterus, tubes, and vagina) and the external genitalia (the vulva and vestibule). (4) The final step occurs after the baby has been born and goes through childhood. At puberty, the appearance of breasts, the development of axillary and pubic hair (secondary sex characteristics), and the beginning of menstruation complete the developmental sequence.

Sex hormones from the ovaries are vital for the formation of the vulva and vagina and influence what they look like and how they function through life. At birth, a baby has no bacteria in her vagina. But shortly after birth, because of high levels of estrogen that she received from the

V NOTE

Appearances are deceiving

In the womb, boys and girls look exactly alike until the ninth or tenth week of gestation. Then the shrimp-sized fetus begins to develop either testes or ovaries, depending on how it's been genetically preprogrammed to evolve. These differences aren't visible on an ultrasound for almost another two months, though.

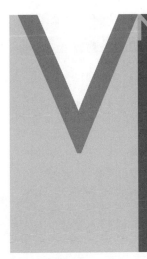

Rare birth defect

It's possible for a woman to be born without a vagina. In some cases, during fetal development the cells in the embryo that are supposed to form the pouch do not. No one knows why. The uterus, tubes, and ovaries develop normally, since they form from a different set of embryonic cells, but only a dimple appears where the vagina should be. A "neo-vagina" can be constructed surgically with a skin graft or by gradually expanding the dimpled area. To date no one has been able to connect the new vagina to the uterus, but in-vitro fertilization and cesarean delivery make pregnancy possible. Most gynecologists have never even seen this uncommon condition.

mother's blood via the umbilical cord, the vulva and vagina of the newborn are similar to the vulva and vagina of the reproductive-age woman. This situation lasts only a few weeks, however, until the amount of estrogen drops after birth.

The skin of a baby's labia majora and the mons are hairless because pubic hair does not appear until the adrenal glands are activated at puberty. The labia majora are plump and tend to hide the surprisingly well-developed labia minora. When the legs are opened up, the vaginal opening is easily seen between the labia. You can't see the urinary opening, but you know things are normal when the baby wets a diaper. Some thick mucus may cover the vaginal opening, and because of the estrogen plummeting after birth, there may even be some vaginal bleeding in the first few weeks of life. This can happen because the uterine lining bleeds anytime estrogen is suddenly withdrawn from it. It's the same reason you get breakthrough bleeding if you miss one or two birth control pills. There are abundant lactobacilli in the baby's vagina.

Childhood

For the most part during childhood, the V area is in a quiet mode; it doesn't need to gear up until puberty for the demands of intercourse and childbearing. Soon after birth, estrogen levels in the little girl drop and stay low until puberty. The fat pads forming the mons and prominent labia majora diminish in size; by comparison, the labia minora and the clitoris appear relatively prominent. Because there is little estrogen during childhood, the surface of all the vulvar tissues is thin with a pale red to pinkish color (from blood vessels showing through). It's possible for the labia to stick together, a condition called labial adhesion, especially in late infancy and toddlerhood. This is because there's no estrogen to produce

COMMON QUESTIONS: Childhood

Q Is it okay to use bubble bath?

A Bubble bath is fine as a special treat as long as it does not cause irritation or itching afterward for your daughter. Daily use, however, exposes your child to unnecessary chemicals, and irritation or allergy can evolve. Choose a product that's formulated for children's use, but even then, use only periodically. Strongly scented soaps can irritate too.

Q At what age should I use words like vulva and labia when talking to my daughter?

A Use them right from the start. Accurate anatomical terms make a girl feel comfortable that this is a normal part of her body and not some anonymous, cryptic, mysterious "down there."

Q My preschooler tries to stick toys in her vagina—what's going on?

A You'd be surprised how often young children put small objects (pebbles, dried beans, bits of Play-Doh, small toys) into their body openings, including their nose and ears. This is perfectly normal exploration at this age, if not such a good idea healthwise. The leading cause of vaginal discharge in little girls is the presence of something pushed up into the vagina. The commonest foreign body is a wad of toilet paper.

Q Do prepubescent girls ever get vaginal infections?

A Besides discharge produced by a foreign object in the vagina, little girls can get vaginitis caused by strep. (Strep is a very rare vaginal infection in adult women, although one kind of strep, group B, commonly lives harmlessly in the vagina.) Streptococcal vaginitis in little girls is easily treated with an antibiotic. Yeast depends on the presence of estrogen, so yeast infections are not seen until a girl is about to start or has started having periods. Little girls with lots of itching need to be checked by their pediatrician. The skin disease lichen sclerosus (LS), for example, produces symptoms exactly like a yeast infection. Untreated, LS can permanently alter the architecture of the vulva. More innocuous things that can cause mild irritation in the area are a wet bathing suit worn too long, not toweling off the vulva after a bath, or not wiping after urinating. (These are not yeast infections, however, and are easily treated or go away on their own.) Pediatricians tell me they've been asked by parents, when little girls show up at the office complaining of itching, whether masturbation can cause irritation. It doesn't.

any natural lubricant to separate them. If the labia stick together, it's painless and usually outgrown without treatment, though you should ask your pediatrician about it if it seems to block urine flow. In the past, some physicians have treated adhesions by pulling them apart in the office without anesthesia. Do not agree to this painful and traumatic practice for your child. If adhesions are a problem, local estrogen may do the

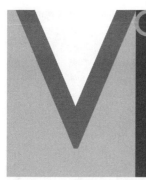

job. Local anesthesia is essential if adhesions are going to be separated any other way.

Without estrogen, the lining of the vagina is thin. The pH level is either neutral or slightly alkaline, and the lactobacilli decrease. Thus the vulva and vagina of the little girl during her childhood years are like those of the menopausal woman. She is especially vulnerable to irritation from chemicals (in bubble bath or the dyes in toilet paper, say) because she lacks the protective lactobacilli.

Puberty and reproductive years

Between the ages of 9 and 16, hormonal activity starts a cascade of physical events in a girl that lead to sexual maturity as a woman. It doesn't happen overnight. On the average, the sequence of accelerated growth, breast development, the appearance of pubic and axillary hair, and the onset of menstruation require a period of four and a half years. At puberty, before a woman has her first period (menarche), the adrenal glands mature and produce male hormones called androgens (adrenarche). That's why, at the age of 9 or 10, girls begin to perspire with body odor and grow hair in the underarms and pubic area. Some develop oily skin and acne. They also begin to be interested in the opposite sex. These functions have *nothing to do with estrogen,* which has not yet appeared on the scene. It's testosterone that stimulates pubic and axillary hair, as well as sweat and

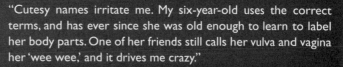

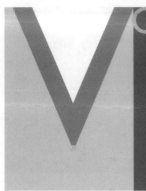

oil gland secretion. There are testosterone receptors in the nipples of the breasts, as well as in the clitoris and in the vagina, making them sensitive to sexual stimulation. And there are testosterone receptors in the brain that provide the libido power of testosterone. For the woman, testosterone in very small amounts is a female hormone. Write that down.

Estrogen doesn't show up until a year or two later in puberty, causing breast and vulvar development, widened hips for childbearing, and menstrual periods.

At puberty, once the estrogen is back, the fat in the mons and labia majora reappears and hair grows on the outer surface of the labia majora. The inner surfaces remain hairless and the skin is softer, moister, and pinker. The labia minora and vaginal opening become less apparent, although there are wide variations in the size and shape of the labia minora.

With the onset of menstruation, the starch content of the vaginal epithelium increases. The increased production of lactic acid lowers the vaginal pH, and this acidic environment favors the growth of lactobacilli and other bacteria that like acid. All of these developments ensure a healthy vagina poised to meet the many challenges it faces at maturity.

As I explained in Chapter 2, the vaginal opening in the virgin is partly covered by the hymen, a delicate, incomplete membrane that has one or more openings to allow the outflow of menstrual blood. Although you

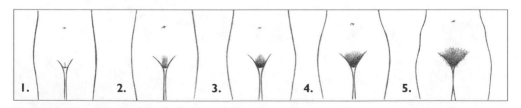

FIG. 26 Tanner stages of pubic hair development
The young girl starts with just a few wisps of hair (stage 1) and advances to hair covering the labia and mons and extending to the thighs (stage 5) at the completion of puberty.

COMMON QUESTIONS: Puberty

Q **At what age should a girl have her first gynecological exam?**

A A girl should be examined by a gynecologist if she has any kind of symptoms such as unusual discharge or bleeding, or after she becomes sexually active, or at age eighteen.

Q **Can using a tampon compromise a girl's virginity?**

A Use of tampons has no relationship to a girl's virginity. (See the section on tampons in Chapter 5, "V Smarts.")

Q **How can I best coach my young teen daughter on how to use a tampon?**

A First, go over basic V anatomy with her. Have her practice with her finger ever so gently so she is familiar with the vaginal opening. Buy the most slender Tampax with the cardboard applicator. Have her lubricate that. Trying after a warm bath might make it easier because the heat will relax all the muscles of the pelvic floor.

Q **Can girls get vaginitis after they reach puberty?**

A Once a woman is sexually mature, yeast may appear. BV is possible, even without sexual activity. Many young women with vestibulodynia think they have constant yeast infections. And then once a young woman starts sexual activity, she is susceptible to any of the vaginal infections.

---

would expect otherwise, not a lot is known about the hymen. There is one study of newborns to age three, but there are none on the development of the labia, vestibule, and hymen during puberty. We do know that the shape of the opening in the hymen varies. There's nothing about a young woman's hymen that reveals her sexual status. There are so many variations in a normal hymen that I can't tell if a patient is a virgin just by looking. A smooth round opening like a ring (annular) is the most common at birth, with gradual change to crescentic in prepuberty. Here's another myth: Despite the folkloric image of enthusiastic villagers waving a stained bedsheet after a wedding night to prove the bride had been successfully deflowered, the hymen has few blood vessels, so bleeding is minimal. Rarely, a woman may have some heavy bleeding.

The hymen easily gives way with sexual activity. It does not have a lot of nerve endings, so it stretches painlessly for most, though some women may have some pain. Reports of pain with first vaginal intercourse vary widely, depending on how ready a woman is emotionally and physically. (A condition called vestibulodynia, extensively discussed in Chapter 17, will cause significant pain.) Young women can prepare for first intercourse by learning all the V parts, mastering the use of a slender tampon, and gently stretching the opening with their fingers after a warm bath.

Very rarely, the hymenal opening may be closed off completely (called an imperforate hymen), leading to the retention of the menstrual discharge. An imperforate hymen, or any hymen that does not stretch open easily, needs a small surgical opening that can be performed in a gynecologist's office with local anesthesia or in an ambulatory care facility with general anesthesia. Please read Chapter 17 and Chapter 18 about painful intercourse before deciding there is a problem with the hymen.

Pregnancy and postpartum

When you're pregnant, you notice physical changes almost immediately, from fatigue to nausea. Well, your vulva and vagina are changing too. After six to eight weeks, blood volume increases throughout the body. In the vulva and vagina, as a result, the mucous membranes take on a bluish-violet color. Pressure from the pregnant uterus and the weight of the baby may cause veins to enlarge, forming harmless but sometimes uncomfortable varicose veins in the V area. The connective tissue in the vulva and the perineum soften so that the tissues will expand more easily during the delivery. The vaginal walls prepare for delivery with thicker mucus, a loosening of the connective tissue, and an increase in the size of muscle fibers. These changes make such an increase in the length of the vaginal walls that sometimes the lower portion of the front wall of the vagina bulges downward slightly.

In the vagina, the lactobacilli reach their highest levels. Bacteria that can live without oxygen (anaerobes with potential to cause disease) decrease. The increase in the lactobacilli from early pregnancy to delivery may help the vagina maintain its acidic pH, which is believed to prevent the multiplication of disease-causing bacteria in the vagina. Here's another example of those "good guy" bacteria, the lactobacilli, at work: They probably protect the baby from bacteria that can cause infection at the time of delivery.

Vaginal secretions are increased considerably during pregnancy, mainly

VOICES

"Crouched on my knees on the little afghan, I caught the infant who rushed from my vagina into the small world between my legs, in the midst of an extraordinary orgasm from the inside out."
—Ruth Claire in *Mothering*

COMMON QUESTIONS: Pregnancy

Q **Why do pregnant women seem to be more vulnerable to yeast infections?**

A Actually, it may be a myth that moms-to-be get more yeast infections; we don't know for sure. The original studies that suggested this were not well done, and we have no recent studies. If yeast occurs in pregnancy, however, it may be harder to treat because of high hormone levels that enrich the amount of starchy food for yeast in V cells, help yeast attach to V cells, and help yeast turn into its invasive (hyphal) form.

Q **What's the best way to handle all the extra discharge I'm experiencing?**

A Additional discharge during pregnancy is normal. But using tampons and pads for discharge day after day can lead to major V irritation. For comfort's sake, one option is to carry extra cotton underwear and change often. You'll need a large bag and several sets, but it's safe and certainly cheaper than panty liners.

Q **Can vaginal infections cause premature delivery?**

A Bacterial vaginosis (Chapter 11) and now trichomonas (Chapter 12) are linked to premature delivery. Many clinicians, and I'm one of them, think that these conditions should always be treated in the pregnant woman, but not all agree. Have a discussion with your health care provider if you're diagnosed with one of these. The treatment for both these conditions, metronidazole (Flagyl), is now considered safe for pregnancy. Another bacterium warranting attention in pregnancy is group B strep (GBS). A normal inhabitant of the vagina in up to 40 percent of women, GBS lives there harmlessly and cannot be eliminated. It is not a common cause of vaginitis and does not cause premature labor. During labor, however, any pregnant woman who is shown by a vaginal culture to be a GBS carrier may be offered antibiotics to try to prevent the GBS from crossing to the baby after the water breaks and causing serious infection (such as pneumonia or meningitis). Antibiotics prevent this early-onset GBS 90 percent of the time, but not all GBS disease can be prevented.

Q **What do I do if the skin around my episiotomy stitches hurts?**

A In the hospital, ice packs and pain pills are provided. At home, soaking in comfortable warm water and using Tylenol or Motrin usually do the job. For severe pain, check with your physician.

Q **Do women really "stretch out" after having a baby?**

A There are definitely changes in the vulva and vagina after delivery, but no one knows exactly what they are or what they mean. Over the years the general medical thinking has been that everything eventually goes back to normal or approaching normal. Yet many women do complain that they feel different, especially during intercourse. In some countries women even choose to be delivered by cesarean section in order to avoid any V changes. There is also vigorous debate in medicine about the role of pregnancy and delivery in incontinence and prolapse (when organs, such as the uterus or vagina, drop from their normal position).

As with most aspects of biology, there are probably individual differences. Your tissue strength, heredity, how long you pushed, and the size of your baby may all be factors. Women who feel stretched out and do not return to near normal in three months may have poor connective tissue or may have sustained injury to the nerves and muscles of the pelvic floor. A specialist called a urogynecologist will know the most about these problems. There are surgical procedures to tighten up the vaginal opening as well as to correct prolapsed tissues. You would not want to do these, however, until childbearing is complete.

from the cervix, making a somewhat thick white discharge. The discharge may have a yellowish tint from the influence of progesterone. If the discharge turns watery, rather than thick and pasty as usual in pregnancy, it needs to be evaluated by a clinician since it may represent premature opening of the cervix (incompetent cervix) or leakage from the bag of waters. It's possible, however, for the secretions of normal pregnancy to roll out of the vagina in a watery fashion. It's also common for pregnant women to lose a little urine and worry that this is abnormal fluid loss. Don't be apologetic about having any or all of these situations checked out by your clinician—better safe than sorry.

Then comes delivery: The simple expansion of that remarkable muscular tube, the vagina, to accommodate the passage of a 5- or 7- or 10-pound baby is simply one of the wonders of the world! Remember, it's the rugae—folds of skin in the vaginal wall that stretch open like so much pleated fabric—and the elastic muscle layers of the vagina that we have to thank for this biological miracle.

The vulva and vagina are understandably altered in the wake of their birth-canal duty. After delivery, the fourchette, the ridge of tissue where the labia meet, is generally flattened. If an episiotomy was made, or if the tissue tears during delivery, there will be a thin scar on the perineum. The hymen now looks like several small tags of tissue around the vaginal opening. The perineum may become shorter from scarring. These changes result in a widening of the vaginal opening and a greater visibility of the vaginal canal because of separation of the labia majora at the back. The exact changes in a woman's vagina immediately after childbirth have not been well studied, though most new moms can sense differences. The rugae, having been stretched to the max, are now smooth and flattened. The vaginal canal is wider. The vagina gradually shrinks over the next six to twelve weeks but may not return to its exact prepregnancy dimensions. The rugae begin to reappear about three weeks after delivery but are less well defined than before pregnancy.

During the days following delivery, there's a spike in the bacteria that can cause disease; this is why uterine infection or endometritis can occur after childbirth.[1] Why this dramatic change in the bacterial contents of the vagina occurs after delivery is not known. Possible reasons include the trauma of delivery, the uterine discharge after delivery *(lochia)*, contamination of the vagina by bacteria from the intestines, or the sudden drop in hormones that also occurs.[2] Estrogen levels postpartum, particularly in breast-feeding mothers, are very low. This causes a corresponding decrease in vaginal lubrication that may make intercourse uncomfortable when it is first resumed.

Clinicians usually advise avoiding intercourse for four to six weeks postpartum. This is largely for V protection but is highly dependent on how delivery went. There may be vulvar or vaginal lacerations, or an episiotomy, or both, to heal. Sex could be painful, introduce infection, or rip out the stitches. The cervix is open and vulnerable to invasion of bacteria into the uterus during the initial postpartum period.

Perimenopause

Perimenopause is a transitional time between the childbearing and the postchildbearing years. There's no exact age or time span for this, but it's roughly in the forties. It can last for four years or more, or only two. Although unusual, some women experience early perimenopause in their twenties or thirties. There is no surefire test to confirm perimenopause. During this time, your ovaries slow—producing less estrogen, releasing fewer eggs—until the time they say good-bye and retire.

The hormone changes of the perimenopause affect not only egg production but also many other body processes since there are receptors for hormones in virtually all your tissues, such as the bones and the brain. So periods change and other symptoms develop. (See the box "Perimenopausal Symptoms.")

The changes in hormones that the ovaries produce (estrogen, progesterone, and testosterone) happen in stages. First, progesterone drops, leaving estrogen to dominate the scene. A woman may experience what seems to be constant PMS, with cramps, bloating, mood swings, and tender breasts. There is the sensation that at any minute her period is coming. In the next phase, estrogen also goes down, resulting in hot flashes, memory loss, heart palpitations, migraine headaches, and vaginal dryness. Finally, in late perimenopause both estrogen and progesterone approach menopausal levels. Many symptoms back off, but some, such as hot flashes and vaginal dryness, may last well into the menopausal years.

PERIMENOPAUSAL SYMPTOMS

If you are bothered by any of the following effects, talk with your clinician about the peri-menopause management options, which may include oral contraceptives, herbals, or progesterone or estrogen preparations in many forms.

Irregular periods	Dry or thinning hair
PMS symptoms: bloating, cramps, breast tenderness	Brittle nails
	Weight gain, especially around the middle
Hot flashes and night sweats	Vaginal dryness or itchiness
Insomnia and fatigue	Pain with intercourse
Heart palpitations	Loss of interest in sex
Mood swings and irritability	Vaginal infections
Migraine headaches	Urinary tract infections
Memory loss	Frequent urination or stress incontinence
Fuzzy thinking or inability to concentrate	
Dry, itchy, irritated skin	Joint pain
	Irritable bowel syndrome

Source: L. E. Corio and L. G. Kahn, *The Change Before the Change* (New York: Bantam, 2000).

Menopause

More than 90 percent of women reach menopause by age 55. With menopause, a woman who does not take estrogen replacement may have some classic changes in her vulva and vagina. The connective tissue and fat deposits under the vulvar skin are reduced, and the skin itself becomes thinner and drier. The labia minora may flatten and shrink, and the vaginal opening may become smaller. Pubic hair turns gray or white and becomes scant. The folds in the vaginal wall flatten as the cells lose their glycogen content, and the vaginal walls become thin and pale in color. Lactobacilli disappear from the vagina, the pH rises, and a variety of other bacteria are found. The thin, dry vagina may be uncomfortable and more vulnerable to injury with intercourse or to the invasion of bacteria that can cause infection. Lack of estrogen also thins urethral and the bladder base tissue with the possibility of urinary symptoms or infection. All of these changes are called *atrophic*.

Postmenopausal changes occur across a range, depending on how much natural estrogen is present in the body. There's no single standard for what happens. Body fat can manufacture estrogen from adrenal sources, for example, so that postmenopausal changes are sometimes minimal in a woman of size. Other factors contribute to how the body changes after the menopause, as well, such as one's genetic makeup, nutrition, and disease

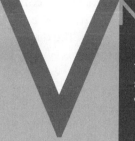

Only halfway to 100

The average age of menopause, defined as the cessation of menstrual periods for a year, is 51. It's held the same since the time of the ancient Greeks.

history. But women who are not taking hormone replacement therapy will eventually have some degree of atrophy.

Most women completely underestimate atrophy. They decide not to take any estrogen without thinking about the Vs. While not a life-threatening problem, low levels of estrogen can make you miserable. It starts with small changes at first, but over the years, without estrogen, you will notice big-time differences. You could develop frequent urinary tract infections. The thin, dry vestibule may feel like sandpaper at each wiping or washing. Sexual foreplay does not feel good and goes nowhere. The thin, dry vagina makes intercourse unpleasant at best and painful at worst. Lubricants help, but it's not the same. After years without estrogen, the labia minora may flatten out and disappear and the vaginal opening may shrink. The Pap test may become painful. A kind of vaginitis common in menopausal women called atrophic vaginitis can cause an unpleasant discharge and even bleeding. These problems can be controlled with the use of small amounts of estrogen vaginally or with hormone replacement therapy (HRT).

Too often, the dispiriting changes in the vulva and vagina that occur with menopause influence a woman who is not on hormone replacement to give up on sexual intercourse. And this is so unfortunate, because it appears that continuing sexual activity may improve vaginal health! One study showed that the vaginal pH in sexually active postmenopausal women is lower than in women who are not active, probably related to the increased blood flow that comes with sexual activity.[3] We also have evidence that sexually active postmenopausal women have less vaginal atrophy than sexually inactive women.[4] One bright spot: The clitoris remains unchanged after menopause.

For those who are taking oral HRT (fewer than one in five eligible women) or those who use local estrogen in some form (cream, ring, or tablet), the added estrogen will prevent the vaginal changes: The vagina stays thick and elastic, the lactobacilli remain, and the pH is normal. Pubic hair is influenced by testosterone rather than estrogen, but the postmenopausal ovary often makes enough to support this.

The decision of whether or not to start estrogen by mouth is a complex one. Your individual health history, family history, and lifestyle must be considered, not to mention the estrogen research article of the day in the local newspaper. You need to think about the breast, uterus, vulva, and vagina, as well as all the other tissues in the body that have estrogen receptors. Mother Nature put them all over the place—brain, gut, bone, genital tract—and when those receptors don't have estrogen on them, you know it! This takes reading and consultation; it's not a simple question that you ask your doctor on your way out the door. Finding a clinician who can work with you regarding hormones, alternatives to hormones, and lubricants is an important part of health for the woman who wishes to remain healthy, sexually active, or just plain comfortable after menopause.

For suggestions to deal with the changes of menopause, see Chapter 7 (on vaginal dryness) and Chapter 13 (on atrophic vaginitis). Don't write off your symptoms as an inevitable part of aging. There are dozens of choices now. And please—know that estrogen works quickly and well. If you're having pain with intercourse at this point in life, in spite of taking estrogen, odds are good that a specific problem is to blame—and can be helped. Check the sections on skin (Chapter 15) and pain (Chapter 17). You're never too old to remedy uncomfortable sex.

Low desire is another thing often written off as part of aging and therefore deprived of the attention it deserves. When perimenopausal and menopausal women tell me they are lagging on the desire front, we discuss all the factors that influence desire (see Chapter 6). If appropriate, I look at their testosterone levels, and if they're low, I prescribe this hormone to improve their situation. Interestingly enough, when it comes to hormones, it's the sex drive of the postmenopausal woman that we know most about. Information pointing to the vital role of hormones for libido in postmenopausal women has been accumulating since 1950.[5] Over fifteen years ago Canadian researchers clearly showed that when testosterone is added to hormone replacement therapy in surgically menopausal women whose ovaries have been removed, there's an increase in libido and intercourse.[6] Desire and fantasies pick up too when testosterone is added to estrogen replacement therapy, particularly in women who have had surgical menopause with removal of the ovaries.[7] There's been a lot of debate, but I agree with the sex researchers (and sisters) Laura and Jennifer Berman: "To us, testosterone is so central to a woman's sexual function that no lover and no amount of sexual stimulation can make up for its absence."[8]

Unfortunately, not all clinicians know about it or work with it. There are limited FDA-approved products to supplement testosterone and few long-term studies of its use in women. What's more, women are scared

COMMON QUESTIONS: Menopause

Q How will I know that I have reached menopause?

A For such a momentous event in a woman's life, it would be nice to have a signal proclaiming, "This is it!" Unfortunately, there's no clear way to know. Traditionally, doctors have said that menopause exists when you have gone a year without a period. But even after a year of silence, the ovaries can kick in again with enough activity to give you another period. Measuring the pituitary hormone that controls the ovaries (FSH) is often done, but can be misleading. FSH can be elevated, indicating menopause, but a few months later the ovary can cycle again. My best advice is to be savvy. Keep a good log of your periods and your symptoms and keep talking with your clinician. If symptoms are making you feel miserable, you should explore the many treatment options. If you're not uncomfortable, there's little need to do more than watch and wait.

Just don't forget: As long as you're having periods, you can get pregnant.

Q What's the story on hot flashes?

A Hot flashes have come to be considered the hallmark of menopause, but like everything else in the body, there is a huge variation. They range from a short period of heat felt in the face and neck to drenching sweat experienced over the entire body. Some women never have them. Hot flashes can begin in perimenopause, long before periods stop. They last on average from six months to two years, but there are women who struggle with them for years longer. No one knows exactly what causes hot flashes, but estrogen therapy is known to lessen their frequency and severity. Nonhormonal options include lifestyle changes (cool clothes, avoidance of spicy foods, use of a fan, sleeping in a cool room), consumption of soy food, and herbal therapy with black cohosh (Remifemin). Herbals that have been shown to not help include dong quai, evening primrose oil, and ginseng. If estrogen alone is not helping, combining it with a tiny amount of testosterone (Estratest H.S.) can do the job.

Q Can drinking lots of water help relieve vulvovaginal dryness, just as it helps the skin elsewhere?

A Unfortunately, no. Vaginal dryness is not a water problem; it's a problem of a lack of estrogen and its effects on vaginal tissues. Circulation decreases because without estrogen, blood vessels constrict (estrogen is a vasodilator) and cells that are normally puffed up and plushy become thin and dry without the blood flow. Circulation also affects lubrication that comes out of the blood plasma through the walls of the vagina. In addition, estrogen has an influence on the vaginal tissue itself; without it, the superficial layer of the vaginal wall thins or disappears altogether.

about using testosterone. They think of it as a male hormone that will give them male characteristics such as a deep voice and a beard. But if you look back to the discussion of puberty in this chapter, you'll be reassured that your ovary makes testosterone naturally in small amounts; it's part of what you need for normal sexual desire. If you replace testosterone when it is gone, male characteristics don't occur any more than they occur the rest of your reproductive years when your ovary is doing its thing.

Testosterone in a woman needs to be about 40–60 ng/dl (nanograms per deciliter, the units labs use to report hormone levels). For comparison, a man's levels run 500–1,200 ng/dl. Men don't lose libido unless their levels drop below 500. But because your range is so much lower and narrower, you are more sensitive to a smaller degree of change. For you, a drop of 10–15 ng/dl can make a big difference in sexual desire.[9] With the dips that begin in the perimenopausal period, libido can start to decline several years before you stop having periods. With surgical removal of the ovaries, levels drop within twenty-four to forty-eight hours after surgery. Besides loss of sex drive, you can experience fatigue, depressed mood, achy joints, and changes in feelings of well-being too.

Here's what often happens when you feel tired, depressed, and disinterested in sex. You're started on estrogen, and it increases a hormone carrier molecule (sex hormone binding globulin) that acts like a street sweeper. It sweeps up any testosterone that might be around, lowering your blood level of testosterone and making your condition worse! Adding insult to injury, some women get depressed because of their hormonal situation and are prescribed a type of antidepressant that may further lessen sexual desire. What a mess!

That's why when perimenopausal and menopausal women tell me their desire is lagging, I look at hormone levels if general health and relationship with partner are good. You have to get the estrogen levels right first. In addition, I use testosterone a great deal. I also tell any woman who is planning to have her tubes and ovaries removed at the time of hysterectomy (removal of the uterus) that without the ovaries, decline in sexual desire is very common. It's really important to understand that major life changes in hormones have correspondingly big influences on so many aspects of our lives.

Replacing testosterone is in its infancy. We don't have a lot of how-tos and we don't have a lot of products. And since sexual desire is complex, we have to remember that hormones aren't the only part. We have learned that the dose has to be right. Only recently we've learned that women need much lower doses of testosterone than men. (I know, you're thinking that this should have been obvious.) And the type of testosterone is also critical. Until recently, the main type given to women has been a manufactured compound not made in the human body, called methyltestosterone. Bad side effects can come from this synthetic and chemically different molecule, which is far more potent than the natural hormone made by the ovary and adrenals. In addition, because of the structure of this manufactured testosterone, measuring testosterone levels becomes inaccurate, so its use can't be monitored without expensive special measurements. It is essential to monitor testosterone blood levels, liver function, and cholesterol when a woman takes testosterone replacement.

A standard oral preparation is Estratest, a combination of 1.25 mg estrogen and 2.5 mg methyltestosterone. Estratest H.S. contains half that amount, 0.625 mg estrogen and 1.25 mg methyltestosterone. Some women report success using the half strength just two or three times a week, though others have unsatisfactory side effects. If you're on it and doing well, don't let me make you think it is wrong or unsafe. (Another treatment, Premarin with methyltestosterone, had 5 or 10 mg of the big guy in it but was discontinued in 1997.)

When we use natural micronized testosterone in teeny amounts (1 to 4 mg per day), women do well, although we still have a lot to learn about what works best. These lower doses are based on what the ovaries and adrenal glands naturally make. You start at 1 to 1.25 mg daily and gradually increase based on how you feel and what a monthly blood test shows. The right balance usually appears at around 2 to 4 mg daily. Oral doses may not be absorbed well or can alter cholesterol levels. A gradually absorbed cream may be the fix for this. Cream or gel forms require much lower doses than the oral route, since more is absorbed through the skin and the liver has no chance to remove any. Some experts suggest starting the cream form at 10 percent of the oral dose that you were taking (0.2 mg in cream form if you were taking 2 mg orally) and adjust by response and blood level.[10] My own experience has been that 25 percent of the oral dose (0.5 mg cream for 2 mg orally) or even 50 percent (1 mg cream for 2 mg orally) works well.

What about DHEA? That stands for dehydroepiandrosterone (say "dee-HIGH-dro-ep-ee-AN-dro-ster-own"), made in your adrenal glands.

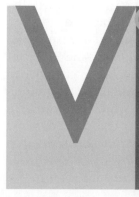

OICES

"After we pass 50 or 60, we've already lost many validations of our femaleness: we don't menstruate, don't have babies, and nobody's after us, trying to get us in the broom closet at a party. But having somebody make love to us keeps us one of the girls. So you have to keep reciting to yourself: I'm a sexual person; I want sex in my life; I deserve it, and I'm not gonna let it disappear."

—Helen Gurley Brown

It's widely promoted in a large variety of over-the-counter products to improve everything from brain function to sexual desire. Unfortunately, there's very little good science behind the claims. Most studies have been done on animals, not women. DHEA isn't regulated by the FDA, and it is difficult for you to know exactly what's in the bottle. And what dose is safe is far from well established. Experts think that the suggested doses on the bottle are much more than women need for daily use.

DHEA is touted as the mother of all hormones, a precursor for the body to make natural estradiol and testosterone, but this won't happen if your ovaries are not working in the postmenopausal years. You may not be able to convert the DHEA to other hormones, and you can have side effects from extra male-type hormones that build up in the conversion process. The only way you'll know is to monitor levels of all the hormones that occur in the pathway of DHEA conversion. Too much DHEA can cause exactly the same side effects as too much testosterone.

DHEA has promising potential, but if you are thinking of taking it, you'll want to work with a physician who will monitor hormone levels, cholesterol, and liver function. Too much DHEA can cause liver damage. You need to pay attention to quality of sleep, any changes in scalp hair, and your weight, all potentially disrupted by DHEA. You need a prescription-grade DHEA from your clinician, not the food-grade stuff you can buy over the counter.[11]

A controversial rite of passage

As a final point in this chapter, I'd like to talk about a controversial rite of passage. Female circumcision is the altering or removal of the external genital organs in girls and women. It may involve partial or complete removal of the clitoris (type I), removal of the clitoris with the labia minora (type II), or removal of the clitoris and the labia minora and partially stitching the labia majora together (type III).

When I first heard of this practice, which is done predominately in parts of Africa and Asia, I was horrified, then enraged. How could people do this? How can this practice continue to go on today? Then I learned that in the areas of the world where female circumcision is practiced, it is considered essential to acceptance in sociey. An uncircumcised woman is considered unchaste and condemned to a life of isolation—ineligible for marriage and facing a life of economic uncertainty. Many circumcised women do not consider themselves mutilated; the use of such terminology can be an insult to the people and cultures from which they come. In fact, although circumcised women may suffer from complications and long-term problems from the surgery, not all do, and sexual enjoyment is possible for a women who has been circumcised.

That information gives me a little glimmer of understanding into this

VOICES

"The feeling of vulnerability and shame I felt lying on my back naked with my legs open and being reduced to a curious spectacle on public display is something I will never forget. It is worse than what I remember of the circumcision."

—Woman who had genital surgery having an office visit in a city-run clinic

long tradition, which is performed by people from a variety of cultures and religions. Knowing the background does not, however, change for me the fact that female circumcision is a form of cruelty and violence against women. Circumcision can cause scarring, cysts, chronic pain, and long-term infections and infertility.

To women who are circumcised, I offer understanding of your position and support of your dignity. But though I recognize the good intention of circumcision in maintaining a woman's position in the society of some cultures, I cannot ignore V destruction—the mutilation of the yoni—with the unique V structure and V function forever ruined. This is not like male circumcision. I want to work for a world where women can make it without regard to their sexuality, where they don't need to be altered sexually in order to survive economically.

Please see the Resources section for information and agencies involved with female circumcision.

▼

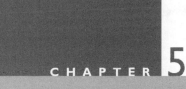

V Smarts

Everyday Habits That Make a Difference

What kind of underwear did you pull on this morning? How did you choose the type of "feminine protection" that's sitting in your bathroom cupboard awaiting your next period? Do you get rid of peekaboo pubic hair in bathing-suit season? Many things that women do routinely, without a second thought, can affect vulvovaginal health. This chapter covers the everyday sorts of things you can do to avoid coming into my office with a problem. I'll explore the medical facts and popular beliefs about all the things that we use or do that alter the V area: tampons, pads, panty liners, douching and other aspects of hygiene, underwear, and pubic hair removal.

Tampons

In the United States in 1933, Dr. Earle Haas patented a vaginal tampon he had devised for his wife. His invention was far from new. Tampons have existed since ancient Egyptian times, when women fashioned their own out of softened papyrus. Roman women used wool. In ancient Japan, women made tampons out of paper, held them in place with a bandage, and changed them ten to twelve times a day. Traditional women of Hawaii used the furry part of a native fern called hapu'u. Grasses, mosses, and other plants are still used by women in parts of Asia and Africa.[1] In 1776, a French physician in Paris used a piece of tightly wound linen cloth dipped in vinegar, inserting it into the vagina to control bleeding and discharge.[2] Tampons of varying size, made of cotton or wool with a short

THE HEART OF V HEALTH: TEN RULES TO REMEMBER

A healthy vulva and vagina don't just happen. It's up to you to actively preserve wellness and prevent problems. Here are some guidelines:

1. *Lay the groundwork.* Good general health is the best defense against infections and problems anywhere in the body, including your genitalia. So it's worth repeating: Eat well, get adequate sleep, and exercise at least a few days a week.

2. *Have smart sex.* That means have one partner, learn your partner's sexual history, and use a condom. You are unlikely to contract a sexually transmitted disease if you have intercourse with only one person who has intercourse only with you. But be aware that a partner with cold sores (herpes simplex virus type 1) can give you genital herpes. A partner who does not know he/she has genital herpes or warts (or has a mild case) can pass genital herpes or warts to you. (See Chapter 20.) This is a common problem. Do not have vaginal intercourse immediately after anal intercourse unless your partner washes first.

   Be aware that the more sexual partners either member of a couple has, the more likely the woman is to develop precancerous or cancerous cells of the cervix. That's because these cell changes are caused by the human papillomavirus (HPV), which is passed around through sexual contact (see Chapter 21).

3. *Do not douche unless your clinician specifically recommends douching.* Although you may believe you need "cleaning out," this practice can destroy the normal bacteria in the vagina, causing infection to occur. Remember that menstruation is not dirty. Everything that makes up the menstrual flow is natural and healthy. The body works so that there are no harmful residues. (Douching is covered in detail later in this chapter, page 100.)

4. *Skip the scents.* Avoid feminine hygiene sprays, scented deodorant tampons or pads, or spraying perfumes in the vaginal area—sure, they smell nice, but all can lead to irritation or allergic reaction. Besides, if you're healthy, your own natural scent is not "bad" or in need of masking.

   If you have sensitive skin or have had vulvar problems, don't even use fabric softener or bleach to clean underwear; they coat every fiber of your underpants with potentially irritating residue. It's best to wash underwear in a mild, fragrance-free soap and rinse thoroughly. If you're vulnerable to vulvar problems, white cotton underwear is your safest bet to minimize irritation.

5. *Don't overprotect.* Do not wear a pad or panty liner every day of your life. Repeated use can be abrasive and irritating. Limit use to a few days at a time. If you have so much wetness that you seem to require daily protection, find a clinician to help you pinpoint the cause.

6. *Use tampons wisely.* Choose the right absorbency for that day of your cycle and change it regularly—every two to six hours, depending on flow. (See "Tampon Tips," page 91.)

7. *Rethink powders.* Talc particles in talcum powder can work their way up the vagina to the pelvis. Talc may be associated with an increased risk of ovarian cancer. Cornstarch is a safe substitute. *Read labels carefully!* Some so-called baby powders contain talc; others contain cornstarch. Some perfumed powders are talc-free, but combined

THE HEART OF V HEALTH: TEN RULES TO REMEMBER   cont.

with the natural oil-like secretions of the vulva, they wind up having the texture of pudding. To avoid this pasty problem, fluff away only on the abdomen, buttocks, and thighs—but note that you still risk developing a skin or V sensitivity to the chemicals in the scent.

8. *Loosen up.* Thongs, snap-crotch bodysuits, or tight spandex garments, such as leotards or tights, can rub back and forth during exercise. They can trap sweat, leading to irritation, even cracking of the skin. Best bet: loose cotton pants, such as yoga pants. The point of exercise, after all, is to keep yourself healthy.

Tight clothes—snug jeans or multiple layers (girdle-style underwear under control-top panty hose under slacks)—can retain moisture and feel abrasive even when you're not working out. Tight layers may also up your risk of yeast infection.

9. *Bathe right.* Frequent, lengthy soaks in very hot water can dry and irritate skin. So can using pure soap, such as Ivory. If you're hooked on really hot showers or baths, limit your time in the water to three minutes. Best advice: Use comfortably warm water with a mild soap such as Dove, Basis, or Neutrogena. Never scrub the vulva with a sponge, loofah, or Buf-Puf—your fingertips or a soft cloth are sufficient. Pat dry gently.

More nos: Do not use other people's towels. Do not overdry; the labia majora and groin folds need to be patted dry, or you could use a hair dryer on low. But the intralabial folds and vestibule are like the mouth, lubricated by little glands and never meant to dry out. Don't use a hair dryer to dry between the lips.

What about bubble bath? It's meant to be a special treat, not a daily ritual. Anyone who's had vulvar problems should skip the suds entirely. But for the rest of the world, an occasional soak in not-too-hot bubbles is fine (and even fabulous). Bubbles form because of chemicals, which is why there's always a chance of irritation. Also remember that natural pure oils such as lavender, rosemary, and clove are highly irritating and must be diluted, just a few drops to a tubful.

10. *Don't stint on birth-control device maintenance.* Wash diaphragms, cervical caps, and spermicide applicators with soap and water after using them. Replace these items periodically as recommended or they can fail to protect. Don't neglect to clean vibrators and sex toys after use either.

string attached for removal, have been used by the medical profession since 1888 for the application of antiseptics. Dancers, theatrical performers, and professional models have long filled the vagina with absorbent cotton to handle menstrual flow.

But the modern era of the tampon began in 1936, when a new company, Tampax Incorporated, bought the Haas patent and started selling the newest form of menstrual protection. The cotton product was an overnight success. Today they are made of cotton or rayon or both, as well as of unbleached cotton, by companies such as Terra Femme and Natracare (see Resources). Millions of women now use them every month without giving them any more thought than they give to brushing their

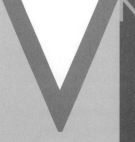

teeth. So welcome was this "feminine protection" product that, although it was invented and marketed with surprisingly little study, it was quickly and enthusiastically endorsed by millions of women who wanted to swim, ride horses, dance, and go about their daily lives free of encumbrance. Tampons have become so ingrained in our culture that large numbers of women continued to use them throughout one of the biggest health panics of the 1980s, the toxic shock syndrome scare.[3]

Tampons are more than a convenience. They're a necessity and, sometimes, a controversy. In addition to having been linked to toxic shock, this method of absorbing menstruation has been accused of causing problems ranging from bleeding vaginal ulcers to the fertility threat endometriosis. They've been suspected of compromising virginity. How safe are they, really, and how are they most safely used?

Being an informed user means separating the facts from the fears.

TAMPONS AND TOXIC SHOCK

One of the main reasons women avoid tampon use is fear of toxic shock syndrome (TSS). It's true that in the 1980s, tampons were linked to this potentially fatal illness, but changes in the manufacture and regulation of this useful product have made such fears almost completely groundless today. Toxic shock is *rare* nowadays, occurring in about 1 in 100,000 menstruating women. TSS is a condition that can make anyone—woman,

NOTE

Protection of choice

More than 63 percent of menstruating women in the United States use tampons exclusively or in combination with pads. Among adolescents, the number rises to nearly three-fourths, though most girls start out using pads. The average age of first tampon use is 14.

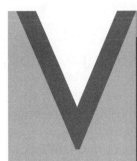

Quick! Get me a Fax

Early tampon brands included Fibs, Fax, Wix, Slim-pax, Nunap, and Holly-Pax.

man, or child, not just tampon users—sick with high fever, a bright red rash like sunburn, and low blood pressure. It affects several body systems at once, so that people may also have other symptoms such as vomiting and diarrhea, severe muscle pain, kidney or liver abnormalities, and disorientation or loss of consciousness. Doctors diagnose TSS when they are sure the patient does not have another disease with similar symptoms (such as scarlet fever and measles) and by showing that a strain of the bacterium *Staphylococcus aureus* that can produce a poison (toxin TSST-1) is present in the body.

Tampons do not cause TSS. Toxic shock is caused by the poison released by the staph bacteria.[4] Tampons themselves are not the source of the bacteria. It may be present normally in the vagina of about 10 percent of healthy women, or staph found on the skin may be introduced by fingers inserting a tampon.

A link between tampon use and TSS was first noted during a big TSS outbreak in 1980. Among the women who had used only one brand of tampon during the menstrual period when they became ill, 71 percent had used a superabsorbent tampon called Rely. In September 1980, Procter and Gamble voluntarily took that product off the market. The number of cases of TSS dropped sharply after Rely was withdrawn. Numbers continued to decline after similar superabsorbent tampons were withdrawn and tampon absorbency was lowered.

What does the absorbency of tampons have to do with TSS? No one's sure yet, because how TSS works has not been fully mapped out by medical researchers. One theory is that the larger, more absorbent tampons introduced more oxygen into the vagina, allowing staph growth and toxin production, and subsequent illness. However, both cotton and rayon tampons have been associated with TSS.[5]

Because of the TSS scare, government regulation of tampons was initiated in 1982. This was the first such regulation since the product was patented nearly fifty years earlier. Manufacturers were required to provide tampon labeling and produce inserts that told women about the association between TSS and tampon use, the risk of TSS, and the importance of using tampons with the least amount of absorbency necessary to control menstrual flow. The warning signs of TSS and what to do if symptoms appeared were included.

Next, standards for absorbency were developed, although it took a long time. It had been difficult for women to choose tampons because absorbency categories varied across different brands. One manufacturer's "regular" might absorb more than another's "super." Finally in 1990, new rules required outer packages to be labeled junior, regular, super, or super plus absorbency, with each category corresponding to specific ranges of absorbency. Tampon boxes now include the standard absorbency ratings shown on the box.

It's too early to determine the impact of the 1990 tampon-labeling governmental regulation, but the number of menstrually related TSS cases in the United States continues to decrease; in 1997 there were six cases, and in 1998 there were just three cases.[6]

TAMPON ABSORBENCY

A menstrual period usually produces around 4 to 12 teaspoons of menstrual fluid, weighing about 20 to 60 grams. (A teaspoon is about 5 grams.) Of course menstrual flow is distributed over several days. You will want to change your tampon long before it is fully saturated (when it will start to leak and feel uncomfortable) while at the same time choosing the least absorbent tampon that works.

Finding the right absorbency is a matter of experimentation. While you are doing your trials you'll want to wear a pad for extra protection. A tampon that's not absorbent enough will allow leakage. One that's too absorbent will be hard to remove—you'll have to "drag" it out. Changing every four hours is a good target. These are the absorbency ratings standardized in 1990:

Ranges of Absorbency in Grams	Corresponding Term of Absorbency
6 and under	Junior absorbency
6 to 9	Regular absorbency
9 to 12	Super absorbency
12 to 15	Super plus absorbency
15 to 18	None
Above 18	None

Source: E. R. Rome and J. Wolhander, Can tampon safety be regulated? in *Menstrual Health in Women's Lives,* A. Dan and L. Lewis, eds. (Urbana: University of Illinois Press, 1992), 265.

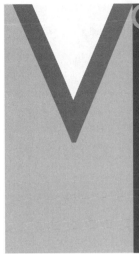

"What would happen, for instance, if suddenly, magically, men could menstruate and women could not? The answer is clear—menstruation would become an enviable, boast-worthy masculine event. Men would brag about how long and how much. Boys would mark the onset of menses, that longed-for proof of manhood, with religious ritual and stag parties. Congress would fund a National Institute of Dysmenorrhea to help stamp out monthly discomforts. Sanitary supplies would be federally funded and free. (Of course, some men would still pay for the prestige of commercial brands, such as John Wayne Tampons, Muhammad Ali's Rope-a-Dope Pads . . .)"

—Gloria Steinem, "If Men Could Menstruate," *Ms.*, October 1978

TAMPONS AND VAGINAL ULCERS

Women sometimes run into another problem related to tampon absorbency—vaginal ulceration. Ulcers are sores where the top layer of skin has been rubbed away. In the vagina, an ulcer can be caused by a number of different things, tampons included, especially if a woman is using them improperly. Examples would be using tampons for weeks at a time because of irregular bleeding or using a product that's more absorbent than she needs for her flow. Vaginal ulcers were unheard of until 1977, then started to rise in the decade after superabsorbent tampons were first marketed.

How can a tampon cause a hole in the vagina? It can draw normal fluid out of the wall of the vagina, crinkling cell membranes and collapsing tiny bridges of tissue between the cells in the vaginal wall. This in turn destroys cells in the top layers of the wall, causing them to erode and, essentially, be rubbed away. Given this mechanism, it's not surprising that

MORE TAMPON DANGERS TO DISCOUNT

Rumors persist that asbestos and dioxin (a by-product of the chlorine bleaching process at paper and wood-pulp mills) pose health risks in today's tampons. Although past methods of bleaching the cellulose fibers in rayon, a common tampon ingredient, could lead to tiny amounts of dioxin in tampons, today's cellulose undergoes a chlorine-free bleaching process. The result: finished tampons that have no detectable level of dioxin.

As for asbestos, the buzz is that it's secretly added to tampons to increase menstrual bleeding and therefore push more product. Ridiculous! Asbestos is not, and never has been, used to make tampon fibers. The FDA has no such evidence and no reports of increased menstrual bleeding following tampon use.

Source: FDA Consumer, March 1999.

Sanitary style

Glamour magazine showcases a lime-and-pink Gucci tampon holder and another model in pewter. Those who feel no need to be coy might prefer Vinnie Angel's cartoony linen sachet. Emblazoned with the words "Vinnie's Tampon Case," it features a grinning fellow in a baseball cap and the motto "One size fits all!"

ulceration is more likely to occur with superabsorbent tampons, especially when they're worn at times other than during active menstruation. One researcher found that applicator-inserted superabsorbent tampons can make ulcers near the vaginal opening on the right in right-handed women, corresponding to the upper resting point of the tampon.[7] These findings suggest that jabbing injury at the time of insertion of the tampon also plays a part in the problem of ulceration.

A vaginal ulcer doesn't necessarily hurt. It might not cause any symptoms—it may be discovered only during a routine exam. Or it could cause some vaginal bleeding or bleeding after sexual intercourse. If an ulcer is found, your clinician will do some tests to make sure you don't have a sexually transmitted disease that could also cause an ulcer, and will recommend that you stop using tampons for a cycle or two. Then you'll be rechecked. Superficial scrapes in the vagina heal quickly, remember—in as little as forty-eight hours. A deeper ulcer may take a few weeks to heal. If the ulcer hasn't gone away after a few weeks, it may be necessary to remove a little sample near the edge of it (a biopsy) to find out what it is. Vaginal ulcers don't increase a woman's chance of getting TSS.

It's pretty easy to avoid ulcers in the vagina. See "Tampon Tips," page 91.

TAMPONS AND ENDOMETRIOSIS

Another, far more serious ailment for which tampons have been blamed—probably mistakenly—is endometriosis, a disease found only in women. Endometriosis occurs when the tissue lining of the uterus, the endometrium, grows outside the uterus in the form of implants, nodules, and cysts. Under the same hormonal influence that stimulates the uterine lining to be shed as menstruation, this tissue found outside of the uterus thickens and bleeds in a monthly fashion too—but because it's not supposed to be there, pain, irregular bleeding, and infertility can result. Endometrial implants are most frequently found on the ovaries, tubes, and the pelvic floor in back of the uterus (called the cul-de-sac). Rarely, implants have been found in such distant locations as the stomach, intestines, lungs, and kidneys. Symptoms include painful menstrual periods (dysmenorrhea), heavy menstrual bleeding (menorrhagia), bleeding between periods (metrorrhagia), pain in the pelvis with intercourse, and infertility.[8] The problem can be confirmed only by seeing the implants in the pelvis through a special instrument called a laparoscope, although increasing numbers of clinicians are starting to make the diagnosis by history alone. Endometriosis is treated by the use of hormones or surgery; it usually becomes inactive during pregnancy. Endometriosis may run in families.

The cause of endometriosis remains unknown.[9] Researchers have suggested that there are some cells in the body that can spontaneously develop into endometrial tissue, or that endometrium may be transplanted through the blood or the lymph. A popular theory suggests that endometriosis is caused by the backward (retrograde) flow during menstruation of endometrial cells through the Fallopian tubes and onto the ovaries or floor of the pelvis.[10] But retrograde menstruation is a common event, occurring in most, if not all, normal women without endometriosis. I see it all the time when we look at the pelvis through the laparoscope if a woman has her period at the time of laparoscopy. Scientists think that some characteristics of the menstrual debris that comes out into the pelvis—how well it can stick to the pelvic tissues or how well it can divide and grow—determine whether endometriosis will develop. There are also differences in how well the immune system cleans up the regurgitated cells in the pelvis, and this may contribute to whether or not this menstrual debris sets up housekeeping outside the uterus.

People have wondered if tampons play a role in the development of endometriosis. There is not a lot of information available. Only one study, done in 1993, showed that the use of tampons for more than fourteen years increased the risk of endometriosis in women under 30.[11] Beyond this single study, there does not appear to be any basis for the concern that exclusive use of tampons for menstrual protection increases the risk for endometriosis.[12]

If you have severe menstrual cramps and/or heavy menstrual flow, you will certainly want to see your physician to figure out if this might be caused by endometriosis. You will want to consider the use of the birth

V NOTE

Not to blame

Tampon use is not associated with yeast infections or other disruptions of the normal bacterial balance of the vagina.

control pill to improve both these problems, since the pill is a standard and effective treatment for endometriosis. But to date, I wouldn't avoid tampons over this fear.

TAMPONS AND VIRGINITY

Tampons aren't only suspected of causing medical problems. They've gotten tangled up in social issues too. Soon after tampons came on the market in the 1930s, people wanted to know whether they could alter the hymen—and, by implication, a virgin's status. The first scientific investigation of this, in 1945, found that the average opening in the hymen of a virginal woman is 25 mm (1¼ inches) and the diameter of a tampon is 17 mm (¾ inch) or less.[13] Thus the researchers concluded that a tampon would not "impair standard anatomical virginity." But since the study's author did not measure the size of the subjects' openings both before and after tampon use, his information isn't terribly reliable.

In 1994, a large study of three hundred young women showed that the median size of the opening in the hymen was slightly bigger in those who used tampons (1.5 cm or ⅝ inch) compared with those who used pads.[14] But once again, it wasn't known what size opening each woman had before she had ever used a tampon—so there's no way to know if the tampon enlarged the opening or not.

The topic of virginity is a highly individual matter, and its definition is open to wide interpretation. To some it means that no penis has entered the vagina; to others it means that nothing has ever entered the vagina. In some cultures and religions, and for some individuals, being a virgin at the time of marriage is a priority. For others, preparation for comfortable sex or pelvic exam is valued, as is the freedom (for exercise, comfort) that comes with tampon use. Whether to put a tampon into your vagina and how acceptable the possibility is that a tampon might alter the opening in the hymen are decisions to be made by every young woman on an individual basis.

V NOTE

Lost in translation

Although up to 70 percent of women in the United States, Canada, and much of Western Europe use tampons, the number drops to low single digits in countries such as Japan, Spain, and India and in much of Latin America. Reasons include the fear that tampon use will compromise virginity, and doctors' refusal to endorse a product they're unfamiliar with. To spur sales, Procter and Gamble, which makes Tampax, hires young women in some of these countries to host in-home "bonding sessions" where they can educate family and friends.

GUILTY OR NOT GUILTY? THE TRUTH ABOUT COMMON TAMPON CONCERNS

The Charge	Key Points to Remember
Tampons are associated with toxic shock.	The entire mechanism of TSS is still not understood. Tampons do not cause TSS; staph-produced toxin does. Women can now compare tampon absorbencies, choosing the lowest level compatible with individual needs.
Rayon or rayon/cotton tampons may promote the production of TSS poison.	A number of studies show that all-cotton tampons may promote poison production; the debate continues.
Tampons introduce bacteria into the vagina.	Tampon use does not significantly alter the population of bacteria or yeast in the vagina.
Tampons promote yeast infections.	There is a moderate association of deodorant tampons with yeast in one study. Tampon use is not generally associated with yeast.
Tampons contain traces of dioxin.	A chlorine-free bleaching process has eliminated dioxin from tampons.
Tampons cause vaginal ulceration.	Proper choice of absorbency and appropriate use prevent this problem.
Tampons may be associated with endometriosis.	Limited information is available. Only one study suggests an association after use for more than fourteen years in women under 30.
Tampons may alter the size of the hymen.	No criteria exist for whether a woman is a virgin or not. No baseline measurement of a girl's hymen is made, and there is wide normal variation. A tampon could enlarge the opening of a girl with a small hymen, or a tampon inserted at a bad angle could change the hymen. No clinician can say for sure if "virginity is intact." Tampons are recommended by clinicians to prepare for sexual activity and to facilitate pelvic exam.

TAMPON TIPS

Tampons are a safe, excellent, and liberating choice for most women. Millions of us have used them successfully without disease. We need to make intelligent choices about their use—to be vigilant but not paranoid. Some advice:

▼ *Choose a tampon that's only as absorbent as you need.* To determine the lowest absorbency needed, note how long it takes a tampon to become saturated. If a tampon is not saturated after four to six hours, switch to one that's less absorbent. During a menstrual period you may need more than one product, to provide varying levels of absorbency for heavy days and lighter days.

▼ *Be gentle.* Go slowly as you insert an applicator or your fingers into the vagina. Fast jabs may injure the vaginal wall. The organ is sturdy, but it's not a battleship.

▼ *Skip deodorant tampons.* Because the flow is absorbed by a tampon up inside, there is no odor. You don't need these chemically treated products, and they might cause irritation.

▼ *Change your tampon regularly.* That's every two hours (for heavy flow) to six hours (for light flow). Do not wear the same tampon all day and all night. But do not change every half hour; this too can be irritating.

▼ *Always remove the last tampon you put in.* A forgotten tampon will create a terrible odor. If you "lose" a tampon, don't panic. Remember that the vagina is basically a pouch. Insert a single finger gently into the vagina and locate the tampon. You may have to reach farther than you're used to, but if you go slowly and gently, you will not hurt yourself and you can usually touch the tampon. Once you have located it, try to free up the string with your finger. If you can't identify the string, work the tampon down with your finger until you can grasp it. If you're just unable to get hold of it, you'll have to go into the clinician's office. (Don't be embarrassed; clinicians see this all the time!)

▼ *Dispose of tampons and applicators properly.* They are not really flushable. Wrap in tissue and put in the trash.

▼ *Use tampons only when you have your period.* They were not designed for vaginal discharge. Misuse can dry out and irritate the vagina.

▼ *Don't endure pain.* If a tampon hurts while it goes in, stays in, or is removed, try a different brand or add a little lubricant. But if the discomfort persists, see a doctor. A tampon should be so comfortable in place that you don't know it's there.

▼ *Don't overdo.* If you have prolonged menstrual flow lasting more than seven days, see your doctor and get it fixed. It's not a good idea to use tampons for weeks at a time. This can cause ulceration and ongoing bleeding.

▼ *Be extra careful if you are postmenopausal.* You may be on hormone therapy that gives a monthly period. If so, choose a tampon with only the absorbency you need, remembering that the vagina may be a little thinner at this time of life.

▼ *If you have a personal history of toxic shock syndrome, do not use tampons.*

▼ *Consider delaying tampon use.* If an intact hymen is important to you because of personal, religious, or cultural reasons, you may wish to postpone tampon use until after you become sexually active. This is a decision that you, not your mother or your friends, make about your body.

▼ *Try tucking the string in to minimize irritation.* If you have vulvar irritation problems but are able to use tampons, you may benefit from their use with the string tucked inside.

Pads

The other common method of absorbing menstrual flow is the pad. Women relied on rags that had to be washed after use until the first disposable sanitary napkin, Lister's Towels, was created in 1896 by Johnson & Johnson. Unfortunately, the product failed to attract many consumers. It wasn't until World War I that nurses found bandages to be an excellent material for absorbing menstrual flow. Shortly after that, in 1921, Kimberly-Clark introduced the first successful disposable napkin, Kotex. Modess from Johnson & Johnson followed in 1927.

Few young women today realize that these early pads were far from the carefree product they know today. The pads had to be held in place with a belt worn around the hips, and fastened with pins. Catalogs and stores also sold a range of other protective gear that women could use to prevent bloodstains when napkins failed, including sanitary aprons, bloomers, and panties. Fifty years went by between the introduction of disposable pads and the next big advance: adhesive backing on pads, which could now be used without belts and pins. Pad modifications accelerated soon after, especially after 1980, when panic over the outbreak of toxic shock

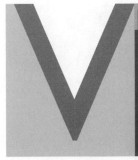

Lost in translation, part 2

Ever wonder what o.b. stands for in the o.b. tampon brand name? Not *obstetrics*. It means *ohne Binde*, German for "without a pad." The manufacturer was originally a German company, later bought by Johnson & Johnson.

DOES YOUR TAMPON FEEL RIGHT?

A tampon should be so comfortable that you're not aware it's in place. Here's a guide to problems with tampon fit.

If you . . .	You should . . .
Are aware your tampon is there	Remove it and insert the next a little deeper or at a different angle
Feel your tampon is too long	Try a brand that expands in width only, such as o.b. or Playtex
Feel irritation and resistance when you remove the tampon	Use a less absorbent tampon
Meet resistance when you insert the tampon	Use a tampon with a narrower applicator; lubricate the tip. Make sure you aim down and back
Feel the tampon is sticking or poking you on insertion	Check for applicator petal protrusion (any product with a misshapen tip should be discarded, as a protruding petal can hurt)
Feel that your tampon is falling out	Check with your doctor about vaginal or cervical tissue sag (prolapse)
Consistently feel pain as you part the labia or try to insert a tampon	Read Chapter 17 about pain

syndrome associated with tampon use caused many women to switch back to pads.

Unlike tampons, pads that do not contain deodorants are not regulated by the federal government. Their descriptions are not standardized. Buying them is a bit like choosing panty hose, because there are so many options. *Maxi* has become a generic term for pads. You can buy plain maxis, winged maxis, curved maxis, super maxis, and double-plus extra-long su-

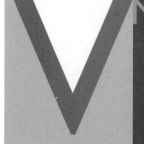

Follow the bouncing ball

In 2000, Kotex began using a big red dot in its advertising— meant to be a new universal symbol for a menstrual period.

per maxis, to name a few of the confusing choices. Most brands also come in three thicknesses: regular, thin, and ultrathin. Within each thickness are assorted lengths (long, super) and adhesive patterns ("wings" or "tabs" that wrap under the panty crotch and stick there). Still others contain deodorant. Even the shapes vary: hourglass, curved, rectangular, and now they're even tapered for thongs. Which you use depends almost entirely on personal preference. Most women keep several kinds on hand—regular for day, long for night, ultrathin for light days.

Pads are made of cotton or synthetics, including rayon. The materials used work remarkably well and cause no problems for most women. If you have vulvar irritation or dermatitis, organically grown unbleached cotton pads (see Resources) without wings are helpful.

Research on the potential effect of pads on the vulva is as scanty as a Victoria's Secret thong. Pads' close contact with the genital area, vulvar skin, perineum, and upper thigh can affect the skin by increasing the amount of dryness or wetness, or by occluding or abrading the skin. One study has shown no pad-related adverse effects in women using deodorant and nondeodorant pads, but this study was sponsored by a company that makes deodorant pads.[15] In the first population-based study specifically designed to evaluate all the standard risks for yeast infections, researchers found that use of deodorant tampons or deodorant sanitary napkins during the last menstrual period had a moderate association with culture-proven yeast infections.[16] When a woman is having problems with irritation from pads, a tampon with the string tucked up may be a helpful alternative.

It's possible for pads to introduce some types of bacteria to the area. Most studies report no difference in the total numbers of bacteria between pad users and tampon users.[17] There seems to be one interesting difference, however: Women using pads have a higher proportion of bacteria from the bowel than do women using tampons.[18] Unlike a tampon, a pad rubs back and forth, dragging rectal bacteria forward to the vagina. But remember, just because bacteria are found does not mean that they are causing trouble. We're dumping the idea that the Vs are dirty. Bacteria are everywhere and are not synonymous with infection. Millions of women wear pads every month without problems.

Panty liners

Among the many refinements to the basic pad was an ultralightweight model that's barely noticeable to the wearer. The panty liner (a.k.a. panty shield) seemed an answer to every woman's prayer not to have to wear a cumbersome thick pad for days on end. Indeed, they are well suited for days of lighter flow, such as a day or two at the start or end of a menstrual period, as well as for a few hours after having sex.

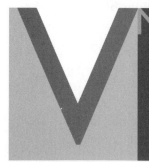

Panty liners have some limitations, though. They hold much less liquid than maxis, though absorption also varies by brand; the Always brand absorbs more slowly than Carefree, for example, so that moisture may stay in contact with the skin for a longer period of time.[19] Panty liners, like pads, can also be abrasive. They are not recommended for daily use; it is far better to change underpants several times a day if you have a lot of normal discharge. This may be the case during pregnancy, for example, or this may be the normal state for you. Remember that a little wetness or a yellowish stain on your underwear is not a sin; it's normal.

If you have had vulvar problems, you will want to minimize your use of panty liners. In one of the few long-term studies of women with vulvar pain (vulvodynia), daily use of panty liners was a common factor.

Alternative protection

Other forms of menstrual collection deserve mention too, although they're far less popular than the ubiquitous tampon and pad. These are a matter of personal preference. To date, no health drawbacks have been found, so if you like one of these options and use them scrupulously, you'll get no objection from me. The menstrual cup, for example, is worn in the vagina, cleaned, and reused. In the 1960s, the first menstrual cup, called Tassaway, was introduced, but it did not catch on.[20] Over the past ten years, newer versions of the menstrual cup, FDA-approved, have been introduced.

The Keeper, a gum rubber cup to be worn in the vagina to collect menstrual fluid, is designed to be washed out and reused. Like the Tassaway, the Keeper is inserted into the lower vagina; a portion extends outside the vagina with a removable pull tab. The Keeper is held in place by suction and is removed by pulling the tab to break suction. Because of the Keeper's position, the wearer is likely to be aware of its presence, but the tab can be trimmed for greater comfort. Drawback: A full bladder or rectum can force the Keeper out of position, causing leakage. Proponents of the Keeper see it as an ecological and less expensive alternative to pads and tampons, since it can be reused.

Another device, Instead, is a disposable diaphragm-shaped cup worn in the upper vagina under the cervix. It rests against the rear vaginal wall and behind the pubic bone. Instead is made of Kraton, a material long used for other medical devices. The rim of Instead softens in response to body temperature and conforms to the wearer's individual anatomy. This creates a gentle seal, effective against dislodging and leakage. Instead is used up to twelve hours at a time and discarded. Instead does not alter the growth of bacteria normally present in the vagina and has no risk of toxic shock.[21] Fans praise Instead for its comfort but acknowledge that it too can leak.

Another new option is the InSync Miniform (initially called Fresh 'n Fit Padette) by A-Fem, a very small rayon pad worn between the labia. It is designed to be used on light days or as a backup for tampon leakage. It absorbs approximately as much as a junior- or regular-absorbency tampon. Physical activity could dislodge the Padette, and leakage is possible. Also, this option would not work well for anyone suffering from pain in the vestibule.

A modern variation on the age-old use of rags is the washable pad. These reusable cotton pads, such as Glad Rags, are held in place by a specially designed piece of cloth that fastens to the underwear, usually with Velcro or by elastic bands attached to special underwear. A bit

V NOTE

More interesting than you might think

There's actually a Museum of Menstruation (MUM). Originally housed in the basement of the Washington, D.C.–area home of its curator, Harry Finley, it's now open to all on the Internet (www.mum.org). The lively museum contains product examples from belts to sponges, old packaging dating to the 1920s, advertisements, medical references, and more—even humor and poetry—and yes, it's all about menstruation.

cumbersome and labor-intensive to care for, they have particular appeal to environmentally conscious women.

Some women use small sea sponges (not the cellulose kind from the kitchen) as a natural tampon. You wet a sponge under the faucet, squeeze the water out, and insert it into the vagina. Sea sponges cannot be sold as "menstrual sponges" because they are not approved for that purpose by the U.S. Food and Drug Administration. Sand, chemical pollutants, bacteria, and fungi have been found in natural sponges. Since sponges are an organic product, the levels of these substances cannot be controlled or regulated. But they can be purchased in health food stores, where they are sold as cosmetic sponges. Some women say they are more comfortable and gentle than tampons. But they are not as convenient; they must be rinsed out (a once-routine household chore we've gotten away from with disposable menstrual products). High numbers of *Staphylococcus aureus,* associated with toxic shock syndrome, have been found in sea sponge users, suggesting that this is not an alternative to tampons for women who are seeking to decrease the risk of TSS.[22]

Underwear

If you have never had any vulvar problems, please wear and enjoy whatever kind of lingerie you wish. But if you have problems, white cotton is the watchword. Why?

Its simplicity is part of the answer. Some women are allergic to dyes used in colored underwear or to synthetic fabrics. And cotton absorbs moisture, wicking it away from the skin.

But most of the women who come to see me with V problems are already wearing white cotton underwear. So white cotton, while safest, is not magic. If this is your experience, take extra measures. Avoid chemicals—perfumed detergents, bleach, and fabric softeners, including dryer sheets. These products coat every fiber of your underwear with chemicals. Avoid tight underwear, no matter what the fabric (but especially the tight weave of spandex), including thongs, snap-crotches, girdles, and control-top underwear. Underpants that bind around the leg openings may also

V NOTE

Fashion faux pas

Too-tight pants or bikini bottoms can leave you with a "wedgie" when the fabric recedes into your Vs and sticks there. Aside from not being the style statement you probably intended, you risk chafing and irritation. Loosen up.

contribute to irritation. So-called tap pants, with no elastic around the leg holes, are an alternative. Men's boxer shorts are another.

If you have a problem, consider going without. Few have the courage, although no one needs to know! It's easiest with long skirts. Or you can, with all modesty, make your underwear the last thing you put on as you leave the house and the first thing you take off when you come home. Nights, weekends, and holidays you could wear long skirts, caftans, or loose pants without underwear. As mentioned, men's boxer shorts can provide a loose and comfortable substitute for women's briefs if you have vulvar irritation.

Consider your bedtime attire too. Many women routinely sleep in underpants out of modesty or personal preference. Once again, if you have no problems, this is your choice. But if you have pain, irritation, or any vulvar skin condition, going bare in bed is helpful. (Exceptions exist if you have been advised to apply an ointment over a large area of the vulva and when you have your period.)

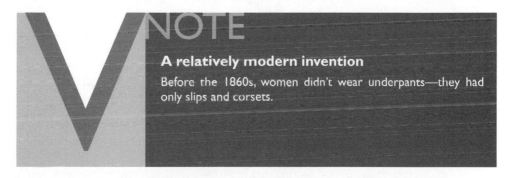

A relatively modern invention

Before the 1860s, women didn't wear underpants—they had only slips and corsets.

Panty hose are not helpful for women with vulvar problems; they are tight and may increase sweating. Changing your lifestyle to avoid these is not easy, but there are options: longer skirts with knee-highs or thigh-highs (which stay up better than ever these days), or a garter belt with stockings. Fortunately, the bare-leg look is increasingly acceptable fashion in many workplaces, especially in summer.

Patients often ask me if tight underclothes can cause yeast infections. In one study, researchers randomly assigned women to wear tight or loose clothing for a two-month period. At the end of this time, 44.5 percent of women were culture-positive for yeast; two-thirds of these were from the tight-clothing group.[23] A follow-up study indicated that yeast was more likely to be present in women who had worn tight-fitting clothing in the previous forty weeks than in the women who had worn loose clothing during the same time period.[24] A recent excellent study of women with culture-proven yeast infections showed a moderately strong association of yeast with noncotton underwear.[25]

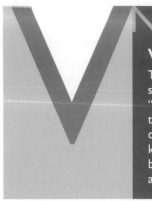

So loose white cotton wins, but only to help prevent or to soothe problems. It's not a cure.

Douching

Medical research is clear that vaginal douching is not a healthy practice. Yet it's incredibly pervasive. Women have done it since ancient Egyptian times. According to a 1988 federal survey, 37 percent of American women of reproductive age reported douching regularly. Half douched once a week. There was a striking racial difference: Two-thirds of African American women douched regularly, compared with one-third of Caucasian women. Overall, women of lower socioeconomic groups (measured by years of schooling and poverty level) were more likely to douche, and this tendency was much more prominent in Caucasians than African Americans.

To douche is to flush a quart or more of a cleansing solution and/or warm water into the vagina under low pressure. The reasons women douche vary. Through the 1970s, women were taught that it provided a necessary form of cleanliness. You douched after your period. You douched after intercourse. Fortunately, this thinking has become passé. Unfortunately, there are still women who persist in douching because they find the normal discharge associated with the changes of the menstrual cycle either abnormal or unpleasant. The practice also continues today as a self-treatment for odor and discharge, as well as an attempt to prevent sexually transmitted diseases. Some women continue to douche as a form of birth control, although (luckily) not as many as there used to be.

When patients ask me about douching, I tell them it's like mouthwash. It feels good for a few minutes and then the effect is gone. Douching is at best ineffective and at worst potentially harmful. But you wouldn't know this from the way commercial douche products are marketed and made so readily available. They represent a tempting prospect—vinegar to promote the naturally acidic environment of the vagina, or Betadine, a kind of iodine known as a powerful germ killer. What could be wrong with these ingredients? Well, neither of them works, and remember, you're not dirty. You don't need iodine! Besides, douching may make things worse.

Here's a quick rundown of the reasons that I encourage women to stop douching—or to never start in the first place.

▼ *Douching is not an effective form of birth control.* Sperm are highly active swimmers that can go through the cervix and into the uterus by the time you get into the bathroom. Anyway, as you douche, you push more sperm into the uterus.

▼ *Douching can't prevent sexually transmitted diseases.* It's a myth that douching "cleans out" harmful bacteria after intercourse, or at any time. Actually, douching devotees tend to have more STDs: Studies show that women who douche often tend to have significantly greater numbers of lifetime sexual partners and more sex partners who have other sexual contacts—both factors that improve your odds of getting chlamydia or gonorrhea. These same women are less likely to use condoms and spermicides, which also help prevent infection.

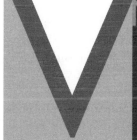

Solutions of choice
Half of douching women use commercial preparations, 30 percent use a home mixture of vinegar and water, 10 percent use water alone, and 10 percent use other preparations.

▼ *Douching can make odor and discharge worse, not better.* The short-lived relief that douching brings if you have irritating symptoms comes at a cost: The douching in turn promotes even more bacteria, so that you wind up ultimately feeling worse than before you douched. This bounce-back effect can create a vicious cycle of discomfort.

▼ *Douching may cause pelvic inflammatory disease.* Pelvic inflammatory disease (PID) is the most frequent serious infection encountered by American women, and it has reached an epidemic level. It's responsible for more than a quarter of a million hospital admissions and 2.5 million outpatient visits each year.[26] PID occurs when bacteria from the vagina travel after intercourse through the cervix and uterus and into the tubes and pelvis, causing infection in all these areas. Such infections can lead to chronic pelvic pain, ectopic pregnancy, and infertility.[27] Women who douche have a 73 percent greater risk of PID in comparison with those who do not douche. A woman who douches once a

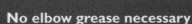

No elbow grease necessary

Remember that the vagina is a self-cleansing organ. It does not require any outside additives—from soap to douching solutions—in order to be clean, even if you are experiencing vaginal infection.

week or more has an approximately fourfold increased risk relative to a woman who never douches.

How would this work? Douching may provide a fluid carrier to transport disease-causing bacteria up into the pelvis.[28] So if a woman had an infection such as chlamydia, which was giving her a discharge, and she used a douche in order to feel cleaner, she could push the harmful bacteria through the cervix into the uterus; from there the infection could travel to the ovaries and tubes.

The occasional high pressure that occurs during douching may push out a plug of mucus that protects the opening of the womb.[29] Timing of the douche may also be important. At ovulation the mouth of the cervix opens gradually and the plug of mucus gives way to thin, clear mucus, which allows sperm to get through in order for conception to occur. Douching at this time could allow fluid that contained bacteria easy access through the open cervix.

▼ *Douching may cause ectopic pregnancy.* An ectopic pregnancy occurs when the pregnancy develops somewhere outside the uterus. This is most often in a Fallopian tube and often occurs because the tube has been damaged by previous infection (PID). Three recent studies have shown a modestly increased risk of ectopic pregnancy among women who douched.[30] A study focusing on African American women found a fourfold higher risk overall, which rose to a sixfold higher risk for women who had douched for longer than ten years.[31] One small study failed to show any association between vaginal douching and ectopic pregnancy.[32] Combining all these results, researchers' analyses suggest that if a woman who douches gets pregnant, she will have a 76 percent higher risk of having an ectopic pregnancy than a woman who does not douche.[33]

Hair removal

Pubic hair is in many ways a nuisance. Discharge gets stuck in it, menstrual flow and semen tangle it, and it sticks out beyond a bathing suit or leotard.

INSTEAD OF DOUCHING . . .

Reason for douching	Alternative to douching
Feminine hygiene: routine cleansing after menses or sex	A bath or shower is adequate; the vagina takes care of itself.
Wetness or vaginal discharge	Normal secretions increase during second half of the cycle, and some wetness is to be expected. Learn what's normal; change underwear as necessary. See your clinician for discharge that irritates.
Birth control	Douching does not prevent pregnancy; see your clinician for all the other options.
Irritation, itching, pain, or painful intercourse	Douching does not help. See your clinician.
Odor	Most odor is caused by bacterial vaginosis or yeast. Douching may worsen these conditions. Read the Odor section of Chapter 7 and see your clinician.

You may want to find ways to minimize these problems, but remember that eliminating pubic hair entirely may make intercourse uncomfortable from friction on your hairless mons. (That protection is a big part of the reason you've got hair there in the first place.) Your partner also may have strong opinions about the presence or absence of pubic hair.

Dealing with pubic hair is a challenge because of the shape of the hair shaft in cross section (round in Asian and Native American women, egg-shaped in Caucasian women, and elliptical in African American women) and because each hair comes from a saclike follicle with hair-generating cells at the base and an opening along the shaft for oil from sebaceous glands. No matter how you choose to remove the hair—shaving, plucking, waxing, laser—you run the chance of inflaming the follicle, thus causing red bumps. These are most likely with shaving (razor bumps) but can be seen to a lesser degree with other hair-removal methods.

If, however, you want to have less hair for whatever reason, you have some options. Perhaps the simplest approach is to use scissors to *carefully* trim the hair as closely as possible. No bumps, no irritation, no product to buy, no expensive visits to professional hair removers—just don't accidentally jab the scissors into the labia. You're also left with some protection of

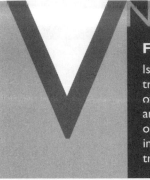

Flash quiz

Is a merkin (1) a type of flyfishing fly, (2) a small endangered Australian rodent, or (3) a pubic wig? All three, actually. In the case of the last of these, they were originally worn in the fourteenth and fifteenth centuries by men to mask signs of syphilis. At least one company, in London, still makes them today—cut and dyed into customized designs, and held in place with adhesive or a transparent G-string.

your pubis, though some women find trimming unsatisfactory because hair may remain visible at the sides of certain bathing suits.

Careful shaving works reasonably well for women with round or egg-shaped hair shafts. For African American women it, unfortunately, often causes bumps. The shape and curliness of the hair make it especially difficult to shave. (Laser, though expensive, is an excellent choice for African Americans.) To shave properly, use a double-edged razor blade. You need good lighting, time, and care to avoid nicks. Wet the skin and lather with mild soap such as Dove. Shave only in the direction the hair grows, down on the mons and labia. You'll have to look at your thighs—you may need to go down and in or down and out.

Depilatories are chemicals to remove hair. Available in gel, cream, lotion, aerosol, and roll-on forms, they dissolve the protein structure of the hair, causing it to separate easily from the skin surface. Many women find them satisfactory, and they can be applied in the privacy of your home. But depilatories take some time to work and can cause irritation and allergy for many. Do a skin test first and follow directions carefully to avoid chemical burns. It's a good idea to make sure the product you're using is recommended (on the label) for the bikini line. Avoid use on inflamed or broken skin.

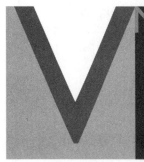

It hasn't always been out of vogue

In 1985, designer Rudi Gernreich unveiled the "pubikini," a bathing suit meant to expose pubic hair. (He's the same fellow who brought us the topless bathing suit.) "Slowly, the liberation of the body will cure our society of its sex hang-up," he predicted in 1970.

Waxing is popular and works well. Because it plucks the hair at the root, it lasts longer. Waxing has to be done every few weeks. (You could be among the lucky few whose hair doesn't grow back, but don't count on it.) The cost is moderate. Home products contain combinations of waxes such as paraffin and beeswax, oils or fats, and a resin that makes the wax adhere to the skin. There are hot and cold waxes. For the hot-wax technique, a thin layer of heated wax is applied to the skin in the direction of hair growth. The hair becomes trapped in the wax as it cools and hardens. The wax is then pulled off quickly in the opposite direction of the hair growth, taking the uprooted hair with it. Cold waxes are pretty much the same. Strips precoated with wax are pressed on the skin in the direction of the hair growth, and pulled off in the opposite direction.

The FDA does not recommend the use of over-the-counter waxes on genital areas, though many women like to remove hair well beyond the bikini zone.[34] In that event, your best bet is to have the job done professionally. Irritation and allergy from waxing are uncommon but possible. Because the wax is pulling the hair out of the follicle, bumps just like razor bumps can develop, I'm sorry to say. These can show up even with professional waxing jobs. Note that your skin may feel more sensitive premenstrually, but that shouldn't prevent you from waxing. You might experience some itching when hair regrows, but it's not usually a problem.

Electrolysis, or electrical epilation, has been around a long time. Successful electrolysis usually requires considerable time for an ongoing series of treatments and costs a lot of money, depending on how large the area is and how thick the hair is. Many women choose this technique for bikini work. It can be done with the needle epilator or the tweezers epilator. Needle epilators introduce a very fine wire close to the hair shaft into the hair follicle under the skin. An electric current travels down the wire to destroy the hair root at the base of the follicle. The voltage and current used are not high. The loosened hair is removed with tweezers. Each hair is treated individually. Because this technique destroys the hair follicle, it is considered permanent. But the hair root may persist if the needle misses the mark or if insufficient electricity is delivered to destroy it.

Tweezer epilators are relatively new. They also use electric current to remove hair. The tweezers grasp the hair close to the skin and the current travels down the hair shaft to the root.

The risks of electrolyis are electrical shock if the needle is not properly insulated, infection if it is unsterile, or scarring from improper technique. There are no uniform standards governing the practice, but thirty-one states require electrologists to be licensed. A list of licensed and certified electrologists is available (see Resources).

Home-use electrolysis devices are available, but I would not recommend them for bikini-line hair removal. You just can't see well enough. If you have time and money for the salon electrolysis, it's fine in licensed and certified hands.

Laser hair removal is the latest and most rapidly growing method of hair removal. It is safe and effective in the hands of a physician, often a dermatologist, or technician trained and experienced in the use of the laser for this purpose. Don't ever let anyone laser anything unless you know that he or she is specifically trained and experienced in laser work and you know exactly what outcome to expect. Laser removal works better for some women than others, depending on your coloring and hair type. The ideal candidate has dark hair and light skin. Pain varies with the type of laser used and may be minimized with a topical anesthetic cream. Ask lots of questions before you proceed: how many treatments are required, the extent of treatment, possible problems, what level of success to expect given your skin and hair coloring, the cost, and the operator's credentials and experience with the procedure.

Remember that laser hair removal is relatively new, so many technicians lack extensive experience with this method, and we don't know what the long-term results are. As of May 2001, the FDA has given several manufacturers permission to claim "permanent reduction"—*not* "permanent removal"—for their lasers. This means that although laser treatments with these devices will permanently reduce the total number of hairs, they will not result in a permanent removal of all hair. (See Resources.)

Other V styles

Let me mention a few more forms of V care that, while not practiced by the majority of women, nevertheless are being done and deserve some fair warnings.

Because pubic hair tends to be darker than one's hair color and grays with age right along with the hair on your head, many women wonder about dyeing it. I'd really rather that you didn't. V skin is so sensitive that even if you have no reactions to using dyes on your scalp, you may have problems here. Your best bet would be to consult a professional colorist;

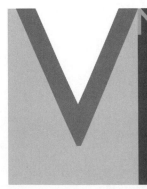

Be careful what you ask for

A bikini wax usually removes extra hair around the bikini line and along the upper thighs, possibly including the edges of the mons. A Brazilian bikini wax (alias the Mohawk or the Playboy) goes much farther—removing all hairs in sight, including those you probably never realized you had, straight back to your rear, sometimes leaving a narrow "landing strip" or other design of the wearer's choice.

some spas and salons that handle bikini waxing will also perform this service. (Most don't advertise, though; you have to ask.) A dye for facial hair, not for the hair on your head, should be used. Only the hair on the top of the mons—not on the labia—should be attempted. If you develop irritation, that's a problem. Stripping the dye with other chemicals is going to increase the irritation. Best to cut the dyed hair as short as possible and use tub soaks until the skin calms down.

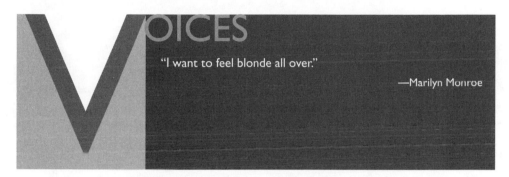

VOICES

"I want to feel blonde all over."

—Marilyn Monroe

Another direction for the style-obsessed is labia décor. Again, proceed only with extreme caution if you must do this at all. Tattooing, piercing, and branding are unlicensed and unregulated industries. In most communities, tattoo and piercing "artists" are not subject to health inspections. Nor are body-art practitioners required to be trained in anatomy ("Where exactly is the labial artery?") or infection control. These are some of the reasons I agree with the American Academy of Dermatology in opposing piercing anywhere but the earlobe. Risks include infection, prolonged bleeding, scarring, hepatitis B and C (which can be fatal), tetanus, and HIV. Also, you should know that both the U.S. Red Cross and the Canadian Red Cross won't accept blood donations from anyone who's had body piercing or a tattoo within a year because both procedures can transmit blood-borne diseases. So that's why I say that while a labia ring or a secret tattoo might seem fun or make a statement about you, they're not worth the risk.

▼

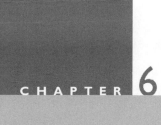

CHAPTER 6

Sex Matters
V Health Facts for Sexually Active Women

nformation about sex is everywhere, it seems: how to spark it, how to do it better, how to have it more often. But I want to talk about sex from a point of view you might not have considered before—the V perspective. What happens inside your body during sexual activity? How does sex affect your V health, and how can V health problems affect sex?

Far from being obscure or unimportant questions, they have a direct impact on your quality of life. It's sometimes implied, for example, that you should respond to your partner's sexual appetite whether yours is whetted or not, that men have a stronger sex drive, that sex is aimed at his pleasure and not yours, that birth control is your problem, and so on. It's all nonsense, of course. Sex ought to be an equal-opportunity event—mutually desired, wonderful for both. Birth control, if it's necessary, concerns both. And if you have a V problem that's causing you pain or irritation, it too can work both ways. Maybe you and your partner will need to abstain or revise your sex life for a while.

Bugs and babies aside, you have a pleasure motive for knowing about the Vs' sexual side. Ever wonder why you often want to tip your hips up during intercourse if you're lying on your back? Why some lubricants seem to feel better than others? Why it sometimes hurts to have your clitoris rubbed directly in the heat of the moment, when you'd think it ought to feel great? The answers have to do with some biological basics.

This chapter maps out what's supposed to happen. For sexual problems or pain, see Part III and the Resources section.

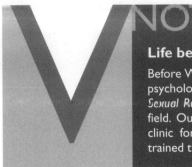

First, desire

Ideally, it all starts with being "in the mood." Sexual desire is a complex brew. It's flavored by both physical factors (such as your general health, state of fatigue, medications, hormonal status) and emotional factors (such as anxiety, confidence, mood, and tension). Desire is further influenced by your sexual attitudes, past sexual experiences, the current environmental setting, the person you're with, and your relationship—to mention only a few.

Right, you might say. Isn't it obvious that you have to want it? As a matter of fact, being in the mood for sex has not always been recognized as one of the basics. In the 1960s, when research on sexual function started to move forward with the famous Masters and Johnson studies, American sex researcher Helen Singer Kaplan introduced the concept of desire for the first time. She considered it an element as important to sex as excitement or orgasm.[1]

Lately researchers wonder whether desire is different for a woman at the beginning of a new relationship—when it's a lusty warm-up to the big heat of sexual gratification—than in a relationship that's a year old or longer. In long-term relationships, it may be that desire and physical arousal occur at a point after these women have *chosen* to experience sexual stimulation. This choice is based initially on the emotional needs (to be close, to bond, to be loved, to please) other than a desire to experience physical sexual arousal and release. Sexual desire, then, may also be a *responsive,* rather than spontaneous, event.[2]

This new way of thinking about desire reveals that a woman who might otherwise be called underactive in sexual desire is perfectly normal. You may not have spontaneous sexual urges, but you become fully responsive after you choose to be turned on.

Now let's look at what happens in the vulva and vagina once desire has been triggered. The four stages of sexual response were first mapped out by Masters and Johnson in 1966 and still hold true today.[3] They are (1) excitement, (2) plateau, (3) orgasm, and (4) resolution. This classic model

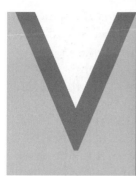

NOTE

The science behind the little blue pills

Nitric oxide, which helps relax blood-vessel walls in a woman's pelvic area during arousal, is also responsible for penile erection in men. The drug Viagra (sildenafil citrate) increases levels of nitric oxide, which is why it holds promise to improve sexual functioning in women as well as men. To date, though, it hasn't been adequately tested in women.

has been criticized because it implies that sexual problems are purely physical. This is certainly not the case. This model also levels the differences among individual women. In fact, all women are not the same, and their sexual needs, satisfactions, and problems don't fit into neat categories. But I like this model as a starting point for understanding in a general way what happens in a woman's body during sexual activity. So let me walk you through these four stages.

Stage 1: excitement (arousal)

Remember that much of the vulva—the labia majora and minora, clitoris, prepuce—is made up of erectile tissue crisscrossed with blood vessels.

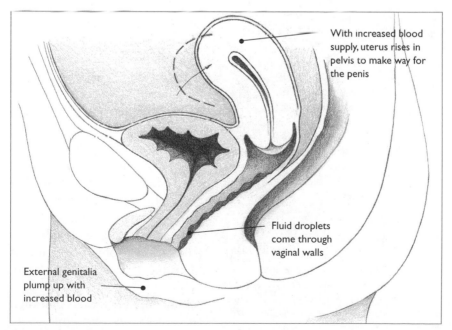

With increased blood supply, uterus rises in pelvis to make way for the penis

Fluid droplets come through vaginal walls

External genitalia plump up with increased blood

FIG. 27 Excitement

Source: W. H. Masters, V. E. Johnson, R. C. Kolodny, *Heterosexuality* (New York: HarperCollins, 1994).

LUBRICANT LOWDOWN

When natural vaginal lubrication is low, using an artificial lubricant can ease the way and boost enjoyment. Lots of different products are readily available right at your local grocery or drugstore. But finding a lubricant that's both effective and nonirritating can be challenging. Petroleum products such as Vaseline and mineral oil weaken the latex in condoms and are not recommended for use with them. In addition, these substances are not water-soluble and are greasy to use. People have tried egg whites as a natural slippery substance, but these can serve as a dangerous culture medium for bacteria to grow in. You may also see mixtures of glycerin and water with poly-carbophil or a cellulose derivative marketed as vaginal moisturizers; an example of these is Replens. Although Replens is a safe and effective alternative to estrogen vaginal cream, a moisturizer isn't the same thing as a lubricant, so it's not recommended for use during sex.

Better choices are the personal lubricants sold over the counter. Read their ingredients carefully, though. The popular K-Y jelly, for example, contains an ingredient called chlorhex-idine that causes burning for many women. What's more, any lubricant containing chlorhexidine should be avoided if you are attempting pregnancy because it's toxic to sperm. Astroglide, another popular over-the-counter lubricant, contains the preservative propylene glycol, which bothers some women. Some women have found vitamin E suppositories or the oil out of vitamin E capsules helpful, but it's possible to develop an allergy to topical vitamin E.

If you have V problems, be careful to avoid lubricants with ingredients such as propylene glycol. Otherwise, experiment with different brands to see what works best for you. Whichever lubricant you choose, use it sparingly. My vote for a handy, safe choice for every woman is ordinary olive oil. It's pure, without added ingredients or preservatives. Vegetable oils work fine too. A little dab is all you need.

Erectile tissue is the same stuff that makes a penis hard. These structures respond to stimulation (sexy thoughts, racy images, a lover's touch, cologne) by filling with blood. A substance even less familiar to most women than hormones has a starring role in this little passion play. Nitric oxide (NO), a chemical found in blood-vessel walls, relaxes the smooth muscle in these walls. Mellow, wide-open blood vessels means greater blood flow—and that, in turn, means the whole area feels fuller and more responsive.

The labia minora, clitoris, and vestibular bulbs plump up. In the vagina, this blood flow causes fluid droplets from the blood plasma to come through the walls in a "sweating" reaction with the wetness that we recognize when aroused. The Bartholin's glands add to the wetness with their lubricating mucus.

The wetness can occur within seconds after stimulation, or it may take a little longer. Initially, the amount of lubrication is slight, but with further arousal, lubrication may trickle out of the opening of the vagina, producing a sensation that some women describe as "gushing."[4] On the other hand, some women have an initial abundance of wetness that then disappears in the wink of an eye. This is perfectly normal; you may want to add extra lu-

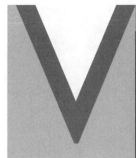

NOTE

An old idea

The ancient Romans used olive oil as a sexual lubricant. In the seventeenth century, honey and different oils not only lubricated the vagina but reduced irritation caused by the brandy and other alcoholic spirits that were used as spermicides.

bricant if this is how your body works. Characteristics of this fluid may vary from colorless to whitish, from runny to slippery to sticky. Vaginal fluid, typical of the marvelous Vs, does more than make intercourse comfortable. It helps to keep sperm alive, helps keep sperm swimming, and decreases genital tract infection from bacteria that might ride in on sperm and be carried through the cervix. The slippery feeling of vaginal fluid comes from the various proteins it contains.

You need to learn about your own patterns of sexual lubrication. Not only does the amount of fluid vary from woman to woman, but also you can lubricate without realizing it. If a woman is lying on her back, for example, the moisture may pool in the back of the vagina too far from the opening to make intercourse comfortable. Before penetration, a finger dipped into the vagina can draw some of the fluid out to coat a dry surface. Frequency of intercourse makes a difference too; when you have sex on a regular basis, you naturally make more lubrication.

With lubrication come other changes. The inner two-thirds of the vagina expand from their normally collapsed walls to a cavity with enough width and depth to receive an erect penis. The color of the vaginal walls changes from normal purplish red to a darker purple—again, from all the blood rushing to the area. Pumped up by the blood, the uterus rises up in the pelvis, and the cervix rises with it. They're getting out of the way.

The labia majora swell slightly. The fattened labia minora push them away slightly from their covering position over the vagina so that it's opened up. The clitoris enlarges. Farther north, increased blood flow contributes to nipple erection and an increase in breast size. The heart rate increases, blood pressure rises a little, and muscle tension increases throughout the body. In some women, the skin develops a mottled, splotchy look.

Stimulation of the clitoris during this phase is for many women one of the most important aspects of lovemaking, but most men (if your partner is male) are far from expert in this art.[5] Our culture teaches that the man is "supposed" to know how to please a woman. Unfortunately, one of

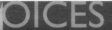

women's most common complaints is that many men (even those who consider themselves skillful lovers) search out the clitoris almost immediately and then stimulate it vigorously and almost continuously in a determined effort to fire up their partner's passion. According to Masters and Johnson, whose research is based on tens of thousands of interviews, many men fail to realize that most women don't enjoy clitoral stimulation until they are more physically involved through cuddling, caressing, and kissing. What men believe is vigorously enthusiastic touching is perceived by many women as too rough. Few women like the "find-it-and-stick-with-it" approach, preferring that their partners move away from the clitoral area entirely for a while after initially fondling it, and then return to it. *Direct* clitoral stimulation is often so intense that it can actually be unpleasant. Many women prefer being touched or rubbed in the area around or above the clitoris. Because there's no source of lubrication close to the clitoris, touching it with dry or rough fingertips may be physically uncomfortable. Lubrication with saliva or another lubricant may be necessary.[6]

One possible explanation for the male reluctance to use a light touch around the clitoris may be that it's not what he prefers on his own genitals. Men tend to find a woman's light touch or gentle stroking of the penis tickling or annoying rather than stimulating. What's the answer? You have to *talk* with each other about what feels good! You have to keep saying it. And sometimes you have to demonstrate. You may need to move your partner's hand to the right place or lift his/her hand if it's too heavy. Likewise, a man may need to show you how to rub more firmly if your touch is too light.

Also, if the clitoris is not the primary source of your pleasure, you certainly need to let your partner know this. If you've located your G spot, you'll need to show your partner where this is. We'll talk more about this below.

Stage 2: plateau

The changes of the excitement phase, when the sensitive tissues fill with blood and muscle tension increases, continue to build and then level off.

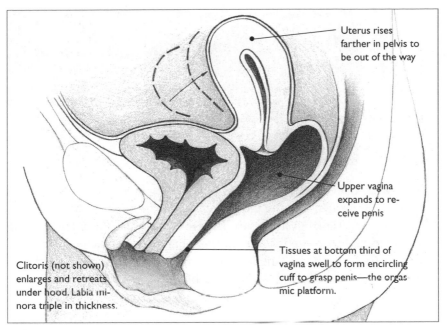

Uterus rises farther in pelvis to be out of the way

Upper vagina expands to receive penis

Tissues at bottom third of vagina swell to form encircling cuff to grasp penis—the orgasmic platform.

Clitoris (not shown) enlarges and retreats under hood. Labia minora triple in thickness.

FIG. 28 Plateau

Source: W. H. Masters, V. E. Johnson, R. C. Kolodny, *Heterosexuality* (New York: HarperCollins, 1994).

Most notably, the tissues surrounding the bottom third of the vagina swell tremendously. This forms an encircling cuff called the *orgasmic platform*. Filled with blood, the tissues of the platform push inward, narrowing, and enclosing the shaft of the penis with a grasp that's pleasurable to the male. And because that part of the vagina where the platform arises is rich in nerve endings, you feel good too.

Natural lubrication may continue during the plateau phase, but if the phase lasts more than a few minutes, fluid production may drop off considerably or completely. Additional lubrication in addition to the natural moisture may be necessary. (See box on page 112.)

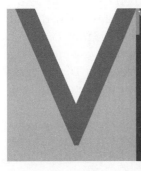

NOTE

Oops

What causes "varts" (you know, those embarrassing little whooshes of noise that sound like gas being passed) during intercourse? They're no big deal. Usually there is no air in the vagina. Any activity—inserting a tampon, sexual practices—can introduce air. And it comes out.

During the plateau, the amount of blood pumped into the area pushes the uterus up farther, and the upper vagina continues to expand. The clitoris enlarges further, but it pulls back against the pubic bone. This pulling back, combined with the swelling of the labia, makes the clitoris seem to disappear under its hood. The labia minora double or triple in thickness and—again owing to vastly increased blood flow—change color to a bright red or deep wine red.

As with everything related to sex, the plateau phase may vary. Sometimes it's a brief moment. Or a couple may go back and forth between excitement and plateau in an extended fashion.

Stage 3: orgasm

It's the briefest—and most pleasurable—stage, marked by contractions of the perineal muscles, of the muscles around the vagina, and of the orgasmic platform.

Some experts believe that no matter how an orgasm is produced (by masturbation, oral sex, vaginal intercourse, or use of a dildo or vibrator), female orgasm always results from some form of clitoral stimulation.[7] The penis in the vagina is not enough for most women to achieve orgasm. In fact, most positions of intercourse fail to usefully stimulate either the erectile tissue around the urethra or the erectile tissue of the shaft or glans of the clitoris.[8] Most women need more—either direct stimulation of the clitoris or friction from rubbing the clitoral hood. (Remember, it looks like a small nubbin, but it's actually pretty vast.) Only then can overall sexual tension build to the point where the orgasmic threshold is reached.[9] The pudendal nerve is the pathway for this sensation. Impulses travel through branches of this nerve to the spinal cord, whence they ascend to the brain. In the brain the impulses are interpreted as pleasure. The pleasure message is sent back down the spinal cord and out the fibers of the pudendal nerve to the vulva.

Others disagree that the clitoris is central to orgasm. Some women describe orgasms that are different from the clitoral model in that they have deep vaginal and uterine sensation.[10] Some women report sexual pleasure

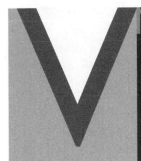

Jolly good vibrations

The portable, mechanized vibrator was invented in the 1880s in England, by a physician. By the 1920s, nearly a dozen manufacturers were producing vibrators in the United States.

and orgasm from vaginal stimulation alone, particularly from an area of sensitive tissue in the front wall of the vagina, under the urethra (a.k.a. the G spot); researchers have also reported this.[11] Other researchers have reported that the G spot is the major source of stimulation for a second reflex pathway in addition to the pudendal nerve; this one's thought to travel through the pelvic nerve and a collection of nerve fibers called the hypogastric plexus.[12]

Who's right? I wish I knew for sure. It's possible that the G spot represents the underside of the clitoris stimulated through the vaginal wall, the bulb of the vestibule, or special vaginal tissue. Only you or your lover, not a gynecologist, can find the sensitive area. That's because it's not obvious in the unaroused state. Nor is it a magic button that turns on

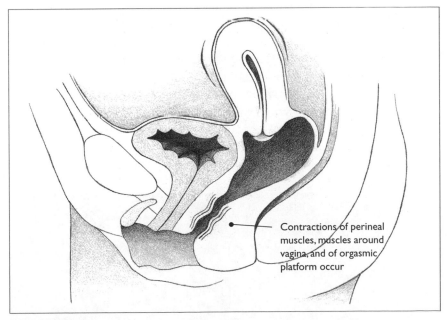

Contractions of perineal muscles, muscles around vagina, and of orgasmic platform occur

FIG. 29 Orgasm

Source: W. H. Masters, V. E. Johnson, R. C. Kolodny, *Heterosexuality* (New York: HarperCollins, 1994).

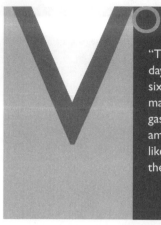

immediate ecstasy when pushed, no more than a single touch of the clitoris releases instant nirvana.

The G spot, if a woman has one, can be found after she's aroused by inserting a finger, penis, dildo, or vibrator into the vagina and exploring along the front wall up and toward the navel. The area is anywhere from a knuckle of your finger to a knuckle and a half inside the vagina, not way up near the cervix.[13] The area is, unlike the rest of the crinkly vaginal wall, smooth. Stimulation of this area may require three or four fingers, but other women say rear entry or the woman on top works well. G spot orgasms are said to be more difficult to achieve than clitoral orgasms.[14]

If the G spot eludes you, don't throw in the towel. Think of it as one of many potentials to explore in enhancing your sexual pleasure.[15] If you or your sexual partner is unable to find it, move on to enjoy the areas that do bring pleasure and don't worry about it.

Clitoral and vaginal stimulation (or some combination of the two) aren't the only paths to orgasm. Some women can climax with imagination as the only source of stimulation.[16] The pathway for this type of orgasm is not understood. An additional sensory pathway has recently been proposed to involve the vagus nerve that extends directly from the cervix to the brain,

VNOTE

O is for optimism

Women who have difficulty achieving orgasm used to be called "anorgasmic." Sex therapists now prefer the term "preorgasmic," in light of the fact that almost every woman can learn how to have orgasms.

bypassing the spinal cord.[17] This may account for sexual responses reported by women with spinal cord injuries.

Over the years women's orgasm has been greatly misunderstood, often with terrible implications for women. From the time of Hippocrates, it was thought that women achieved orgasm only when the vagina was penetrated by the penis—forget the clitoris. The problem is that intercourse fails to produce orgasm in more than half the female population.[18] Back then, alternatives were not discussed and, presumably, not widely practiced. Masturbation was considered unchaste and possibly unhealthful. As a result, many sexually frustrated women developed symptoms of anxiety, insomnia, depression, irritability, nervousness, sensations of heaviness in the abdomen, lower pelvic swelling, and vaginal lubrication. Collectively these complaints were termed "hysteria." The treatment: marriage and vigorous vaginal intercourse. Failing that, women sought medical assistance for their "disorder." The genitalia were massaged with fragrant oils until the afflicted woman was aroused to a "paroxysm" (that is, an orgasm). Amazingly, medical massage wasn't viewed as sexual since no penetration was involved, and that was the only definition of sexuality that

DO WOMEN EJACULATE?

Amazingly, no one's sure. Release of fluid from the urethra at orgasm occurs in a small percentage of women, who experience it as extremely pleasurable. Some suggest that women can learn how to ejaculate. If it occurs, the ejaculate is about a teaspoon of fluid similar to watery skim milk. Some chemical analyses suggest that this fluid is urine, while others show that it's different from urine.

Above all, release of fluid is a normal function for some women and does not require surgery or medication to make it go away. Some women report that they stopped having orgasms to avoid wetting the bed. No man would say that! This sounds like an example of a cultural obsession with cleanliness overwhelming what is natural and wonderful. Change the sheets! Use an underpad. Find a towel or some disposable underpads. Fluids and moisture are part of nature, part of womanhood. Fluid represents one of our essential essences, from the lubricating mucus of the cervix and the moisture that comes through the vaginal wall during sexual arousal to the bag of waters surrounding our babies. We are often wet. We don't need to stop it, to get rid of it, or to hide it. Whether a woman ejaculates or not is less important than the fact that sex bring joy and closeness to both partners.

Sources: B. Whipple and B. R. Komisaruk, Beyond the G spot, *Med Aspects Human Sexuality* 1998:1(3):19; J. Berman and L. Berman, *For Women Only: A Revolutionary Guide to Overcoming Sexual Dysfunction and Reclaiming Your Sex Life* (New York: Henry Holt and Company, 2001); H. Alzate, Vaginal eroticism: a replication study, *Arch Sex Behav* 1985:14; D. C. Goldberg, B. Whipple, R. E. Fishkin, et al., The Grafenberg spot and female ejaculation: a review of the initial hypothesis, *J Sex Marital Ther* 1983:9:27; F. Addiego, E. G. Belzer, J. Comolli, et al., Female ejaculation: a case study, *J Sex Res* 1981:17:13; M. Zaviacic, S. Dolezalova, I. K. Holoman, et al., Concentrations of fructose in female ejaculate and urine: a comparative biochemical study, *J Sex Res* 1988:24:319; E. G. Belzer, B. Whipple, W. Moger, On female ejaculation, *J Sex Res* 1984:20:403.

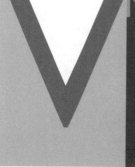

counted. Bringing countless women to orgasm, however, was not a job that the medical profession wanted. Midwives were pressed into service, but ultimately the job was facilitated by various devices, including the vibrator. Office treatments of this nature continued until the early 1920s.

Hysteria wasn't dropped from psychiatric terminology until 1952.[19] As late as the 1970s, medical authorities assured men that a woman who did not reach orgasm during heterosexual coitus was flawed or suffering from some physical or psychological impairment. The problem was automatically assigned to her, since any fault in the theory of vaginal orgasm by penile penetration was unthinkable.[20]

There are, as I've said, many routes to sexual orgasm for women. And orgasm is not essential to sexual enjoyment or fulfillment. We must never again fall into the trap of having anyone give us "the rules." For years women were told that the only way to climax was mutually, with penetrative penile intercourse. We must never again listen to someone like Sigmund Freud. In the nineteenth century, he maintained that vaginal orgasm was "mature" and clitoral orgasm was "infantile." He caused a lot of confusion and misery when he said that only by shifting her focus from her clitoris (vestigial phallus, he called it) to her unmistakably feminine vagina could a woman find psychosexual fulfillment. Now that we know

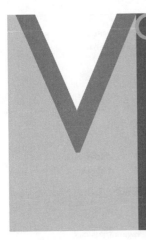

better about the beauty and versatility of V structure and V function, there's no looking back.

There's no "right" orgasm. Rather, orgasm seems to vary immensely from one woman to the next and from one time to the next. Sometimes it is a fleeting wisp of a sensation; at other times it can be an intense and sustained physical pleasure. With continued stimulation immediately after orgasm, women can have additional orgasms within a short period of time without ever dropping below the plateau level of sexual arousal.

All women have the physical capacity to have multiple orgasms. Yet not all women do. A reason for lack of success may lie in the mechanics of the process. If clitoral stimulation after the first orgasm is too immediate or too intense, it can result in something like a spasm without the pleasure sensation. You need to learn by experimentation (often by self-stimulation) how quickly a very light touch will feel stimulating again and how many seconds are required to bring another orgasm of the same intensity as the first wave. You then need great communication with your partner, who needs to be aware of the timing. With the proper understanding and sensitivity on his or her part, it's possible for a woman to have twelve or more successive orgasms once the correct rhythm of stimulation is discovered.

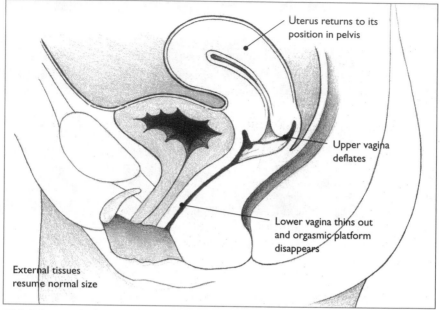

Uterus returns to its position in pelvis

Upper vagina deflates

Lower vagina thins out and orgasmic platform disappears

External tissues resume normal size

FIG. 30 Resolution

Source: W. H. Masters, V. E. Johnson, R. C. Kolodny, Heterosexuality (New York: HarperCollins, 1994).

Stage 4: resolution

In the last stage of sexual response, the body returns to its baseline, unaroused state. The orgasmic platform disappears very rapidly after orgasm, and the clitoris returns to its normal position within five to ten seconds. As blood drains from the genital area, the labia minora revert to normal color within ten to fifteen seconds. The uterus goes quickly into its standard position, and the vaginal walls collapse inward.

Masturbation and V health

Everybody thinks about masturbation. Sometimes women "confess" to me that their V problem developed shortly after self-stimulation. They worry that they've injured themselves by masturbating. Or women who can't have vaginal intercourse during a particular treatment will want to know if masturbation is okay. Still others, suffering from the chronic pain of vulvodynia, firmly inform me that self-stimulation is all they have left: "The only touch I can count on not to hurt is my finger."

The vast majority of women masturbate—it's just another expression of sexuality. It's as healthy and normal as the toddler who holds on to her labia while Mommy sings to her in the tub. Adolescents learn that self-stimulation relieves the potent sexual tension that hormonal and other changes bring at this time of life. For young women there are other benefits too: You can develop a positive self-image by becoming comfortable with your own body as well as discover that there are more ways to be sexual than through having intercourse. In fact, masturbation may actually keep a young woman from having sex before she is ready. Not least, you can pleasure yourself no matter what your age.

I "give permission" all the time in my office to patients who ask if it's okay. So it's worth repeating here: I hereby declare for women everywhere that there is absolutely no evil consequence, no illness or disease, no character weakness or moral decay, that comes from fingering the Vs. Self-stimulation does not cause vulvodynia or any other V problem. Their development would only be coincidence. The only rule to apply to self-stimulation is the one that applies to any activity involving your body: You must never do anything that hurts. If it causes pain, stop.

So explore your Vs. Enjoy them. The response mechanism works just as I've described in this chapter whether sex is penile, oral, through a vibrator, with a partner, or on your own. And an added benefit to masturbation is that it's a splendid way to really find out how you work.

VIBRATING WITH CARE

Are vibrators safe? They're certainly popular. I'll bet if *Consumer Reports* did a survey, they'd tell you that there are 2.9 vibrators in every American household. They're widely used to enhance sexual pleasure. A vibrator produces a level of stimulation that no human can match (one reason they're frequently used in sex therapy). It's a misconception, though, that if you use one, you won't want a real penis or won't be able to become aroused or reach orgasm on your own without the device. Orgasm may be easier for some women to reach with the help of a vibrator, but it's only a small piece of the action. Nothing you can buy in a sex shop (or discreet mail-order catalog) can replace the joys of intimacy with another person.

Vibrators aren't regulated by the FDA, and there are so many different shapes, sizes, and materials available that I can't offer any one-size-fits-all recommendations. They also vary in electrical and mechanical activity; some are actually heavy, powerful massagers. That leaves us in the common sense department. A vibrator is meant to enhance pleasure. It's possible for a vibrator to be too big, too heavy, or too powerful. It should not hurt against the clitoris. Nor should it hurt as it stretches the vagina or rectum. The vagina was meant to accommodate the smooth and cylindrical penis. The rectum is accustomed to smooth stool. A vibrator that is too large can damage the anal sphincter. Don't use anything that could catch or cut the vaginal or rectal wall. At the first bit of pain, stop. You absolutely must not do anything to your body that causes it pain.

Passion's pests

No discussion of sex and health is complete without considering two of its biggest implications: sexually transmitted diseases (STDs) and pregnancy. First, the former.

Just as there are many different kinds of STDs, they make themselves known in a myriad of ways. One might appear as anything from a skin

AT-A-GLANCE GUIDE TO STDS

Name	Cause	Symptoms	Diagnosis	Treatment
Gonorrhea	Bacterium: *Neisseria gonorrheae*	Often none. Urinary burning, frequency; vaginal discharge. Pelvic inflammatory disease.	Culture of pus or secretions/DNA test	Ceftriaxone injection and doxycycline tablets
Syphilis	Bacterium: *Treponema pallidum*	Primary: painless ulcer on genitals. May not be obvious; comes and heals after four weeks. Secondary: fever, swollen glands, rash. Tertiary: cardiac or nervous system abnormality.	Blood test	Penicillin
Chlamydia	Bacterium: *Chlamydia trachomatis*	Often no symptoms. Urinary burning; cervicitis and discharge. Pelvic inflammation.	Culture/DNA test	Doxycycline tablets or erythromycin tablets
Chancroid	Bacterium: *Haemophilus ducreyi*	Genital ulcer; swollen glands.	Culture	Ceftriaxone; erythromycin
Genital herpes	Virus: *Herpes simplex*	Often no symptoms. Irritation and burning; blisters or cracks (fissures).	Culture and blood tests; exam by clinician	No cure; antiviral drugs help reduce intensity and duration of symptoms
Genital warts	Virus: human papillomavirus	Warts ranging from tiny single dots to large irregular rough surface masses that protrude from labia, vagina, or cervix.	Exam by experienced clinician; biopsy; DNA test	No cure; chemical, laser, or freezing treatments
Hepatitis B	Virus: hepatitis B	Fatigue, fever, gastrointestinal symptoms, jaundice.	Blood test	No treatment; vaccine can prevent
Hepatitis C	Virus: hepatitis C	Sometimes none. Fatigue, fever, gastrointestinal symptoms, jaundice.	Blood test	Interferon with antiviral drug ribavirin. No vaccine exists.
Trichomonas	Protozoan: *Trichomonas vaginalis*	Profuse malodorous discharge, itching, and pain.	Microscopic exam of discharge; culture	Metronidazole (Flagyl)
Acquired immune deficiency syndrome (AIDS)	Virus: human immunodeficiency virus	Often no symptoms for years. Fever, weight loss, various infections, and skin problems.	Blood test	No cure; course can be slowed by numerous antiviral drugs

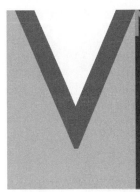

A long way from Pinocchio

In 1993 women's health advocate Dorrie Lane created a line of hand-sewn, anatomically accurate vulva puppets fashioned from velvets, silks, and satins, filled with fragrant flowers and herbs. Her Wondrous Vulva Puppets have since developed a cult following among sex educators and rape/sexual abuse counselors, who use them as a nonthreatening way to explain erogenous zones, safe-sex techniques, and the basic beauty of vulvar design.

problem (ulcers, blisters, pimples, and rashes) to vaginal discharge and pelvic pain. There is no "classic" finding, no one way to tell if you have a sexually transmitted disease or whether your partner has one. You cannot tell by talking with someone or knowing his background or character or social class whether he carries bacteria or viruses that could change your life forever. The worst news of all is that while men often have symptoms that reveal a problem, for women many STDs work silently, producing no symptoms until a woman is unable to become pregnant and tubal scarring is found. But even in men, symptoms may not be obvious; for example, we are learning that for both sexes genital herpes can be a completely undetected disease. And now, with the onset of the AIDS epidemic, we are faced with an STD that can kill. Never before has safe sex been more important! The chart on page 124 summarizes STDs.

Safer sex

What makes sex safe? It's not a question with a quick, glib answer. The only completely safe sex is no sex, but we all know that complete abstinence is not realistic for most humans. Masturbation is safe and often all that is available to someone without a partner, but self-stimulation is limited by the lack of joy that comes from sharing pleasure with a partner. The next choice is safer sex: a mutually monogamous relationship be-

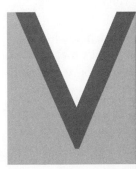

Olde-tyme STDs

The outdated term for sexually transmitted diseases is "venereal disease," named for Venus, the Roman goddess of love. "Clap," a common slang term for gonorrhea, comes from the Old French word *clapoir*, meaning a swelling in the groin that is characteristic of the disease in men.

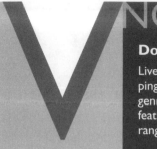

tween two uninfected partners. Yet that too can be a tall order. There's no single test that can be done, no all-encompassing question that can be asked, no test of time or relationship to guarantee that an individual is faithful to the other and free of disease.

Women and men don't need to worry about STDs if:

▼ Neither partner ever had sex with anyone else

▼ Neither partner ever shared needles

▼ Neither partner has ever been infected with an STD

Of course, partners who have never had sex with anyone else are not always the ones we meet. Most of us have more than one sex partner during our lives. As a result, many of us get some kind of infection from a partner who:

▼ May not have known he/she was infected

▼ May have hoped he/she wouldn't infect us

▼ May not have been honest about his/her sexual history

As a woman, you are at greater risk than a man is. The vagina, the cervix, and the rectum are more easily infected than the penis. Tiny cracks (microabrasions) in the vaginal walls that may occur with normal sex may be a source of infection. Infection of the vagina and cervix can ascend silently, without symptoms, through the uterus to the tubes to infect and scar, and even wipe out fertility. A woman's risks are huge!

What can we do?

Establishing trust in a sexual relationship is important. Sexual activity doesn't have to make up the first part of a relationship. It's meant to be something that evolves as a relationship develops. Talk openly and honestly with a partner about your sexual histories and theirs prior to a sexually intimate relationship. Discover as much as possible about a partner first. You need to learn about other sex partners and any STDs they might have had as well as the sexual history of your present partner. Unfortunately, you can't blindly believe everything you're told. People often don't reveal how many sex partners they have had.[21] And many people don't reveal the truth about STDs they have had. Or they may truly not know that they have genital warts, herpes, or HIV.

Choose your sexual partner carefully. There is no way to judge someone's health just by looking. You need to go with the statistics: People who have had a large number of sex partners and people who inject drugs are more likely to have been exposed to and infected by STDs. About 80 percent of people who have had five or more sexual partners have evidence of HPV. Men who have had same-sex contacts are also more likely to have HIV. It's also generally true that relationships that are secretive, have little open communication, or lack equality or respect are at risk for STDs.

Here are some questions you might think about in your relationship:

▼ Do I know how my partner spends time away from me?

▼ Is my partner always open about everything with me—including the past?

▼ Does my partner get upset if I want to have a serious talk about our relationship?

▼ Does my partner keep secrets from me?

▼ Does my partner ever say, "I'm just going out" or "It's none of your business"?

▼ Is my partner always respectful to me?[22]

Safe sex is possible if there is no exchange of body fluids. This eliminates sexual intercourse and oral sex, though. A woman can become pregnant if a man ejaculates at the vaginal opening without penetration. HIV can be transmitted in preejaculatory fluid and vaginal secretions. Any practice that can cause injury or rips in tissue is not safe. Massage, use of vibrators, and mutual masturbation do qualify as safe sex.

Proper and regular use of condoms greatly lessens the risk of STDs. The condom has to be made of latex to prevent the passage of tiny viruses that can get through condoms made of natural membrane or animal skin. The

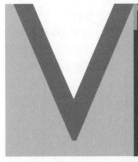

Chaste but probably not clean

Chastity belts were in vogue during the Middle Ages to ensure wifely faithfulness during a husband's long journeys. The "partial pudenda" covered the vulva with a metal plate, leaving only a small slit for urination. The "full pudenda" also blocked access to the anal opening, except for a second small slit for defecation.

CONTRACEPTION AND V CONSIDERATIONS

Your choice of birth control can affect your V health, sometimes depending on your individual situation. If one form is causing V problems, you may want to discuss other options with your clinician.

Contraceptive	Possible V Effect
Breast-feeding	Low estrogen causes dryness, painful intercourse
Condom	Possible latex allergy
Diaphragm	Possible latex allergy; spermicidal jelly may irritate; increases risk of UTI
Foam, jelly, cream, suppositories	May act as irritants
IUD (intrauterine device)	Promotes yeast infections; increased menstrual flow may lead to irritation from pads
Birth control pill	May affect sexual desire; may increase dryness; may increase risk of yeast infection
Depo-Provera	Low estrogen may cause dryness, painful intercourse

condom has to be put on properly before any sexual contact. Rather than pulling it all the way on the penis, the man should leave a little looseness at the tip to catch the ejaculate. The penis and condom should be withdrawn immediately after ejaculation. Use of a spermicide with a condom may offer additional protection. The female condom Reality is unfortunately less effective than the male condom, with a failure rate of more than 25 percent.[23] But condoms work! In a 1993 study, using condoms every time prevented HIV transmission for all but 2 out of 171 women with male partners with HIV.[24]

Birth control and V health

Most American women spend some thirty-six years in the reproductive stage of life. Three-quarters of this time, or twenty-seven years, is spent trying to avoid pregnancy.[25] Birth control is more important than ever. The average age at marriage has risen substantially for both men and women in the past few decades, so many people are sexually active for a longer time before wanting to have children.

Although a variety of safe and effective birth control methods are available to Americans, fewer than two-thirds of reproductive-age women use contraception.[26] Astonishingly, about *half* of all pregnancies in the United States—some three million a year—are unplanned and unwanted.[27] More than half of unintended pregnancies are terminated; in 1995, 1.2 million legal abortions were done.[28]

The bottom line is that the average woman who has unprotected sex will become pregnant. If you don't want to be pregnant, you must do something to prevent it.

You can become pregnant even if:

▼ You are a virgin (sperm ejaculated at the vaginal opening even if there is no penetration can swim up to fertilize the egg)

▼ You have never had a period (you still can have made an egg)

▼ You are having your period (depending on cycle length, some women ovulate before the flow has ended)

▼ He pulls out (preejaculatory fluid is rich with sperm)

▼ You didn't enjoy it (pleasure has nothing to do with conception)

▼ You douched (sperm can reach the egg by the time you reach the bathroom)

▼ You are over 50 (if you are having periods, you are never too old to get pregnant)

▼ You are sick (whether you have heart disease, diabetes, lupus, multiple sclerosis, cancer, whatever, you are never too sick to get pregnant)

Most women, particularly young women, feel that it is better to be swept away by passion than to "plan" to have sex and do something to prevent pregnancy. Passion is something we all desire, and our minds let us sweep details such as pregnancy into the corner. Unintended pregnancy, however, can be terrible. There are only three ways out: keeping the child, giving the child up for adoption, or terminating the pregnancy. Most women would prefer not to choose among those three.

Birth control is the answer. Although there are many different kinds, there is no single "perfect" method. Women can choose based on their individual needs what is best for them. Whatever you choose, realize that the use of birth control is healthier for women than use of no birth control. It is far more dangerous to be pregnant than to use most kinds of birth control.[29] And most birth control methods offer both protection from pregnancy and additional, noncontraceptive benefits. These include protection from STDs by condoms and prevention of ovarian and uterine cancer by the pill.

▼

When You Need Help

CHAPTER 7

The Most Bothersome Symptoms

Possible Causes and Cures

An aggravating, can't-take-your-mind-off-it irritation begins. Or you notice that your vaginal discharge has a funny scent and is more profuse than normal. Or you feel uncomfortably, even painfully, dry, so that intercourse or even inserting a tampon hurts.

One or more of these symptoms may represent a V problem, either on the vulva, in the vestibule, or up in the vagina. A variety of harmless scenarios also may be to blame. To help you evaluate the situation, here's a detailed tour of some of the most common—and annoying—vulvovaginal symptoms women experience: odor, itching, unusual discharge, and dryness.

Odor

Almost every woman worries at one time or another that she has an unpleasant odor associated with vaginal secretions. Yet this is one symptom that my patients are especially reluctant to admit to because they believe that odor implies poor personal hygiene. Inadequate washing is almost never the cause of a V scent. Remember that some scent is to be expected from all activity in the Vs. As I mapped out in Chapter 2, the vulva has many sweat glands, and sweat produces odor. Normal secretions from the vagina may not be noticeable at all or may smell faintly like sour milk. Then there are the secretions, discharge, and menstrual flow that stay on a pad or underwear and are exposed to bacteria normally present, producing an odor. Not least, you should realize that every woman has her own unique scent. Most women are especially sensitive to this personal scent, which may not be detectable to others.

If the same odor that you've had for as long as you can remember is suddenly bothering you or your partner, first consider whether anything simple discussed in this chapter—sweat, a new vitamin pill—might be responsible. If not, it should be checked out by your clinician. You want to rule out a vaginitis such as BV, yeast, or trich. You'll need to be as specific as possible describing what the smell is and when you notice it. Be brave and go to the clinic when the odor is present.

You don't ever need to douche or use an antiperspirant or vaginal spray to remove or improve vaginal odor. Yes, I know these products are advertised everywhere with visions of clean waterfalls and fresh-scented flowers. That doesn't mean you have to buy them. They're unnecessary.

Vaginitis is the number-one reason behind an unpleasant odor. More specifically, the leading culprits include the following types of vaginitis (for details on these conditions, see their specific chapters as well as the following chapter):

1. *Bacterial vaginosis (BV).* Of all the causes of odor, BV is the likeliest suspect. The leading cause of vaginal complaints in the United States, BV is not an infection but an imbalance in the bacteria normally found in the vagina. Instead of being the most predominant bacteria, the lactobacilli disappear. In their place large numbers of other bacteria overgrow. They can wax and wane during the menstrual cycle, and are often worse after intercourse. These huge numbers of bacteria cause a heavy discharge and change the acid-base balance of the vagina to alkaline. With the elevated pH come increased concentrations in the vaginal fluid of proteins that tell you how bad they smell: putrescine and cadaverine. In mild form the odor is like ammonia; a bad case smells like dead fish.

2. *Yeast infection.* Yeast can also cause bad-smelling discharge, which women often variously describe as "sour-smelling," "yeasty," or even "putrid." Generally, yeast is a much less common cause of odor than BV. Sometimes, however, yeast occurs with BV, causing a mixed bacterial and yeast infection with odor.

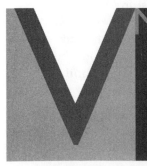

VNOTE

Leave the evidence

If you are going to see a clinician about an odor problem, don't take any medications, use any products, wash, or douche before the visit. It may feel difficult to have a pelvic examination while feeling unclean, but you're putting the clinician at a big disadvantage if he/she can't even detect the symptom.

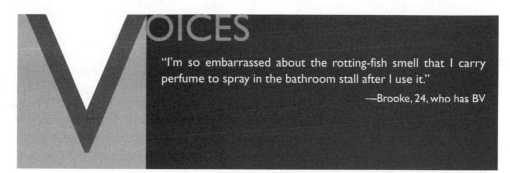

OICES

"I'm so embarrassed about the rotting-fish smell that I carry perfume to spray in the bathroom stall after I use it."

—Brooke, 24, who has BV

3. *Trichomonas.* Like BV, trich will also cause a fishy odor accompanied by discharge and itching.

What if a thorough workup rules out vaginitis as the cause of an odor problem? Then there are other possibilities.

4. *Sweating.* We all worry about our underarms producing odor from sweat, but the vulva is just as relevant. Ordinary sweating is a common cause of vulvovaginal odor. Remember that the genital region contains numerous apocrine glands, which produce sweat, as well as oil glands and glands associated with each hair follicle. Odor from sweat happens for one reason: Sweat includes the waste product urea, filtered from the blood (it's actually dilute urine), and the resident bacteria in the region interact with sweat-gland secretions, giving the external genitalia its odor.[1]

Treatment of a problem with odor from sweat involves (1) washing daily with antibacterial soap such as Dial, Lever 2000, or pHisoHex, then drying well, and (2) applying Zeasorb powder, which is available over the counter.

ODORS THAT TALK

One interesting side note is the role of odor as an essential communication tool. Pheromones are odor-containing substances that are released by one individual and produce a change in behavior or physiology of an individual of the same species. In the animal world, mating habits are virtually ruled by pheromones, but work on human pheromones is just getting started. In women, sweat and oil glands under the influence of estrogens produce pheromones responsible for sexual attraction. You may have heard about how women in close quarters seem to menstruate in sync. One early study shows that some component of women's perspiration could affect the timing of other women's menstrual cycles. The significance of vaginal fluid odor on human sexuality is not known. But consider this: The pubic hair serves to trap and concentrate pelvic odors, which can be quite attractive to a mate.

Sources: C. Arimondi, G. B. Vannelli, G. C. Balboni, Importance of olfaction in sexual life: morphofunctional and psychological studies in man, *Biomed Res* (India) 1993:4:43; G. Preti et al., Determination of ovulation and alteration of menstrual cycle by human odors, abstract, 188th National Meeting of the American Chemical Society, 1984; J. Paavonen, Physiology and ecology of the vagina, *Scand J Infect Dis* 1983:40 (suppl.): 31.

Antibacterial soaps can be drying to the skin. You'll note elsewhere in this book that I usually suggest a superfatted soap, such as Dove. But if you have an odor problem from sweat, the action of antibacterial soaps is important.

For women of size who have thick skin folds of the groin and abdomen, strips of plain white cloth such as old sheeting or handkerchiefs may be placed between the skin folds along the panty line and under the abdominal fold to help absorb sweat.

Another helpful product is an antiperspirant called Drysol (aluminum chloride). It is helpful when applied daily at bedtime to the groin and labia majora. Once daily is usually enough. Drysol is available by prescription or by purchase from Canada via the Web. See Resources.

There are also prescription medicines, available either by mouth or to apply topically, to help control sweating. They will help cut down sweating everywhere in the body; it's not possible to take a pill that works only on V sweat glands. Dermatologists who are interested in the problem can prescribe these antiperspirants when a chronic condition known as hyperhidrosis, or excessive sweating, is thought to be the cause of odor.

5. *Urine.* Substances in the urine are another potential source of odor. When evaluating an odor problem, specify for your clinician whether the odor comes out of the toilet bowl after you have used the toilet or whether the odor is present at times unrelated to the bathroom. Urinary odors are produced by foods such as asparagus, certain vitamins (especially B complex) and herbs, and medications, especially antibiotics such as ampicillin and nitrofurazone.[2] Urinary tract infections can cause foul-smelling urine. So can a host of uncommon diseases that alter metabolism, such as liver failure—but they make people so sick that urinary odor is much less important than other related problems. One aptly named disorder that is diagnosed because patients complain of urinary and body odor is fish odor syndrome; people with it can't properly process a protein called trimethylamine. This condition can develop in adulthood.

Loss of urine (incontinence) can be another source of odor, as bacteria act on even small amounts of urine in the underwear. Sometimes a

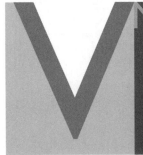

NOTE

Never let 'em see you sweat

Ever wonder why your crotch sometimes turns damp when you're in a tense situation? It's because your labia majora sweat when you're nervous, as well as when you're exercising—just like your palms or underarms.

woman may be losing urine in small quantities without even being aware of it. To check, a clinician can give a substance that colors the urine orange (Pyridium); then the woman can see if there are orange stains on a pad that she wears after taking the medication. Some women are afraid to ask their clinicians about incontinence, thinking that surgery is the only cure for urinary loss. Fortunately, we have nonsurgical ways to help with this problem, such as exercises and the use of vaginal weights. But even if you need a surgical remedy, these procedures are becoming faster, better, and smarter each year. For example, a sling of tape or mesh can be put into place to support and stabilize the bladder neck and urethra; this can now be done as day surgery or in the office.

6. *A retained tampon.* A tampon forgotten in the vagina long enough after a menstrual period will create a very bad odor. Check by feeling inside the vagina to make sure no tampon has been left behind. Even if it seems high up, you can reach up with your finger to find the string and tease it down to the point where you can grasp it. Don't panic—just persist slowly and gently. Once the tampon is taken out, believe it or not, you don't need any other treatment such as douching or antibiotics. The odor—having been provoked by the tampon—disappears along with it.

7. *Your own individual differences.* Not only does each woman have an individual scent, but it's also possible for that odor to change, possibly leading you to suspect a problem when none exists. Odor in body fluids is very complex, since hundreds of ingredients present in the fluids contribute to the odor. Familiar food examples with complex odors include coffee, cocoa, strawberries, and roasted nuts.[3] In some cases, one or more of the ingredients evaporating easily from these mixtures may resemble the overall aroma (often referred to as "top notes," to borrow a phrase from the perfume industry), but none is the same as the entire bouquet. Research on human body fluids such as urine, saliva, and blood has shown that they, like foods, contain complex mixtures, or chemical compounds, that contribute to their characteristic odors.[4]

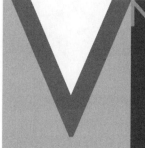

NOTE

Oui!

Alluring French women are reputed to drink special beverages to improve the scent and taste of their vaginal secretions. I don't know of any research on this and can't give you any recipes, although it certainly makes sense that certain foods could work in this way.

Not a lot of work has been done on vaginal odor. There seem to be two distinct types of women, those who produce large amounts of a certain kind of acid (short-chain aliphatic acids) and those who produce little or no acid other than the weak acetic acid of vinegar.[5] Acid producers seem to have a stronger and more distinct odor. The top notes of this odor result from the acids with a cheesy smell. In both the high acid producers and the low acid producers, the most common acid was lactic acid, one of the components of milk. It's assumed to be the principal cause of vaginal acidity.[6] The odor of lactic acid is almost identical to that of sour milk or yogurt and is often the top note in secretions from women who are non-acid-producers.[7] If you are a high acid producer, you may have secretions that have a slight cheesy kind of smell, and if you are a low acid producer the faint odor of sour milk may predominate.

One interesting study on vaginal fluid found big variations in vaginal odors during the menstrual cycle. The testers weren't told what they were smelling. Odors from the secretions were generally rated as unpleasant, with the menses odors having the highest intensities and least pleasant ratings. Odors from the preovulatory and ovulatory phases were the least unpleasant.

These odors reflect the complex biochemistry always going on to keep the vagina healthy. To date science does not know how to alter these chemicals—and in fact altering them is probably undesirable. Sweat, urine, and vaginal secretions are part of the great design. In the absence of another physical problem, they're not something that needs fixing.

So if you are concerned about odor, rule out vaginal infection. Deal with sweating and urinary causes as suggested. In addition, you can use a plastic squeeze bottle filled with warm water to rinse vaginal secretions from the vulva after using the bathroom, and you can change underwear (carry extra sets) two or three times a day.

Itching

It's become one of the biggest knee-jerk reactions in gynecology: You experience vulvovaginal itching, you immediately suspect a yeast infection.

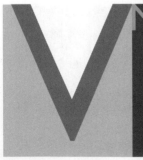

NOTE

Blooming marvelous

The flowers most often used to represent the vulva in art and literature all smell sweet: the multipetaled lotus (India, China), the lily (Europe), and the rose (Arabia).

VOICES

"I'm not having much sex these days because I can't seem to achieve vaginal harmony. Something's always wrong. First it's discharge. Then it's odor. Then my period comes for two weeks. Can you give me a new vagina?"

—Faith, 35

So you go to the nearest drugstore to purchase a tube of over-the-counter antiyeast cream (e.g., Monistat, Femstat, Gyne-Lotrimin). If the problem is indeed yeast, the cream will usually work. Unfortunately these antifungal creams are of little value against itching from other causes.

And in the vulvovaginal area, everything itches! That's how most problems first show up. Correctly pinpointing the source of this annoying symptom is important, because misdiagnosis can prolong or even complicate it. Say the problem is something as simple as a sensitivity to bath salts. If misinterpreted by the woman as a yeast infection, she'll start with yeast cream. Then, when there is no improvement, she'll visit a clinician, who may prescribe antibiotics. At that point, she will truly develop a yeast infection. But even when the yeast is treated, the original problem, sensitivity to bath salts, will still be there—and the itching will go on.

What causes itching? The possibilities can range from the truly benign (and easily remedied) to more serious conditions that require a clinician's care.

1. *Clothing.* The simplest reason for itching comes from moisture trapped under tight layers of clothing. I've mentioned this before, but it bears repeating here because my patients are surprised to discover that some irritation problems can be eased simply by changing the way they dress. Just think about how many layers could cover your vulva in a given day. Many women wear a panty liner, with a moisture-trapping adhesive backing,

VOICES

"No one talks about these things. You feel very alone, like no one has your problem."

—Rosemarie, 43, who has long-term itching

every day. On top of this go underpants, which may be synthetic or fit snugly. On top of these may go panty hose (perhaps a tightly woven control-top kind) and a skirt or jeans or pants. Bodysuits go in and out of style, but that's another layer. Ditto for body shapers, hip slips, and girdle-style foundations. These may be replaced during the day with tights or other exercise clothes of spandex for vigorous activity.

Remember, the V area is one of the key places on the body where we perspire. If locked under many layers, this moisture has nowhere to go. Moisture alone, or the combination of moisture plus friction plus chemicals left in the fabric after laundering, may irritate the skin and leave you feeling the need to scratch. The problem may develop suddenly, after years without being bothered—the Vs are rebelling! It's not easy to change your lifestyle. But following the V-smart guidelines in Chapter 5 will help you avoid or ease a fair amount of misery.

2. *Bathing.* Another common cause of itching is the way you bathe. How could keeping clean have unpleasant consequences? Being overly enthusiastic or obsessive about bathing can lead to drying and irritation of the vulva. When some women wash, they use the hottest water they can stand, scrub vigorously with pure soap, and even turn a hair dryer on the vulva. Others wash the vulva with soap and water after every urination. Hot water is particularly drying; pure soap, such as Ivory, is too. Fatted soaps, such as Dove or Basis, with warm water are preferable, along with gentle blotting to dry. Recognize that while moisture is not desirable in the groin folds, the area between the thin inner lips (the vestibule) is part mucous membrane, like the mouth. It does not need to be dried out.

3. *Irritants.* Many women are sensitive to products available for personal care. The advertising world has done a great job of convincing American women that they smell bad and that the way to avoid unsuccessful relationships and acute embarrassment from their odors is to douche with, bathe in, or spray on fabulous-smelling "feminine" products. I've already explained that these products don't keep the vagina clean. Now here's another reason to avoid them: They can cause irritating or allergic reactions.

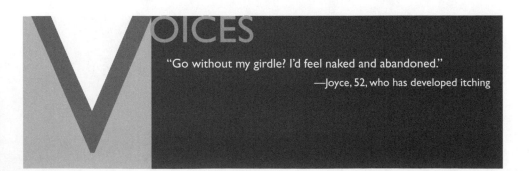

VOICES

"Go without my girdle? I'd feel naked and abandoned."

—Joyce, 52, who has developed itching

ITCH RELIEF DOS AND DON'TS

If you are plagued by itching, no matter what the cause, you should simplify your vulvar hygiene.

	Recommended	Avoid if possible
Clothes	Loose underpants that do not bind in the groin, knee-highs and thigh-highs, going without underwear at home; fragrance-free detergents	Girdles, tummy-control pants, panty hose, bleach and fabric softener in underwear
Bathing	Dove bar soap, Basis, Neutrogena	Bubble bath, very hot water, scrubbing hard, drying with hot hair dryer, washing with soap after every urination
Toiletries	None on the vulva; use soft white unscented toilet paper	Products with fragrance, sodium lauryl sulfate, propylene glycol
Menstrual products	Natural-fiber pads; tampon use as recommended by manufacturer (choose the right size for amount of flow, and change as directed)	Daily use of pad or panty liner, deodorant pads and tampons, douches
Exercise gear	Loose, baggy sweatpants	Tight spandex, snap crotches, thongs, remaining in sweaty clothes, prolonged wearing of wet bathing suits

Irritants are limited to the skin only; true allergies start with itchy skin and then may proceed to systemwide reactions, from watery eyes to trouble breathing to, in severe cases, drop of blood pressure and shock. Allergic reactions to personal products are rarer than irritations.

A substance that causes a skin reaction is called a *contactant*. Contact (irritant) vaginal dermatitis can come from anything that touches your skin: cleansers, abrasive clothing with chemical residues in it, beauty products, topical medications, products that have been dyed or colored. You probably have several of the most common contactants around your house right now. The offending agent may be the substance itself. For example, lavender oil and oil of clove are highly irritating to the skin, despite the fact that they are pure and natural. (They have to be highly diluted for safe use.) As I have mentioned several times, pure soap, such as Ivory, even though it's pure, can be irritating because its alkalinity is drying. Or the offending agent may be something added to the product, say, perfume to make it smell nice or a preservative such as propylene glycol, which is added to many lotions and creams (including the over-the-counter antiyeast creams). Other chemicals such as alcohols or sodium lauryl sulfate can also cause irritation. There are zillions!

An irritant reaction produces immediate stinging and burning upon application of the agent. Women often decide that they are "allergic" to a product—say, estrogen cream—because it stings immediately on application. This is not an allergic reaction, but irritation from something in the cream base, probably propylene glycol.

Given how universal these potential irritants are, what are you supposed to do? If you're healthy without V problems, don't worry about it. But if you have sensitive skin and you're having V symptoms, read labels and avoid the worst offenders. Generally speaking, medication in an ointment of pure petrolatum is unlikely to cause trouble. When I need to prescribe a topical medication for a woman who has burning and itching with everything she applies, I have a compounding pharmacy make up the prescription in a neutral base such as petrolatum or natural vegetable wax. Consult the following list of common irritants and allergens, but remember—just to remind you that the human body isn't easy—some items can be both an irritant and an allergen, and an individual can be sensitive to or allergic to anything.

Women often fail to nab their beauty or hygiene habits as the source of an itching problem if they haven't used any new products lately. Yet sensitivity develops through exposure over time to chemicals. *This is very important*—it's the product used repeatedly that finally gets to you.

Irritant reactions can be soothed by stopping the use of the irritant and bathing in comfortable (neither hot nor cold) water. Problems with irritants can be further assisted by working with a dermatologist who is expert in these areas.

4. *Allergy.* Coital allergy, which is sensitivity to your partner or his semen, is another possible cause of itching. It's one of several different kinds of allergies that show symptoms in the V area. These are discussed in detail in Chapter 14, "Could You Be Allergic?"

5. *Skin disorders.* Skin disorders are a cause of often intense itching. Eczema, psoriasis, lichen sclerosus, lichen planus, and lichen simplex chronicus are examples of such conditions. Properly diagnosed, they can be controlled with cortisone ointment, but they usually do not go away entirely. (These conditions are discussed in Chapter 15, "When Skin Gets Sick.") Problems such as warts and herpes may also begin with itching. (See Chapter 20, "The Lifetime Virus.")

COMMON VULVAR IRRITANTS AND ALLERGENS	
Irritants	**Allergens**
Soap, bubble bath, detergents	Benzocaine
Sanitary pads, adhesive on pads	Neomycin
Nylon underwear	Chlorhexidine in K-Y jelly
Secretions, sweat, and urine	Ethylene diamine in neomycin
Tampon strings	Fragrances
5-FU cream, other HPV medications	Propylene glycol, preservatives (this is also an irritant)
Fragrances, natural oils	Nickel
Douches, yogurt, deodorant hygiene products, alcohols	Tea tree oil

6. *Low estrogen.* As levels of estrogen drop in a woman approaching menopause, she may experience a dry and itchy sensation. Untreated estrogen deficiency progresses to burning for many women. Small amounts of estrogen cream solve the problem.

7. *Vulvar skin cancer and precancer.* Skin cancer is a rare vulvar problem, but it may show up as an itchy bump that does not go away. Skin cancer is completely curable when diagnosed early. Precancerous skin changes will also cause itching with bumps.

8. *Pinworms.* The microscopic pinworm can lead to itching around the vagina, although it's mainly a cause of anal itching. In order to diagnose, a clinician would have to suspect it was present: Maybe another family member has the problem. Pinworms are diagnosed by finding them under the microscope on a piece of Scotch tape that has been plastered against

VOICES

"Itch, itch, itch, itch. I am tired all the time because I do not sleep through the night—I always wake up scratching!"

—Laura, 37, on her severe itching

the perineum or anus; the pinworms' eggs are easily visible. The problem is treated with drugs active against worms.

9. *Vaginal infections.* Finally, of course, vaginal infections—bacterial vaginosis, yeast, and trichomonas—all cause itching.

Unusual discharge

Remember that all women have discharge. It's useful to be familiar with what's normal for you so that you can use a change from that baseline to help figure out what's wrong if you develop a problem. The appearance, texture, scent, and amount of discharge differ for different women; what's normal for you can also vary depending on where you are in the menstrual cycle and your stage of life. Maybe your version of normal is clear and slight, or maybe it's whiter. It may smell a bit like sour milk or have no odor at all. There may be enough of it to cause wetness or stain your underwear. It may leave small, dry clumps in your pubic hair. Not only do secretions vary by individual, but they change during the menstrual cycle, becoming more milky white and slightly clumpy. If you're pregnant, your discharge is apt to be thicker than usual. If you're postmenopausal, it may not be very noticeable at all.

Individual women tolerate widely different amounts of secretions—another reason to cue into what is normal for *you.* I see women all the time who have a vagina full of secretions when the speculum goes in. But if I ask about discharge, they say they have no problem at all. On the other hand, I also see women who are hypersensitive to discharge, noticing just a few drops of fluid. Though it doesn't sound very aesthetically pleasing, I sometimes end up looking at women's underpants with them and telling them whether the amount of discharge they have is okay. Or sometimes I draw diagrams of how much stain normal secretions can leave on panties.

Here's what normal discharge is *not:* It does not itch, irritate, or burn. It does not smell like fish. It does not smell like ammonia.

Abnormal discharge usually occurs when there is an infection. There's no single variation to look for. Abnormal can mean many things: The discharge may vary from scant, to more than usual, to quite profuse. Its color may be gray-white, yellow-white, or yellow-green. It might be blood-stained if the inflammation is severe.

If you notice any of these things, or if there is suddenly a marked change in the amount of discharge and it bothers you, you'll want to have it checked out.

Among the possible causes of unusual discharge:

1. *Vaginitis.* The most common reason for a change in discharge is some kind of vaginitis. Remember, that's just a catchall word to characterize vaginal itching and burning. The root problem may be a yeast infection,

bacterial vaginosis, trichomonas, or another kind of vaginitis. (Follow-up tests can help determine this and direct you toward the proper treatment.) Some yeast infections cause cottage-cheese-like curds, but it is entirely possible to have a yeast infection accompanied by no discharge at all. Look for symptoms along with suspicious discharge, including mild to severe itching of the vulva and vaginal opening, a burning sensation, and frequent urination. Often these symptoms can be quite uncomfortable. Actual pain, however, is not usually a feature of vaginitis.

2. *A sexually transmitted disease.* Persistent vaginal discharge always signals for your clinician to check for some very common sexually transmitted diseases (STDs). The most prevalent is chlamydia, but gonorrhea shares similar symptoms. They cause a yellowish-white discharge, perhaps a little itching, and, sometimes, constant pelvic pain. These infections affect the cervix but give vaginal symptoms. (See "The Silent STDs Worth a Routine Test" in Chapter 9.) Herpes, before the blisters appear, may cause vulvar stinging and burning along with discharge, as well as muscle aches and general discomfort with fever.

3. *Vulvodynia.* Excess discharge may be associated with this pain problem. See Chapter 17.

4. *Cervical ectropion.* Sometimes you might experience normal discharge in greater-than-usual amounts because of a condition in the cervix. The cells that line the cervical canal (endocervical cells) can grow out onto the surface of the cervix, creating a condition known as an *ectropion.* The ectropion has a characteristic reddish, slightly raised appearance, and the cells are glandular, so they may make mucus. This leads to an increased amount of ordinary cervical mucus. A cervical ectropion develops because there is enough estrogen present to cause this outgrowth of cells. Until twenty years ago, clinicians thought the ectropion was abnormal and recommended freezing or destruction by cauterization. We now know that it's a perfectly normal occurrence. Common among women taking oral contraceptives, it's also seen in normal women not on the pill. This is not a condition that needs treatment, and freezing or cauterization may alter the cervical production of mucus considered necessary for fertility.

5. *A problem with the uterus, tubes, or ovaries.* Less often, but particularly in postmenopausal women, discharge that doesn't fit any other category may be coming through the vagina from a place above the vagina. This is true especially if red blood cells are seen in the discharge under the microscope. If the discharge has your clinician stumped, ask if there's any possibility your discharge might be coming from higher up. Sometimes other tests, such as a check of the uterine lining (an endometrial biopsy), are done.

6. *A fistula.* A fistula is an opening between two places that isn't supposed to be there—like a chink in a wall. In gynecology, the best known of these chinks are tiny holes between the vagina and the rectum (called *rectovaginal fistulas*) or between the vagina and the bladder *(vesicovaginal fistulas).* A rectovaginal fistula often happens after an injury related to a complicated labor. As a result, gas and stool in tiny amounts can come out of the vagina. As you might imagine, this fistula is quickly recognized and repaired. Vesicovaginal fistulas result chiefly from obstetrical injury, complications of hysterectomy, radiation treatment for cervical cancer, or after surgery for incontinence. With a vesicovaginal fistula, urine may leak out of the vagina, but it may be small in amount and, mixed with other vaginal secretions, may seem like discharge. So this kind of fistula can be harder to recognize.

Modern obstetric methods have greatly reduced this problem, but it is still common in Asia and Africa as a result of prolonged obstructed labor—after days in labor, the baby's head literally wears a hole in the wall between the vagina and rectum or bladder.

While a rare cause of vaginal discharge, it's something for your clinician to explore if you have significant discharge that does not fit into the usual categories. Have you had any pelvic surgery or bladder work? Did you have a complicated delivery with forceps, or a bad infection after a cesarean delivery? Have you had gyn cancer surgery and radiation treatment? Once recognized, the fistula can be surgically closed off.

A condition similar to a fistula may occur after surgery for incontinence with placement of a sling to hold up the urethra. Material used to make the sling can erode through the wall of the vagina, and a constant discharge develops. I worked with one woman for months, treating her for desquamative inflammatory vaginitis with antibiotics and cortisone. One day she was actually able to feel the mesh that had worked through the front part of the vaginal wall. The material was defective; it was removed and successfully replaced with another sling, and she is now continent and free of vaginal discharge.

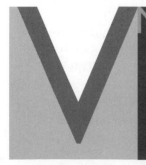

NOTE

Another change in pregnancy

Noticing thicker discharge while you're pregnant? Before you panic, remember that changing hormone levels are responsible—it's perfectly normal and, in the absence of any other symptoms, no sign of a problem. Plan on changing panties more often to feel fresher.

Dryness

V lubrication is one of those things you don't think about until it's gone. Normal secretions from the vulva, vestibule, and vagina keep you comfortable. Their amounts vary from woman to woman, with a wide range of normal. During sexual arousal, a clear and relatively odorless fluid adds to the normal secretions as the perfect natural lubricant. When normal day-to-day V lubrication is present, you may not notice, but when it's absent, you may start to feel dry and uncomfortable. Sexual intercourse can be painful. V dryness is a problem that plagues women of all ages from time to time. Fortunately, it can usually be remedied fairly simply.

What causes vulvovaginal dryness? A number of things can, many of them the same causes of V itching. The delicate V chemistry may react to chemicals or water temperature. Allergic reactions, hormone levels, and skin problems may interfere with lubrication. And when it comes to sexual lubrication, the problem isn't always purely physical. If there is conflict and lack of love in the relationship, no woman will lubricate well.

Key causes of dryness include:

1. *Bathing practices*. All you really need to clean your V area is warm water. If it's too hot, your vulva will dry just like the rest of your skin. Soap isn't necessary on the vulva, but if you use it while bathing or showering, choose a superfatted hypoallergenic soap with no dyes or fragrances—one that is nonalkaline and pH balanced. (Dove is a good example.) You need to read labels. If you're using an antibacterial soap to help combat an odor problem, be alert for possible dryness in the vestibule. If it occurs, confine that antibacterial soap to your mons and labia majora and wash the vestibule with plain water.

2. *Irritants and allergy*. If your skin is reacting to a substance that is irritating or to which you are allergic, you may have to do some work to find the problem. See the list of culprits in this chapter's section on itching as well as Chapter 14. The treatment for allergy can also cause drying. Older antihistamines (called first-generation H1 blockers), prescription or over-the-counter, if taken on a regular basis can dry out all tissues, including the Vs. These include Benadryl, Dramamine, Chlor-trimeton, Atarax, and Vistaril, but not the second-generation H1 blockers such as Claritin, Seldane, and Hismanal. You probably wouldn't notice, however, if you used them only for a couple of days during a cold. Other medications can also have drying effects. Read the package inserts; they are not going to talk about V dryness, but look for the word *anticholinergic*. This means the drug dries up respiratory secretions, causes constipation—and may contribute to V dryness.

3. *Chronic conditions*. The fluid that lubricates the vagina comes through the vaginal wall from the bloodstream. Diseases that affect blood vessels

make them less flexible and less able to act as a conduit, possibly contributing to a dry vagina. Such diseases include high blood pressure (hypertension), hardening of the arteries (arteriosclerosis), diabetes, and some connective-tissue diseases. Vaginal dryness combined with pain at intercourse may be the first signs of a connective-tissue disease called Sjögren's syndrome.[8] A wide range of skin conditions can cause vaginal dryness too.

Unfortunately, the Vs often get left out of medical discussions about the impact of these chronic problems. One of my patients who has had Sjögren's syndrome for years, with arthritis, dry eyes, dry mouth, and dry skin, was furious when she started having V problems. No one had prepared her for this likelihood.

4. *Vulvodynia.* Vulvodynia, pain believed to develop when nerve fibers are not working as they should, can also lessen lubrication in some women; for others, secretions may actually increase without the proper nerve controls. (See Chapter 17 for a full discussion of this problem.)

5. *Breast-feeding.* If you are breast-feeding, vaginal dryness and even painful intercourse can be troublesome. Estrogen levels are low during lactation, so the vagina becomes thin, inelastic, and dry. Your clinician can give you some estrogen cream to use vaginally every night for a week or two and then once or twice a week. This will improve your symptoms without affecting your milk supply. Breast-feeding women vary in how quickly the dryness resolves. For some it is with the return of menstrual periods; for others dryness lasts a longer period of time.

6. *Birth control pills.* Some kinds of combination estrogen-progestin birth control pills change the secretions of the cervix, making them scanty and thicker. For some women, this reduced contribution of the cervix to V moisture can be a noticeable change. The influence of the pill on cervical secretions depends on the type of progestin, and the balance between the progestin and estrogen. If you are on the pill and dryness is a problem, talk with your clinician. A different pill in which estrogen is a little more dominant than progestin may help. If you are going to go off the pill because of a dryness problem, be careful to plan another method of birth control.

7. *Lack of menstrual periods from low body weight.* Low estrogen can also develop if body weight drops to a low level, usually less than 100 pounds (depending on height and frame). Controls in the hypothalamus (a part of the brain) shut down the hormones to the ovaries, and menstrual periods stop (amenorrhea). Hypothalamic amenorrhea can be seen in athletes, especially runners whose high levels of exercise drop weight below the level that the brain thinks is safe for reproduction. This type of amenorrhea is also seen in women who have anorexia.

Restoring the weight will usually restore menstrual function. Vaginal estrogen helps with the dryness.

8. *Perimenopause and menopause.* With the decline in estrogen that occurs during late perimenopause and menopause, significant V changes occur, including dryness. I am a big proponent of supplemental estrogen, not least to relieve the annoying vaginal dryness these natural changes inevitably bring. In Chapter 4, "At Different Ages," I describe the most popular current remedies for vaginal dryness caused by menopause. Explore the options with your clinician.

To date, while there are some herbal alternatives to estrogen to treat hot flashes and maintain bone strength, there has been no such luck for vaginal dryness. Vitamin E oil and lubricants help, but it is estrogen that keeps the vagina thick and elastic. We don't have a good substitute for that. And don't forget that even when you're menopausal, taking a little extra time with foreplay and lovemaking can be as helpful as many tubes of cream.

▼

CHAPTER 8

Now What?

How to Proceed When There's Trouble

S o you think you have a V problem. Now what? Perhaps you dread the idea of discussing it with anyone, even a clinician. You don't have time for a doctor's appointment, anyway. You let it ride—maybe the problem will just go away.

It doesn't, though, so you try to handle it at home. You change soaps, wash a little harder. You pick up a tube of yeast cream at the supermarket or some herbals at the health food store. Sex is painful, but you grit your teeth. Sometimes the problem really does vanish on its own. Often it persists or gets worse.

You have no idea what's wrong, so you make an appointment to see a clinician like me. Day after day I listen to a familiar litany of complaints: itching, burning, discharge, pain that's present all the time, pain that comes and goes, pain only after sex, pain only around menstruation. Then I'm almost always asked the same two questions: "Have you ever heard anything like this before?" and "What do you think is wrong with me?"

I usually reassure patients that I hear about similar symptoms all week long. What I don't tell them is that I almost always have a good idea of what's wrong. That's because without an exam and some lab info, I'd be talking out of turn. So I always say the same thing: "If it's okay with you, I'd like to do an exam and look under the microscope to get the whole picture. Then I'll be back to talk with you."

My gut instincts are often confirmed. But I'm frequently surprised too.

Women who sound as if they have vaginitis don't, and women who seemed to be describing a problem in the vestibule or on the vulva turn up with vaginitis. V problems aren't as straightforward as you'd think.

Why you can't tell by looking

Vaginitis may be the most misunderstood word in the V lexicon. It's the general term for a vaginal infection, which happens when the normal balance of bacteria goes out of whack. When the symptoms of itching and discharge occur, most women automatically dub their problem "vaginitis" (or "vag itch"). When doctors too hear of such symptoms, they instantly think, "Ah, yes, vaginitis." (More specifically, they suspect yeast.) To be sure, almost every woman gets a vaginal infection at some point in her life—three-quarters of us will get at least one yeast infection, and bacterial vaginosis is diagnosed more often each year than yeast.

But V means vulva and vestibule as well as vagina. And all three areas can have problems that create itching and discharge that feel exactly like vaginitis. Symptoms can sometimes be similar whether caused by irritation from clothing or care products, allergic reactions, skin diseases, lumps and bumps, vaginitis, sexually transmitted diseases, low estrogen, or even vulvodynia.

My life (and yours) would be lovely if I could give you a chart that says, "If you have X symptoms, it's vaginitis, and if you have Y symptoms, it's vulvar this or vestibular that." But V itching, irritation, discharge, or painful sex can represent a problem in any of the V areas—a vulvar condition, a problem in the vestibule, or the familiar catchall vaginitis! There are too many gray areas for a simple chart. In fact, some of the reasons that V problems go on for so long stem from the fact that women do a lot of things wrong when they have V symptoms. They remain sexually active in spite of failing to become aroused, failing to use lubrication, and experiencing great pain. And they engage in potentially harmful genital hygiene, such as using commercial douches or taking homeopathic or herbal preparations that have not been tested or are not manufactured with any kind of quality control.

VOICES

"I was so miserable this weekend that I would have gone to the emergency room. But I knew I would just get someone who would have no ideas about vulvovaginal problems and who would just give me antibiotics."

—Claire, 36, who has undiagnosed vulvar complaints

V complaints, just like those anywhere else in the body, require the steps of a formal diagnosis. As I'll describe in the next chapter, a clinician must take a history and do a physical exam and some simple laboratory tests. He or she can't be sure by just listening to your story. He can't only look through the speculum.

WARNING SYMPTOMS NOT TO IGNORE

If you have fever, vaginal discharge, and pelvic pain, you need to see a clinician right away. If you have an open sore or blisters or a lump or bump that is bleeding or enlarging or painful, you need to be seen. If you have a new mole on the vulva or a long-established one that is changing, you need to be seen.

Now let's talk about what you might do as you decide whether to make an appointment.

Evaluating your symptoms

Nobody wants to see a doctor for every little itch or pain. Before you pick up the phone, it's worth following a few simple steps.

▼ *If you develop V symptoms and discharge is not a feature:* First, check a few things out. Have you perhaps added a new product, piece of clothing, or custom to your life? Those are possible sources of irritation. Most likely, though, some established practice is the problem. Follow the hygiene and lifestyle customs in Chapter 5—looser clothes, cotton underwear, and so on—and give it three to four weeks. If you've done all this and still experience uncomfortable irritation, itching, or burning, you need to determine if this is an unusual problem with yeast, another kind of inflammatory vaginitis, a skin problem, or a form of vulvodynia (a pain disorder). To figure things out, you need to be seen by a clinician at a time when you have your worst symptoms.

You will also conduct a self-exam, as described in Chapter 2, to see if there is anything visible. The goal isn't self-diagnosis but information gathering. You may be able to see or feel the source of your discomfort, making you better equipped to accurately describe what's going on to your clinician. Use a bright light and a large mirror. Maybe your partner can help. *Note:* Women often get upset when the vulva or vestibule appears red. To a clinician, redness (known as *erythema*) does not mean much. Certainly many problems can lead to redness, but so can tight clothes, sitting positions, and recent activities such as sexual intercourse. What is far more important than skin coloration is whether there are any other changes in the skin, such as cracks, bumps, blisters, sores, or raised areas. It is also important to know if the areas are tender to touch.

▼ *If you have unusual discharge:* Vaginal discharge that doesn't seem normal may be a hallmark of vaginitis, but self-diagnosing *which kind* of in-

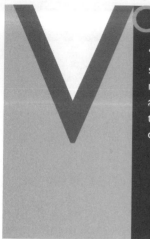

fection is a tricky undertaking. Not all infections produce discharge, and not all discharge points to an infection. If this is your first time with odd discharge plus itching or irritation, it's best to be evaluated, even if you suspect it's a garden-variety yeast infection. Trying a single seven-day course of over-the-counter yeast cream is also reasonable (read Chapter 10, "Yeast Infections"), but if after seven days you are still not comfortable, it's unlikely you have a common yeast problem. *Using another tube of cream is not going to help.*

If you have had a yeast infection in the past, diagnosed by a clinician who looked under the microscope, and you feel the same way again, it's also reasonable to try a course of nonprescription antifungal cream. If your symptoms do not improve after a few days, make an appointment.

▼ *If you experience sporadic itching and irritation:* Irritation that lasts only for a week out of each month, leaving you comfortable the rest of the time, suggests a kind of recurring yeast infection. You need to be seen at a time when you are having symptoms and have a yeast culture done on Sabouraud's medium, a special broth used specifically for diagnosing yeast.

If you have itching, burning, and irritation that come and go but are unrelieved by yeast cream, you need an exam at the time of the symptoms. You may need to have a special skin test (a biopsy) done to find out exactly what is going on. Most skin diseases can be kept in control, but left unchecked, they can alter your skin permanently. You want to get a skin disorder diagnosed promptly so you can manage it and get on with life.

▼ *If you have pain only with intercourse or when using a tampon:* In other words, if it hurts only upon being touched in the vestibule outside the vaginal opening, it's likely you have a kind of vulvodynia (vulvar pain condition) called vestibulitis. Yeast cream, antibiotics, or cortisone cream is not going to help. When you look with a mirror, there's not much to see except a little redness, but it will be painful to the touch in one or several areas in the vestibule between the thin labia minora. It's best to find a clinician who is experienced in working with this particular problem.

Why telephone diagnosis doesn't work

It would be handy if you could give your clinician a quick telephone call to describe what you feel and see, without having to come into the office. In fact, much of health care is now moving toward phone-based management—that is, screening patients' problems and answering common questions over the phone before automatically advancing to an in-office appointment. Unfortunately, when it comes to V problems, expecting an answer about what's wrong with you over the phone is unrealistic. It's simply impossible to figure out all the causes of itching and/or discharge over the phone.

This was strikingly demonstrated in a study done in the Denver area to see if nurses could arrive at an accurate diagnosis solely on the basis of a telephone report of a group of symptoms.[1] The nurses were given a standard group of questions to ask when a patient called with vulvovaginal complaints. Based on those histories, the nurses made a diagnostic assessment and drew up a treatment plan. They did not share their diagnoses or treatment plans with the patients, who instead were invited to come in

Warning signs of a mediocre gyn

- ▼ Diagnoses freely over the phone to "save you the trouble" of coming in
- ▼ Suggests first trying OTC antiyeast cream every time you have a complaint
- ▼ Doesn't explain what's happening during an exam
- ▼ Doesn't ask you questions or doesn't listen to your answers
- ▼ Doesn't want to hear your opinions because he/she is the expert

- ▼ Is hard to reach (whether you have a question or need emergency care)
- ▼ Seems disorganized (doesn't always know which tests you've had when; doesn't follow through to inform you about test results)
- ▼ Frowns on second opinions
- ▼ Doesn't use microscope; uses routine bacterial cultures of vagina

and see either a nurse-practitioner, a physician, a physician's assistant, or a certified nurse-midwife.

When the patients came into the office, they completed the same form that the nurses had used during the phone interviews. This meant that the clinicians providing face-to-face care in the office received the same information the nurses had. The clinicians did a physical exam, measured vaginal pH, and took specimens for culture.

There was no correlation between the phone nurses' answers and those of the clinicians who conducted comprehensive evaluations of the same women. The only agreements were those that would emerge by chance. In other words, a woman's story and what was actually found on exam were very different, suggesting that phone diagnosis is not appropriate.

Which doctor to see

Even though phone diagnosis is not a good idea, not every woman needs to advance immediately to a vulvovaginal expert for every little V issue. Standard vaginal infections or simple vulvar irritations are often handled by a visit to your primary-care practitioner. If the problem doesn't clear up or come under control within an appointment or two, a gynecological exam is necessary. With the proper testing and treatment, your gynecologist should be able to handle a wide range of problems. Give it a little time.

If, however, the condition isn't in control after a couple of visits, it's time to seek expert help. Unfortunately, getting the help you need to pinpoint a V problem isn't always easy. *V clinicians are hard to find.*

Here are some suggestions for tracking down a good V specialist:

▼ Ask every physician and nurse-practitioner you know. Someone may have a connection or know a patient with a V problem who found good help.

▼ Consult your female friends and female relatives. This is not a topic we usually discuss over tea, but if you do not ask, you cannot find out.

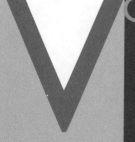

VOICES

"I've had irritation, itching, and burning for years. Sometimes there is discharge. I've seen one doctor after another. After the antibiotics and the antifungals didn't work, I was told everything—you have poor hygiene, your husband is unfaithful, you need to see a psychiatrist."

—Cindy, who has undiagnosed vulvovaginal complaints

▼ Call local gynecologists and speak with their office nurses. Ask if the physician or nurse-practitioner does a lot of V work or has any experience with vulvodynia. If they don't, ask where they refer their V patients.

▼ Call the ob-gyn department of a large hospital and ask for a V clinician referral.

▼ Surf the Web. There are chat rooms on many Web sites. You have to be careful here, though. If you obtain a physician's name, you can check his or her license and board certification through the American College of Obstetricians and Gynecologists or the American Medical Association. There is no good way of learning about his or her V abilities, however.

DON'T BELIEVE THESE MEDICAL MYTHS

The following "truisms" are still widely believed by physicians today, but don't believe them!

▼ If it itches, it's yeast or trich; if there's discharge and odor, it's BV.

▼ You can diagnose yeast by history or by just glancing through the speculum.

▼ If the patient isn't red, raw, and inflamed with a curdlike discharge, and if you can't see yeast under the microscope, it isn't yeast.

▼ If one yeast cream doesn't work, prescribe another.

▼ There are several itchy skin diseases all called lichen something-or-other and you have to use cortisone cream for them, but cortisone is dangerous and you shouldn't give much of it.

▼ Pain with intercourse may be caused by endometriosis; women with other pain related to sex or women with vulvar pain probably need counseling.

▼ Contact the National Vulvodynia Association or the Vulvar Pain Foundation (see Resources) and ask for a referral.

▼ Contact the International Society for the Study of Vulvovaginal Disease (see Resources) and ask for a member gynecologist or dermatologist in your area.

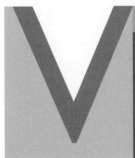

NOTE

Not my way of practicing, but I like the name

In the form of holistic healing that reads the body's energy patterns, or chakras, the V area is known as the second chakra.

You need to find a clinician who is willing to work with you in a team approach to solve your V problem. Many are open to suggestion and willing to try something that is reasonable. Be sure you ask for some simple tests described in the next chapter: a vaginal pH measurement, a wet mount, and a special yeast culture on Sabouraud's medium. If you have read portions of this book that seem to fit your picture, share them with your clinician. The medical references from texts and journals are all included.

▼

CHAPTER 9

The Ideal V Exam

What to Say, What to Expect, and a Guide to Tests

Effie complained of a yeast infection that wouldn't clear up. Her itching had gone on for twenty years. I asked if her doctor had examined material under the microscope to make the diagnosis.

"Oh, no—he just always said I had yeast."

"Did he ever take a yeast culture?"

"No. He just did an internal exam and said it was yeast."

Effie didn't have yeast. She had eczema. Her vulvar skin was red, yes. But it was thickened, with very tiny cracks in some areas. She also had seen a dermatologist for itchy patches on her scalp and had a history of asthma and hay fever—more red flags for eczema. Some cortisone cream did wonders to end the itch.

V complaints, just like those anywhere else in the body, require the steps of a formal diagnosis. When you go to see a clinician about a V

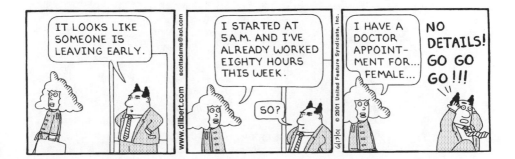

complaint, you should expect that he/she will take a history, do a pelvic examination, and run some simple tests. Anything less cheats you of the full effort that should go into the diagnosis and treatment you need. It's not enough to just listen to your story or glance inside your vagina. Vaginitis may be common, but that doesn't mean that all vulvovaginal complaints are vaginitis. Nor is pinpointing the cause of your symptoms always simple. Sometimes a bit of sleuthing is involved.

Why timing is everything

Schedule an appointment with care. Ideally, you should be seen at a time when you have your worst symptoms. (Remember, some worsen at different points in the menstrual cycle, for example.) It's best if you do not have your period at the time of the visit; it's hard to evaluate the vagina and study a slide under the microscope if there is a lot of blood around. For similar reasons, it's also important not to have intercourse or douche within twenty-four hours of your exam. Finally, and most important, you should be off all medications and creams before the visit. If you have used yeast cream or taken a Diflucan tablet in the past three weeks, for example, it won't be possible to figure out if yeast is or is not part of the problem. Being partially treated at the time of evaluation is a leading reason for missing yeast infections. And figuring out whether yeast factors into your problem is essential!

Admittedly, such scheduling can be challenging. It may be that you have to make two visits: one to start on the history and exam, and another at a time when you have the worst symptoms and are medication-free.

If you are uncomfortable off medications while waiting for the appointment, you may find comfort in frequent soaks, ice packs, and a topical anti-itch such as Vagisil (OTC) during the day and Dramamine at bedtime.

If you have previously been seen by other clinicians for any V problem, their records are important. Your current clinician will want the details of your history, your test results, and the names of medications or treatments that were used. A woman named Irene once came to see me, explaining she had had vulvodynia for more than eighteen years. She had seen a number of physicians, taken many medications, and tried numer-

V NOTE

Man or woman?

Half the women surveyed in a 2001 Gallup poll said they prefer a female ob-gyn; 15 percent preferred a male. Only about a third of practicing ob-gyns are women now, but that number is expected to rise to two-thirds within a little more than a decade, according to the American College of Obstetrics and Gynecology.

HOW TO TALK TO YOUR GYN

An appointment is ideal for me when as much information as possible is exchanged in a comfortable way. Here's a list of things you can do to make the most of your visit:

▼ *Be prepared.* Bring a list of symptoms or questions if you think you might forget something. One of my patients comes with an artist's sketchpad covered with questions—that's so helpful.

▼ *Keep track.* Maintain logs or charts of symptoms and their timing and bring them to me.

▼ *Don't be embarrassed.* There's nothing you can say that your gyn won't have heard before. And he or she is there to help, not make judgments.

▼ *Speak up before you lie down.* Describe your problem before your exam begins so the doctor can take those clues into consideration as he or she works.

▼ *Show and tell.* If you can point to the exact areas of discomfort during the exam, please do. If you can't localize the discomfort, though, that's important information as well.

▼ *Be physically comfortable.* If you need to discuss something in detail after your exam but aren't comfortable doing so in your little gown, ask to get dressed first.

▼ *Use proper terminology if you can.* Not only does it show that you know your stuff and are ready to be an active partner in your care, but precision can help your clinician better pinpoint the problem and its treatment.

▼ *Be brutally honest.* Your doctor isn't there to judge your lifestyle or your life choices. He or she simply needs to know about every factor that may have influenced your condition. Don't leave anything out.

▼ *Ask away.* If you don't understand something about a test or treatment, don't act as though you do. Get clarification.

▼ *Ask for a handout.* Your clinician may have detailed material you can read when you're more relaxed at home in order to better understand a problem or test.

▼ *Ask for records.* Just as I want to see your full medical history, other doctors seeing you (a dermatologist or your regular ob-gyn, for example) may appreciate the same. Records are critical. When a patient asks me to send copies to four different consultants, it's no problem. I want her to feel satisfied that she's come to the right place.

ous treatments. She had even been to a pain clinic. But she came to her appointment with me without a scrap of paper to tell me what had been tried. Help your clinician help you. Obtain a copy of your records and carry them to the appointment, or request that your records be forwarded. Be sure to check before your visit that the records made it.

The vulvovaginal history

A history of your health and your current problem is probably the most important part of your visit. A history includes questions about your specific problems as well as all the details of your health. Before I see them, I ask my patients to fill out a questionnaire. This saves me a great deal of time asking about routine stuff and allows me to focus on pertinent details. A brochure that accompanies the questionnaire assures patients that I am interested in their whole story, short or long. It invites them to describe any information they feel is relevant.

Here's a set of questions I ask as I figure out a V problem. You can use them to prepare an accurate description of your own situation before your history is taken.

THE BASIC PROBLEM

▼ What is the main problem (chief complaint)? Itching, burning, soreness, pain? Constant irritation and rawness? Discharge, bleeding? Bumps, rash, cracks?

▼ What else is going on (associated symptoms)? Urinary problems, bowel problems, skin problems elsewhere, gynecological complaints?

▼ Where is the problem? One little spot, a larger area, several places, the whole vulva? Over the bladder, up in the pelvic area, or around the anus?

▼ How bad is the problem? On a scale of 1 to 10 with a 10 the worst, where does it rank?

▼ When did the symptoms start? Days, weeks, months, years ago? Was there any other illness when the symptoms started?

▼ What's the timing? Constant, comes and goes, has a pattern, associated with menstrual cycle, related to sex or physical activity?

▼ What helps? What makes the symptoms worse?

PAST VULVOVAGINAL HISTORY

▼ Have you had yeast infections over the years? How often?

▼ Have you had other vaginal infections?

▼ Have you ever had any genital injury such as a straddle injury or any other trauma to the vulva or vagina?

SEXUAL HISTORY

This is vital information. I'm not trying to snoop or make judgments about you. I just need to know what's happening with the Vs. I need to know whether you have never been sexually active, have been sexually active with women or men or both, and how many partners you have currently.

▼ Is there a new partner?

▼ Were you ever hurt or abused with sex, and if so, have you dealt with the emotional consequences or not?

- ▼ Do you have a history of STDs?
- ▼ What sexual practices are used—oral? anal? vibrators? sex toys?
- ▼ What do you use for contraception?
- ▼ Above all, are you able to have receptive, lubricated, orgasmic, comfortable sex?

MEDICAL HISTORY

It will be important to know any significant medical problems that you have or surgery that's been done. Gynecological problems, urinary issues, bowel disease, and skin diseases elsewhere in the body are all important. Any history of back injury, slipped disc, back surgery, or orthopedic problems may relate to the V pain condition vulvodynia. Many medical problems, such as diabetes and Crohn's disease, have connections to the vulva. There are even some vulvar skin diseases that tend to run in families.

MEDICATION HISTORY

I really need to know what medications you have taken, both prescription and over-the-counter, the doses, and how long. Women often tell me, "Oh, I tried amitriptyline [Elavil]. It doesn't work." But then I find out that they took it for only a few weeks at a minuscule dose. Some V problems need time and a decent dosage for improvement. Other common complaints: "I'm allergic to cortisone" or "The doctor gave me a strong topical cortisone but I couldn't use it because it burned so much." It may be that the medication is right for you but not in the form you tried. Knowing these details can help me find the right remedy for you. Please try to tell about everything you have used, whether it's your own prescription or a medication you obtained from a friend or family member. Don't forget to include herbal products, vitamins, and homeopathic programs—all these are types of medication that represent part of your story. I'll also want to know whether each seemed to help or not.

URINARY ISSUES

Since the urethra is part of the vestibule, and the urinary tract is so closely allied with the Vs, I will want to know about any urinary symptoms you have had.

- ▼ Have you had frequent bladder infections? Were they proven by culture? Often vulvodynia can feel exactly like a UTI, for example, but the culture is negative.
- ▼ Are you troubled by pain with urination or frequent urination, or do you get up at night more than once or twice to urinate?
- ▼ Do you sometimes lose urinary control (such as when you cough)?

▼ Do you wear protection for urinary leakage? Vulvar irritation may follow. I can put you in touch with experts who can give you options about gaining control again so you won't have to wear pads.

LIFESTYLE CUSTOMS

Lifestyle, employment, athletics, and travel may all be relevant. All the nerve supply to the vulva originates from the spine and can be influenced by your activities. Vulvar skin can also be damaged.

▼ What kind of activities do you do, and what do you wear while you are doing them?

▼ Are you in a swimming pool for long periods of time?

▼ Do you have an old back injury, or skate and frequently fall on your tailbone?

▼ Do you have a job where you sit for hours slouched down or curled around in a poorly designed chair?

I end the history portion of an appointment by asking if I know everything I need to know about your health and vulvar problem. You need to speak up and add anything that might have been overlooked.

From these questions, the clinician receives a clear idea of what you need to have fixed. For example, a particular patient's answers may have run like this: The main problem is itching. Nothing else bothers her. The itching is in one spot in the middle of the left outer lip (labium majus). The itching rates a clear 10. It even awakens the patient from sleep. It's been there off and on for years; it started in grad school during examinations. It's always worse just before a menstrual period. Patient can't think of any bothersome products or activities that seem to affect the itch. The primary-care practitioner prescribed a cortisone cream that really helped, but when she stopped using it the itching returned.

This is a classic story for a chronic itchy skin condition, the type that is easily treated with cortisone cream but never goes away completely; the pelvic exam and maybe other testing will pinpoint which disease it is.

Ancient origins

There is a brief description in the Talmud in which a woman was instructed to introduce a cylindrical leaden tube in her vagina to distinguish uterine bleeding, which was considered "unclean," from vaginal bleeding, which was considered trauma from intercourse. A Roman speculum of 79 CE was found in Pompeii.

The pelvic exam

Once your story is complete, it is time to move on to the examination and lab test part. I always ask two questions at this point: "Do you need to use the bathroom?" and "Will you be more comfortable if we have a nurse with us during the exam?" It's a policy of my practice (and most others) to offer a chaperone whether the physician is a man or a woman, mostly for our own legal protection. A few women do want the nurse, usually as a hand holder.

> **WE ALL FEEL WEIRD**
>
> I won't sugarcoat it: This is the most despised exam there is. It's an unusual patient who doesn't have something derogatory to tell me as she maneuvers into stirrups: "I hate this!" "Why do I have to be a woman?" "I don't know who invented this, but I'm gonna get even!" "I know, you're going to tell me to just scoot down to the edge of the table." Actually I've never used the term *scoot* in my life, and I never will. But I do tell patients that I dislike having the exam myself. Everyone feels awkward or tense to some degree during an internal exam.

Most, however, assure me that they are seasoned veterans of pelvic exams. "I'd be uncomfortable if any more people than absolutely necessary looked at me," as Mary put it. Tonya just laughed: "Need a nurse? Honey, at this point I've had so many pelvic exams that I could have one without a problem in Times Square!"

Many women come with their partners, mothers, or friends, whom I always invite to stay. Putting their own needs second, women often shoo their male partners or husbands into the waiting room, since they know how uncomfortable it is for some men to be around a pelvic exam. But I love it when a partner is present for this part of the appointment, since I think it shows investment in the relationship.

My suggestions for making things easier:

▼ Do everything you can to cut down on your anxiety. Tell me beforehand if you have had painful experiences with exams. Parts of the exam can be modified or omitted. We can use some antianxiety medication beforehand. In some cases, the exam may be omitted entirely until work with counseling or other therapy is done. I always use the smallest possible speculum, and I have little, gentle hands. I also always tell patients what I'm going to do.

▼ Don't tense your muscles. Before the exam, locate your pelvic floor muscles and then relax them by doing a Kegel exercise or two (see Chapter 3).

▼ Do practice taking slow, deep breaths from your abdomen—like Lamaze breathing, if you've had childbirth training.

▼ Do close your eyes if it helps you relax. Think of something distracting. I invite patients to look at the cartoon on the next page, which I have taped on my ceiling.

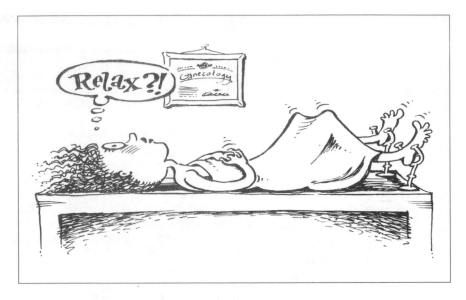

- ▼ Don't raise your arms over your head or make any sudden moves that will tense up your abdominal muscles.

- ▼ Do expect a slight pinch or pressure with the speculum, and some awkward sensations during the bimanual exam, but nothing should produce pain.

- ▼ Don't keep quiet if you are experiencing pain. Tell me!

- ▼ Do go ahead and ask questions. You don't have to keep silent, and we need to make the most of our time together.

The pelvic exam includes looking at all the tissues of the vulva, a speculum exam of the vagina, and a bimanual exam of the uterus and ovaries.

Examination of the vulva may include a plain visual inspection, the use of a simple magnifying glass, or colposcopy, which is a special way of looking at the vulva with a magnifying lens and a bright light. For better visualization, the clinician may first wash the vulvar area with dilute vinegar.

The only way to see the vagina is to use a special device called a speculum. The vaginal speculum spreads open the walls of the vagina, which

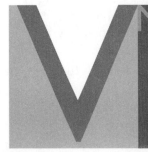

NOTE

Inspecting the speculum

The small metal or plastic instrument uses a front and a back blade to push the walls of the vagina apart for viewing. Rest assured, though, that despite the word *blade*, nothing about the instrument is sharp!

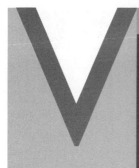

Sex toy?

The vaginal speculum was thought capable of stimulating orgasm in women, and by the end of the nineteenth century it was controversial as a medical instrument. Elaborate tales were told of women and girls lusting after vaginal examination and climaxing on the examining table the minute the speculum was inserted!

normally touch one another, so that the clinician can see what they look like, see what the cervix looks like, check the pH level, view any discharge present, and collect samples for culture or testing.

Use of the vaginal speculum can be very uncomfortable or even painful, especially if the vulva or vagina is inflamed. Fortunately, these devices come in a variety of shapes and sizes; for women with a lot of tenderness or inflammation, a pediatric (child-sized) speculum may work, or there is a very narrow adult speculum called a Pederson speculum. If the speculum causes pain, let your clinician know immediately. Use of the speculum is not pleasant for any woman, but it should not cause pain. If you know of a speculum that has worked well for you, be sure to tell your clinician.

The bimanual exam involves the use of both the clinician's hands to evaluate the pelvic organs. One hand in the vagina identifies and pushes up on the cervix while the other hand outlines the top of the uterus by pressing down through the abdominal wall just above the bladder. In that way, the clinician can feel the size and shape of the uterus. The ovaries can be felt in a similar fashion.

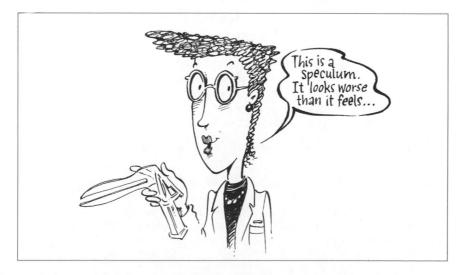

NAGGING LITTLE QUESTIONS ABOUT PELVIC EXAMS

Q *What if my period just started the day of my appointment?*

A Appointments are so hard to come by that I ask women to come in regardless, but it's much easier for me (and you) if you can avoid period time. Keep a record of your periods so you know when you're due, and consult it before making an appointment. (In the regular gyn office, thirty to forty-five minutes are usually reserved for annuals. If you cancel at the last minute, your gyn is left with a large block of unfilled time.) But in order for your Pap smear to be read accurately, it helps if there is no blood. If the exam is for discharge, it's really hard to evaluate it during your period, so that's one appointment you probably should reschedule.

Q *Can you tell if I've had sex recently?*

A Yes. If you had sex without a condom, the pH will be elevated and I will see sperm in the wet mount. For the most accurate evaluation of vaginal discharge, you should not have vaginal intercourse for two days before your appointment.

Q *Am I the only one who shaves my upper thighs before exams? It just seems tidier. Do you care?*

A Many women scrub and shave before pelvic exams. Recently the other clinicians in my ob-gyn group put in place a system called Easy Access, which includes same-day appointments. But we found that women tended to decline them; they felt they needed to "prepare" and, yes, shave their legs, for a pelvic exam. Preparations are not necessary! I don't care whether your legs are hairy or not. In fact, if there is a problem such as odor or discharge, too much scrubbing can make it impossible to evaluate.

Q *I'm too embarrassed to have a checkup because I recently got rid of all my hair—should I wait until it grows back?*

A Believe me, nothing will surprise me, whether your mons is hairless, heart-shaped, pierced, or tattooed. The important thing is that you're coming in because you think you have a problem. If you're not too embarrassed to wear a certain look in front of a sexual partner, you won't bother me a bit. My daughter-in-law Diane told me a funny story about a friend of hers whose longtime gynecologist uttered only one word during the exam: "Fancy." Her friend was puzzled until she got home and realized that the can of feminine deodorant spray she'd reached for that morning was, in fact, gold glitter spray!

Q *Should I say something by way of warning if I smell really bad?*

A If you think you have an odor problem, it really helps me to know up front—as a useful piece of medical information, not as a social warning. There will be a bunch of questions I'll want to ask. Try not to feel embarrassed about vaginal odor. I know I keep repeating myself, but it's so important: Don't wash, douche, or use vaginal spray before an appointment in an effort to mask the scent. Certain odors signal certain types of infection to a clinician.

NAGGING LITTLE QUESTIONS ABOUT PELVIC EXAMS   cont.

Q *Why don't you heat up the speculum?*

A Doing so is not as easy as you might think. The government arm that regulates office safety (OSHA) doesn't allow heating pads or devices in the drawers of exam-room tables because of the danger of shocks or burns. Some offices get around this by using a separate table from the exam table to hold the heating pad with the specula. The speculum can also be warmed with hot water, but alas, many exam-room taps are tepid and inadequate.

Q *Why are those little exam rooms so cold?*

A Room temperatures vary from office to office. But the fact that you're wearing a thin cotton or paper gown while everyone else is in street clothes may make you experience the temperature differently.

Q *Can I ask you questions during the exam, or does that ruin your concentration?*

A Ask anything you like. But it's most helpful if you let me know what your issues are before we get started on the exam part. It's really hard if you bring up a symptom such as discharge or odor after I think I have completed my evaluation.

Q *Is it okay to take my feet out of the stirrups before we start talking?*

A I may ask a quick question while you're in this awkward position. But for anything more, I want you to be comfortable—which usually means sitting up with your legs closed and the drape in place. For initial appointments, I always ask women to get dressed again after the exam. Then we talk. I think that trying to carry on a conversation while your feet are in the stirrups is humiliating. If you have a clinician who routinely expects you to do this, you'll want to find another.

Q *How do you stand doing this all day?*

A Because it's such important work! There's not a woman alive who enjoys a pelvic exam. But look at it from the other end of the speculum: I do this work because of the satisfaction I get from all the questions I can answer and the problems I can solve.

Three important in-office tests

If a V workup stopped with just a history and a physical exam, essential information would be missing. Three simple procedures can be performed in the office to find out what is going on in the vagina: (1) pH determination (acid-base balance), (2) the whiff test, and (3) the wet prep, which is the microscopic examination of vaginal secretions. These tests take just a few minutes. Some physicians send the wet prep to an on-site lab and have results before your visit is over. Without these tests, it is not possible to say what is happening vaginally. *No one can merely listen to a history and make a diagnosis; no one can just look through the speculum and say what is happening.* That's the way doctors were taught fifty years ago; it's out of date now.

These tests have shortcomings, as do any tests, but the main shortcoming is that some clinicians don't use them.[1] Finding one who does is an important job for you to do as you try to figure out what's wrong. Not only are the pH, whiff, and wet prep tests readily available and very useful, but they cost virtually nothing in time and expense.

THE ACID-BASE BALANCE (PH)

Once the speculum is in place, the pH (acidity) of the vagina is measured by placing a piece of chemically treated paper against the lower wall of the vagina. Remember, the healthy vagina is acidic; the reading after sixty seconds should be 3.5 to 4.5. This simple test gives worlds of information: If the pH is normal (acidic), that means that a healthy estrogen level is present. Normal lactobacilli are in the vagina, causing the release of lactic acid. Bacterial or trichomonas infection cannot be the problem, since the lactobacilli predominate. The only *vaginal* problem (remember that many other problems besides vaginitis can cause symptoms) that can exist with a normal pH is yeast, which can grow whether the vagina is acidic or alkaline and even though there are plenty of lactobacilli around.

What a great test! In sixty seconds, a clinician can say that estrogen balance is present, lactobacilli predominate, and that vaginal infection other than yeast is not the source of the V problem.

If, on the other hand, the pH is elevated (alkaline), many possibilities exist to explain the elevation. If the test is done at the cervix or on fluid on the lower blade of the speculum that has been next to the cervix, the pH will be alkaline because that is the nature of cervical secretions. If a woman has had recent intercourse, the pH will be alkaline because semen has a high pH. If there is any menstrual blood in the vagina, this too can raise the pH. The pH also tends to be elevated in breast-feeding mothers or postmenopausal women, who have lower estrogen levels.

But elevated pH can also mean that a vaginal problem, either inflammation or infection, has wiped out the normal lactobacilli that create the acid environment (low pH) in the first place. So an elevated pH tells a clinician trying to solve a V problem to look for inflammation or bacterial vaginal infection.

THE WHIFF TEST

For this test, a drop or two of vaginal discharge is mixed with a drop of a strong chemical base, potassium hydroxide. The mixture is then smelled

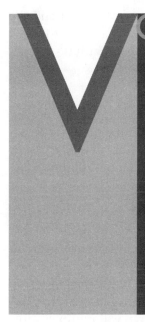

Women on gynecologists:

"I like that he asks me not whether I have any questions but rather what's on my mind that I'd like to talk about—it's a more welcoming invitation."

"I like that he never looks at his watch."

"I have to ask very specific questions to get anything out of her."

"My ob/gyn is more important for me than my primary-care physician."

"She looks at the whole patient—always takes time to inquire about diet, exercise, stress levels—without driving me crazy with too much New Age stuff or unrealistic suggestions."

"I feel my ob-gyn is a baby doctor, not a gyn. I think as I head toward menopause I might switch to a woman, to a caregiver who knows what's going on and will listen."

(whiffed) by the clinician to find out if strong-smelling proteins are present. A positive whiff test is indicated by the presence of a fishy odor released by bacteria present in the vagina when there is bacterial vaginosis. The whiff test may also be positive if there is infection with trichomonas.

THE WET PREP (ALSO CALLED WET MOUNT OR VAGINAL SMEAR)

When a few drops of vaginal secretions are mixed with a few drops of salt water (saline) on one slide and a few drops of potassium hydroxide on another, this is what's known as a wet preparation, or wet prep.

The slide with the potassium hydroxide (the same mixture used for the whiff test) can be examined under the microscope to see if yeast hyphae or spores are present. These will not dissolve in the strong potassium hydroxide, but other cells and bacteria will.

Then a drop or two of vaginal discharge is mixed with a little saline for examination under the microscope. In this sample the clinician can see if yeast or trichomonas is present. He or she can look at the type of vaginal cells present; if there is plenty of estrogen in the body, the wet prep will show many squarish superficial cells from the vaginal wall. If bacterial vaginosis is present, the square cells of the vaginal wall will be covered with bacteria. These are clue cells. Finally, in the wet prep the clinician can see what bacteria predominate.

FEMEXAM

A newer test you might encounter called FemExam also measures vaginal pH. Specially prepared circles of chemical reactants on a card are covered with vaginal fluid; the chemicals change color to reveal the pH and the presence of proteins (amines) associated with BV. It's a great test for BV, but you still need information about yeast, trich, and other causes of vaginal problems.

Other testing methods

You may also encounter some other tests during your workup. Unfortunately, some of these tests are misused or ignored in the quest for an accurate diagnosis of a V problem. It's a good idea to always ask your clinician to explain a test before it's done and what kind of finding is being looked for.

VAGINAL CULTURES

A vaginal culture consists of swabbing the vagina with a dry cotton-tipped applicator. The swab is then sent to a lab, where technicians smear it on culture medium to identify the bacteria that grow.

Vaginal cultures are as inaccurate to diagnose most V complaints as Pap smears are to diagnose anything other than cervical precancer and cancer. Bacteria such as *E. coli,* gardnerella, and group B strep will routinely grow because they are normal inhabitants of the vagina. Despite this basic fact, thousands of doses of antibiotics are handed out each year because a woman with a complaint is cultured and found to have bacteria that, although normal, are thought to be the cause of the problem. (Please read Chapter 13, "Vag Itch, Continued," to understand the limited circumstances under which these bacteria might cause vaginitis.)

So a plain vaginal culture is usually not a helpful test and can in fact be misleading. Sometimes yeast will grow from such a culture, but the yield is low when just a dry swab is transported to the lab. If yeast is a possibility, you need a very specific yeast culture (see below).

YEAST CULTURES

A yeast culture consists of swabbing the vagina and then, while in the exam room, putting the swab directly into a special substance called Sabouraud's medium. Sabouraud's is a special combination of ingredients (called a culture medium) that yeast loves to grow in. The yield from a yeast culture on Sabouraud's is high, meaning that a culture done on this medium is more likely to tell you if yeast is present than a culture done on a medium for growing bacteria.

Yeast cultures, in contrast to vaginal bacterial cultures, are very helpful in the evaluation of vaginal discharge. When a woman has itching and yeast cannot be seen on the wet prep, a yeast culture can determine for sure whether or not yeast is present. Unfortunately, many clinicians do not do yeast cultures. *Note:* A yeast culture won't be of any value if it's taken at a time when the woman does not have symptoms or if the woman has recently treated herself with a night or two of antifungal cream or a Diflucan tablet.

TRICHOMONAS CULTURES

Though as helpful as yeast cultures, these are infrequently done because the clinician can usually see trich under the microscope. When a clinician suspects that a woman has trichomonas because she has marked itching with discharge and an elevated vaginal pH, he/she may not be able to see evidence of trichomonas if there are many white blood cells on the wet prep. A culture for trichomonas will give the answer. The culture may also be helpful if a woman has been treated for trichomonas but her symptoms persist. A swab of vaginal secretions is put into a special broth that trichomonads will grow in, triticale soy.

SKIN SCRAPINGS

The skin of the vulva can be affected by a kind of fungus other than candida that produces itching and a rash. This fungus is called a dermatophyte because it is specific for skin (*derma* means "skin"). To find out if it is present, the clinician scrapes off some cells from the surface of the labia, the groin, or wherever the rash is and applies some potassium hydroxide or a special purple stain called Schwartz-Lampkin. Under the microscope the clinician can see the fungus if it is present. This is important because some yeast creams treat dermatophytes and others are of no value.

Vulvar biopsy

In order to find out exactly what a lump, rash, or ulcer might be, the clinician may need to take a very small sample of skin called a biopsy. This is a simple, safe, and important procedure to obtain precise information that will guide your treatment. The area to be sampled is made completely numb. Then a few millimeters of skin are removed, and medication or a tiny stitch is placed to prevent any bleeding. The area heals in a few days; ibuprofen or Tylenol with soaks in the tub keep you comfortable afterward. The biopsy material is forwarded to a lab, where it typi-

VOICES

"You know, I know my doctor takes a Pap smear during my checkups but I have no idea what it's for. I kind of take it for granted and hope that I don't hear any more about it afterward."

—Joyce, 32

THE SILENT STDS WORTH A ROUTINE TEST

Many health care providers—but not all—now routinely screen young women for two rampant sexually transmitted diseases, chlamydia and gonorrhea. Although not strictly V problems (they affect the cervix), they can create V symptoms. Tests for these STDs are easily done with a swab of the cervical canal.

Many clinicians still wait to test until a woman complains of symptoms, which include yellow-white discharge and possibly itching or pelvic pain. But you can have chlamydia or gonorrhea and be symptom-free. Men can get these STDs too. In fact, these bacterial infections are spread precisely because many men and women have chlamydia and gonorrhea without knowing it.

The danger is that these diseases can spread up through the uterus and into the tubes, causing infection there and on into the pelvis. The net result can be scarring of the tubes and infertility. Each is treatable, but you have to know you have it in the first place! That's why, especially if you are under 30 and sexually active, I think it's smart to ask for a chlamydia and gonorrhea screen as part of your annual exam.

cally takes a week or so to examine it and make a diagnosis. The biopsy may not always give a specific diagnosis; it may just show inflammation or thickening of the skin, for example, but it is as helpful to know what is *not* present as it is to know what is there.

The thought of having some tissue removed from a sensitive area such as the vulva is frightening to many women. They may have had a painful experience with biopsy before. They may have a very tender inflamed area that needs to be sampled, or they may have an area that is not tender but is located in a sensitive area near the clitoris. There are, however, excellent ways to make the procedure virtually painless. EMLA (it's short for "eutectic mixture of lidocaine and prilocaine") is an anesthetic cream that can make the inner labia, the labia minora, the hood over the clitoris, or any part of the vestibule numb in just a few minutes so that an injection is not necessary. Or EMLA can be used to reduce sensation so that a needle stick will scarcely be felt.

Injections of lidocaine often hurt because a large needle is used or because the lidocaine is injected without buffering it to reduce its sting. Lidocaine mixed with a little sodium bicarbonate (for your clinician, that's 0.1 cc of $NaHCO_3$ for 1 cc of lidocaine) and injected with a fine-gauge (30 g) dental needle causes minimal discomfort.

The Pap test

One familiar test deserves special focus because it's often misused and misunderstood. Nearly every woman I see for a V problem says, "I've had this itching [or burning, or pain] and I saw my gynecologist—but my Pap came back normal, so I don't know what the problem can be!" The Pap smear is a means of evaluating cells removed from the cervix to see if there are any

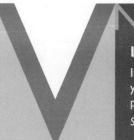

Lifesaving track record

It has been estimated that with Pap test screening every three years, death from cervical cancer can be reduced by at least 70 percent.

Source: Mortality and Morbidity Weekly Report 1989:38:650.

changes in them that signal cancer or a precancerous condition. It's the single most cost-effective disease screening test known to modern medicine.[2] Since the introduction of the Pap smear, cancer rates and death rates from cervical cancer have drastically dropped. While the Pap smear is a lifesaver when it comes to identifying abnormalities of the cervix before they develop into cancer, it's not a test for anything else. A normal Pap doesn't mean everything is all right with the Vs; it only means no precancer cells were found in the cervix.

Many clinicians still assume too much about the Pap as well. For example, they may rely on the other information that is occasionally reported on Pap smears as definitive evidence of vaginitis, even though the Pap is not considered reliable for indicating anything other than precancer.[3] What the lab may report as trichomonas may in fact be a vaginal or cervical cell that looks similar. The Pap smear may report a "bacterial shift" thought to represent bacterial vaginosis, but this finding does not accurately indicate BV; it might instead reflect other disturbances of the bacterial inhabitants of the vagina. When the Pap smear suggests vaginitis, a woman should be evaluated with a vaginal exam, a pH reading, and a wet prep. Because of the possibility that an infection with many inflammatory white blood cells may make it difficult to see the cervical cells to be studied, most clinicians refrain from obtaining a Pap smear when they think you might have an active vaginal infection.

You should also realize that the Pap is only a screening test; it can't diagnose cancer. A screening test gives you information about your risk. Screens require ongoing follow-up or other tests in order to provide a fuller picture. No test, screen or otherwise, gives you all the information you want about a condition; this is why understanding what a test can and cannot tell you is important. The Pap's effectiveness lies in sampling the cervix at regular intervals.[4] No one single normal Pap guarantees anything, but a string of normal Paps year after year is very reassuring. Even if you have a suspicious Pap, there's seldom cause for five-alarm panic, because cervical cancer evolves very slowly and the precancerous changes, known as *cervical intraepithelial neoplasia* (CIN), are highly treatable.

All cervical cancer and most of the cervical changes found on a positive Pap are caused by human papillomavirus (HPV) (see Chapter 21, "The Crafty Virus"). The Pap doesn't test for HPV, which you can have without showing any symptoms at all; the Pap looks at the cells for evidence of changes caused by HPV.

GETTING A GOOD PAP

An optimal Pap test depends on several different elements: a good sample, proper interpretation of that sample, a good screening lab, and an accurate reading. Each aspect along the way holds opportunities for error.

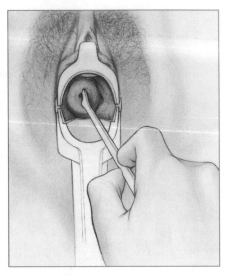

FIG. 31   The Pap Smear

Taking the sample from the cervix as seen through the speculum.

Source: K. J. Carlson, S. A. Eisenstat, T. Ziporyn, *The Harvard Guide to Women's Health* (Cambridge, MA: Harvard University Press, 1996).

A Good Sample

As with any good testing, the expression "Garbage in, garbage out" prevails. A poor-quality Pap may miss disease or lead to errors in interpretation. Your clinician has certain guidelines to ensure a good sample. Here are some things you can do:

▼ Don't use intravaginal medication or douche for twenty-four hours before the sample is taken.

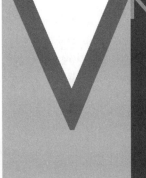

V NOTE

Pain-free Paps?

A Pap smear is normally not painful, though many women note a strange sensation as the sample is taken. Pain is a flag signaling a V problem. If the speculum hurts, there may be vestibular and vaginal atrophy from a lack of estrogen or from vestibulitis. A Pap might be uncomfortable if you have a yeast infection or other vaginitis, but it still should not cause significant pain. If you have never had intercourse, tell your clinician and ask for a narrow speculum.

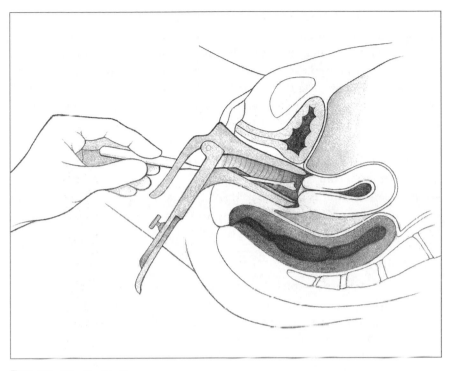

FIG. 32   **The Pap Test**

You can see how a clinician reaches through the speculum to take a scraping from the cervix to look for precancerous cells. This is the only information the Pap gives.

▼ Don't have intercourse or use contraceptive jelly or cream for twenty-four hours before your Pap.

▼ Don't schedule a Pap when your period is due. Small amounts of blood will not interfere with evaluation of the cells, but large amounts during the menses are likely to make the smear impossible to interpret.

▼ Don't wait until after your Pap is finished at an annual exam to tell your clinician about other V symptoms you're having. Talk about your problem first and let her/him decide whether to go ahead with the Pap.

Proper Interpretation of the Smear

The study of the cells on the Pap smear is called cytology. In the lab where cells are studied, slides are stained with a special substance by a technician who then protects the cells on the surface of the slide by applying a glass cover slip. After drying, the slides are forwarded to a screener, who is either a cytotechnician (someone with an associate degree and twelve months' experience in cytology) or a cytotechnologist (someone with a bachelor's degree and twelve months' clinical training). The screener is required to review the entire surface of the slide, viewing every cell on the smear and marking representative abnormalities. Any slides that appear atypical must be reviewed by a doctor with special training in abnormal tissue (a pathologist). Slides without atypical cells are designated negative and may then be signed out of the lab without a pathologist's review.

This system is far from foolproof. The average slide contains from 50,000 to 300,000 cells; the variety of abnormalities is large, and there are many mimics of cancer that turn out to be nothing. The issue of workload volume per screener is a major concern in quality assurance. Ideally, you want your Pap read by a cytotechnician who is board certified and required to do continuing education to keep up with the field.

The Right Laboratory

Your clinician chooses which lab to send your Pap to. Odds are good today that you will get a fairly accurate reading. In the 1980s, reports surfaced of "Pap mills" where unreasonably large numbers of smears were found to be interpreted by undersupervised and overworked cytotechnologists. As a result, federal regulations have been set up that specify workloads, documentation, standards for rescreening slides and slide storage, unannounced proficiency testing for both cytotechnologists and pathologists, procedures for detecting and dealing with inadequately prepared smears, and periodic inspections of the facility.

In addition to state and federal rules about standards for rechecking Pap smear slides, each lab has its own standards. These depend on the clientele. If—just for an example—you ran a lab in a nunnery, where the chance of finding HPV (which is contracted through sexual activity) was low, you wouldn't double-check many slides because it would be a waste of time. On the other hand, if your lab were in an area of a big city where there were a lot of sex workers, you'd expect a lot of HPV, and rescreening slides would

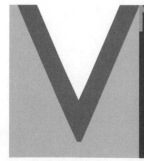

No good memory required

Pick a memorable day to schedule your annual Paps, like your birthday. The College of American Pathologists runs a free e-mail reminder service. You pick the date, they send the reminder to call your health care provider to schedule an annual exam. Check out www.papsmear.org.

COMMON QUESTIONS: PAP TESTS

Q **Are there symptoms I should look for to indicate it's time to have a Pap?**

A Cervical precancers are not associated with symptoms. One of the miracles of the Pap test is that it can detect a disease that is completely silent. That's why it's wise to be tested regularly even if you feel fine. If you have itching, burning, discharge, or painful intercourse, look for other causes. Cervical cancer also may produce no symptoms, but when it does, usually in the late stages, it tends to cause bleeding after intercourse or between periods, pelvic pain, or foul discharge.

Q **Who should have a Pap test?**

A Every woman. Get one annually starting at age 18 or when you become sexually active, whichever occurs earlier. Continue to get them regularly after menopause. You should have regular Paps whether or not you are in an active sexual relationship, and whether you are lesbian or heterosexual. Your clinician— whether an ob/gyn, an internist, a family practitioner/general practitioner, a nurse-practitioner, or a physician's assistant—should do it routinely at an annual exam.

Q **How often should I be tested?**

A After three or more consecutive negative tests, many doctors recommend a Pap about every two years. I say take the safest road and get one every year.

Q **Who is most likely to have an abnormal Pap?**

A Risk factors for the precancerous conditions of the cervix that show up on Paps include having had more than five sex partners or a male partner who has had more than five sex partners, first intercourse before age 17, a male partner who has had a sex partner with cervical cancer, a history of HPV infection, genital herpes, smoking, regular use of illegal drugs such as cocaine, a history of abnormal Pap smears or reproductive cancer, infection with the human immunodeficiency virus (HIV), a suppressed immune system because of organ transplant, low economic status, exposure to diethylstilbestrol (DES), and being over 65 without ever or rarely ever having had a previous Pap.

Q **Why do I have to have a second test sometimes?**

A A Pap test should include cells from both the outer surface of the cervix (squamous cells) and the cervical canal cells (endocervical). Women are often asked to return for repeat testing if the endocervical cells are not seen on the smear or if the smear is unsatisfactory. A thick normal vaginal discharge, vaginal infection, or menstrual discharge can also prevent accurate reading of a Pap.

You may also have a second test if the first one was abnormal. See "Repeating the Pap," later in this chapter.

Q **How do I find out the results?**

A The results of your Pap analysis are sent from the lab to your clinician. As a patient, you have the right to know the results of every test taken, and you need to make sure that your Pap test is normal. If your health care providers do not routinely inform you of the result, call to find out. You don't want the results of this important test to fall between the cracks. Some clinicians contact you only if the test is suspicious and requires further investigation; you're told that no contact indicates a negative result. Follow up yourself anyway. It's smart to be proactive about all test results. Never assume anything is normal. We health care providers are human, after all.

Results can take one to three weeks. Why so long? Remember that cytologists are now strictly limited in how many Paps they can read in a day—this is a good thing, so be patient.

Q Should I get a Pap if I'm pregnant?

A Part of the first prenatal visit is a Pap smear. Abnormal Pap smears occur frequently during pregnancy. This is not surprising because abnormal Paps are common in all women, pregnant or not. Cervical precancer is usually not treated during pregnancy since it is slow-growing and clinicians know that there is plenty of time to treat it afterward. The main goal of evaluating a pregnant patient is to make sure that actual cancer is not present if the Pap is abnormal. Another test, colposcopy (see page 183), can be easily performed, and an experienced clinician can determine if there are areas on the cervix that must be biopsied (a cervical biopsy is safe in pregnancy) or whether the biopsy can wait until after pregnancy. If the colposcopy is satisfactory, the Pap and colposcopy can be repeated as the clinician thinks necessary based on the severity of the abnormality. If there is an abnormal area that extends up the canal, a limited cone biopsy can be safely performed in pregnancy by an experienced clinician. In such cases, it is important to obtain a second opinion with review of the Pap test and any biopsies before proceeding to cone biopsy.

pay off. The best method of evaluating quality is for a pathologist to look at the abnormal Pap smear slide along with the slide of any cervical biopsies that were done to evaluate the abnormal smear. Unfortunately, many labs that read Pap smears do not receive cervical biopsies.

Ask your clinician about his/her comfort level with the lab used. Or you could call the lab yourself and ask about the technicians and pathologists and about the standards for double-checking slides (they should be rechecking 10 percent or more). The one I use puts out excellent information for patients. If you have big questions about a lab result (such as whether something is cancer or not), you can always ask for the slides to be transferred to another lab, ideally at a big teaching hospital, for reevaluation. (But be sure to find out about your insurance coverage for this second opinion.)

Please see the Resources section for obtaining more information about lab standards.

The Accuracy of the Pap Smear

So how reliable is your test? If your Pap is normal (negative), can you rely on this? If your test is positive, does that mean there is something really wrong? Generally accepted figures are that a negative Pap is right 99.4 percent of the time, and a positive Pap is right 80 percent of the time.[5] But some recent studies have found lower accuracies: A negative finding is accurate only 69 percent of the time, and a positive finding is right just over half the time (58 percent).[6] These are troubling figures.

About two-thirds of false negative results (the test is negative but the woman has cervical disease) are caused by problems in the way the Pap smear is taken (sampling error). Another reason for a false negative Pap is misinterpretation or failure of the lab to detect abnormal cells on the Pap slide (detection error).

Sampling error occurs when abnormal cells are not collected or are not transferred to the Pap slide. To reduce this problem, a relatively new technique, called a ThinPrep, is gaining ground. The sample is collected as usual. But instead of smearing a glass slide, the clinician swirls the spatula and the brush in a jar of special fixative solution. In the lab, the cells are collected in a filter and transferred to a microscope slide for interpretation. Twirling the spatula and brush in the fixative lessens the amount of material lost when the implements used to smear the sample on the slide are discarded. The process also reduces the amounts of blood and mucus that might get onto the slide to obscure the cells, and deposits the cells on the slide in a single clear layer. ThinPrep Paps make good sense, but they cost more and aren't always covered by insurance. I always use it in follow-up Paps after a patient has had an abnormal Pap, or if a patient asks for it.

To reduce detection error, labs can look at the positive slides again (rescreening, as mentioned above) or double-check a randomly chosen bunch of all smears. Rescreening can be done on a bigger number of slides through the use of two computerized technologies, AutoPap and PAPNET. AutoPap uses a decision tree to identify slides that go over a certain threshold for the likelihood of abnormal cells. PAPNET identifies cells or clusters of cells that need to be looked at more carefully. The computer then displays from the Pap slide up to 128 images that are likely to contain abnormalities. A cytotechnologist reviews these images and decides whether to review the actual slide under the microscope. These methods are not routine; you need to ask your clinician about their use in your area.

High technology aside, the time-honored way to reduce errors is to repeat the Pap test on a regular basis. The proportion of false negatives drops to fewer than 1 percent for the patient who obtains three consecutive annual Pap smears. Two-thirds of all women who develop cervical cancer have not had a Pap test in five years, or ever. So get your Pap every year and you can rest a lot easier.

IF YOUR PAP IS ABNORMAL

Your Pap smear is read as negative (normal) or positive (abnormal) and graded according to what the abnormal cells look like. Practically every patient I see who has an abnormal Pap asks, "Does this mean I have cancer?" When Dr. George Papanicolaou, the test's namesake, designed the smear in the 1940s, he did not know about the preliminary cell changes (known as *cervical intraepithelial neoplasia,* or CIN) that exist for years before the cancer invades. We do. If your Pap smear is abnormal, reassure yourself with the following facts:

- ▼ There is a low probability of finding invasive cancer.
- ▼ There is a high probability of finding curable CIN, which only means precancer.
- ▼ CIN represents abnormal cells but not cancer. Nor does precancer necessarily progress to cancer.
- ▼ CIN can be treated by simple office methods without hospitalization or surgery.[7]

"Abnormal" simply means that some different-looking cells have appeared on the slide containing your Pap smear. When abnormalities are found, the Pap is then graded as one of the following three simple categories: ASCUS, LSIL, or HSIL.

Here's what they mean:

- ▼ *ASCUS (atypical squamous cells of undetermined significance):* Unusual cells were seen, but the cause isn't clear.
- ▼ *LSIL (low-grade squamous intraepithelial lesion):* The unusual cells suggest the precancerous condition CIN 1, mild dysplasia.
- ▼ *HSIL (high-grade squamous intraepithelial lesion):* The unusual cells suggest the precancerous condition CIN 2 or CIN 3, moderate or severe dysplasia.

Remember that a Pap is only a screening test, and if it is abnormal, you need more information about what's going on in your cervix. Before I tell you about how each of these three categories of abnormal Pap is evaluated, let me first explain some additional procedures used to obtain that information.

THREE MORE WAYS TO FIND OUT
WHAT'S HAPPENING IN THE CERVIX

Colposcopy

A Pap smear consists of a group of cells scraped from the cervix. The laboratory evaluates the cells and grades them, but the relatively few cells collected this way represent a limited amount of information. Atypical cells could come from an inflammatory condition affecting the cervix such as vaginitis, or they could come from precancerous changes in the cervix. That's where colposcopy comes in.

The colposcope is a magnifying lens with a bright light. It is designed so that a clinician can look carefully at the cervix and search for abnormal areas that the abnormal cells might have come from. First the cervix is washed with vinegar to get rid of the mucus covering it. Abnormal areas will then turn white, and abnormal blood vessels associated with growths can be seen. These areas can be sampled (biopsied) so that the lab receives a little piece of tissue that can give a lot more information about what is going on. This part of the cervix is not sensitive. Most women say that the biopsy feels like a pinch. The biopsy can cause some cramping that can be lessened by taking ibuprofen before the procedure. Anesthesia is not necessary; it's usually done right in the office.

Scrapings taken from the endocervical canal (ECC) are another way to check for disease in the canal. Most colposcopists recommend routine ECC sampling during colposcopy except during pregnancy.

Colposcopy and cervical biopsy are the gold standard for evaluating an abnormal Pap smear. But when should colposcopy be done? Anytime there is a question? For every atypical Pap? The sections on evaluation of the abnormal Pap will tell you about the standards in medicine.

Cervicography

Another test that is available but rarely used because it doesn't provide much better information than the Pap is cervicography. Cervicography is a way of evaluating the cervix by taking a photograph of the cervix after a speculum has been placed in the vagina and the cervix has been washed with vinegar to get rid of mucus and make abnormal areas visible. The photographs are often used in areas remote from medical centers. A nurse or technician can do the photograph of the cervix and send it to a center where physicians are able to read it. Cervicography has correctly identified lesions that were then confirmed by colposcopy and biopsy 90 percent of the time.[8]

So why don't we use more cervicography? Because it's so sensitive that it picks up abnormalities that would go away on their own, abnormalities that are not really precancerous conditions.[9] As a result, this may give us information that really isn't helpful, leads to increased anxiety for both

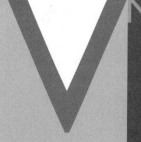

the woman and her clinician, and may result in tests and procedures that really aren't needed.

Repeating the Pap

When a Pap test comes back abnormal, my patients often react in disbelief and think that there must be some kind of error. They want the test repeated immediately, hoping to get a normal result. If the test has shown early stages of abnormalities (conditions known as ASCUS or LSIL—see below) for the first time, then yes, repeating the Pap is appropriate. However, you need to wait three to four months before the repeat test to allow a new crop of cervical cells to mature on the surface. A Pap that is repeated too soon may be falsely negative and therefore falsely reassuring.

It's never a good idea to repeat a Pap that shows a greater degree of abnormality (HSIL or suggestive of cancer—see below), though, because waiting can lead to missed diagnoses and treatment delay.[10]

EVALUATING THE DIFFERENT GRADES OF ABNORMAL PAPS

With repeating the Pap and colposcopy and cervicography in mind, now let's walk through how each grade of abnormal Pap is further evaluated.

Abnormal Pap #1: ASCUS (Atypical Squamous Cells of Undetermined Significance)

This is sort of a catchall category for when odd-looking cells are seen but the problem is not immediately clear. Many V problems that cause inflammation in the vagina will lead to atypical cells in the cervix. These include yeast infections, trich, desquamative inflammatory vaginitis (DIV), and lichen planus (LP) (see Part III). Also, if you're postmenopausal and there's not much estrogen around, guess what? Paps can look atypical. Once any of these conditions is treated, a repeated Pap will become normal. No cancer worry whatsoever.

ASCUS may also be the earliest evidence of human papillomavirus (HPV) infection, which may go away on its own.[11] (For more on HPV see Chapter 21.) Alternately, the atypical cells that show up on your Pap can

---

ALL ABOUT AGUS

I want to tell you about an abnormal Pap that can be scary and often comes to nothing. Not every cell that is found on the Pap smear comes from the top layer of the cervix. Cells from *glands* in the cervix, in the uterine lining, or even in the tube or ovary can appear. If these glandular cells are present on a Pap smear and they look different or atypical, the Pap is classified as "atypical glandular cells of undetermined significance" (AGUS).

AGUS is not a common finding. When possible, the lab tells your clinician whether these are glandular cells from the uterus (endometrial) or glandular cells from the cervical canal (endocervical). The finding of AGUS on a Pap smear always deserves careful investigation to find out why such cells are there in the first place.

There are a number of harmless conditions associated with AGUS. These include previous cone biopsy, endometriosis of the cervix, and endometrial polyps. Often, AGUS just turns out to be one of the precancers (CIN) described in this chapter and Chapter 21.[12] Less often, AGUS can signal a problem with the glands of the uterine lining or, rarely, cancer in the glands of the cervix or outside the uterus, such as the ovary.

When a Pap smear shows AGUS, the test is not repeated. Instead, clinicians do tests to make sure there are no abnormalities in the areas that the glandular cells came from. They obtain an endometrial biopsy as well as colposcopy and scraping (curettage) from the cervical canal. An ultrasound examination of the upper genital tract may be ordered.

---

come from a patch of low-grade or high-grade dysplasia somewhere in the cervix. This patch needs to be hunted down and, depending on what it is, either treated or monitored. So we can't just ignore an atypical Pap.

With all of these possibilities, further evaluation of the ASCUS result will depend on your history and your clinician's opinion. Everyone agrees that any vaginitis or vaginal inflammation, or a lack of estrogen, needs to be treated. Then, if another Pap is still atypical, evaluation of the cervix with colposcopy is often done as a first step. Other safe approaches for evaluating what's behind an ASCUS Pap include:

1. Repeat the Pap every three to six months. If the results of two consecutive tests are negative, a return to yearly Pap testing is indicated.
2. If either of the test results indicates ASCUS or a more severe classification, the woman needs colposcopy.
3. With the first ASCUS Pap test result, the woman could have cervicography or HPV testing. If either test is positive, colposcopy should be done. If negative, yearly screening is resumed.

We don't yet know how to predict what will happen if a woman has ASCUS on her Pap. Often it just goes away, so many women prefer simply to be monitored with Pap and colposcopy every four months. If the problem

THE FIRST V EXAM

Now I'm going to backtrack and provide a little background for girls and young women who have not had a V exam yet. Gyn doctors and nurse-practitioners have special training to take care of women and their problems. They are the clinicians to see when you have medical questions about breasts, sexual organs, your period, having sex, using birth control, or, of course, a V problem. What gyn clinicians care most about is helping you stay healthy. No question is too weird, embarrassing, naive, outrageous, or dumb.

A pelvic exam is the way the clinicians examine both external and internal sexual organs. Nobody likes the idea of a stranger staring at her vulva and up her vagina. But if you understand what it's all about, it can be easy. It may feel a little uncomfortable, but it doesn't hurt. Gyn doctors and nurse-practitioners understand that most women find having a pelvic exam sort of embarrassing. The best thing to do is to find someone you like and feel comfortable with.

First, you'll be asked to lie on your back with your feet resting in holders called stirrups and your legs apart. The clinician will look at the outside parts, then put an instrument called a speculum into the vagina to spread apart the walls and look at the opening to the womb, the cervix. Your Pap test is done by taking some gentle scrapings of the cervix with a wooden spatula and spreading them on a laboratory slide. The speculum is taken out, and the first part of your pelvic exam is over.

Since the clinician can't see past the cervix, he or she uses another way to examine the uterus and ovaries in the second part of the exam. The clinician puts a finger into your vagina and then presses gently over your lower abdomen with the other hand. This allows him/her to feel your uterus and ovaries in between the hands. You may feel pressure but should not feel pain.

A good time for a first pelvic exam is after your first period. You should definitely start having pelvics when you become sexually active, or by age 18, or if you think you have a problem.

persists more than a year, treatment is recommended since it seems unlikely that the lesion is going to go away on its own. Immediate treatment may be in order depending on what's seen on a colposcopy.

Abnormal Pap #2: LSIL (low-grade dysplasia, or CIN 1)

Most Pap smears showing LSIL represent activity in the cervix that will go back to normal without treatment.[13] It disappears on its own in 84 percent of women under 34, and in 40 percent of women over 34.[14] But a few women in this group will have a lesion that will progress. The evaluation of a Pap showing LSIL is straightforward:[15]

1. Most clinicians will do colposcopy to evaluate the cervix and take biopsies for more information. They want to rule out more severe disease than the Pap smear suggested.
2. It is also acceptable to repeat the Pap smear in four to six months and have colposcopy if the LSIL persists.
3. With biopsy proof that a low-grade lesion exists, and if the entire abnormal area can be seen, the lesion can be treated, or the woman can be followed with Pap smears and colposcopies.

Whether to treat or just monitor it at this point depends on the woman's wishes and how willing and likely she is to keep appointments for Pap smears and colposcopies. About 15 percent of women with low-grade dysplasia will move on to high-grade dysplasia because they have an aggressive, active kind of HPV virus.[16] But since most cases will just go away on their own, it's also appropriate to simply monitor the condition without treatment. Then, if the abnormality continues after a year, treatment is indicated.[17]

Abnormal Pap #3: HSIL (high-grade dysplasia, or CIN 2 or CIN 3)

Everybody agrees that any woman with HSIL needs colposcopy and cervical biopsy.[18] With this more complete information about the location, nature, and extent of the problem, treatment can be planned.

For more detailed information about the treatment of CIN and about the virus that causes it, please see Chapter 21.

▼

PART III

V

Problem and Answer Guide

Now it's time for the nuts and bolts of my practice. Every week I see dozens of women with the common V conditions high-lighted in depth in this section (along with some of their rarer cousins). You'll want to turn here to help you figure out what might be wrong, as well as to follow along with your clinician during your care. I'll walk you through the symptoms, the diagnosis process, the common concerns patients have, and the most current treatments. All the latest medical knowledge is included. In fact, because this is such an unexplored terrain in medicine, in many cases this information will be ahead of the curve to clinicians who are not V specialists.

The information is not just thorough but also presented in the same way I treat the patients in my office: with lots of facts but also with lots of empathy and reassurance. The fact is, almost every vexing V condition can be managed effectively. I want you to be concerned but not to panic. I want you to understand your condition so that you're better prepared to heal, and I want you to know that I understand how it makes you feel. I want to help.

But don't save these pages for when you have a problem. I've also included lots of important prevention advice. Such common situations as yeast infections, BV, painful sex, and the human papillomavirus are things that no savvy, sexually active woman today ought to have her head in the sand about. Familiarize yourself with them now and perhaps you'll be spared them later—or at least you'll know the smart way to handle them. It's all part of being in touch with your body, of knowing yourself, of being a woman.

Problem finder

You can read up on some of the most common symptoms in Chapter 7, "The Most Bothersome Symptoms," which catalogs possible reasons behind them. Supplementing that, here's a shorthand guide on where to turn for help. (Notice that almost every chapter in the book turns up under itching— remember, everything itches!)

Bad Itching

Chapter 10: Yeast Infections

Chapter 12: Trich

Chapter 13: Vag Itch, Continued

Chapter 14: Could You Be Allergic?

Chapter 15: When Skin Gets Sick

Chapter 17: "It Hurts"

Mild Itching

Chapter 16: V Bumps and Color Changes

Chapter 11: BV

Chapter 20: The Lifetime Virus

Chapter 21: The Crafty Virus

Chapter 22: V Cancer and Precancer

Odor

Chapter 11: BV

Discharge

Chapter 10: Yeast Infections

Chapter 12: Trich

Chapter 13: Vag Itch, Continued

Chapter 15: When Skin Gets Sick

Chapter 17: "It Hurts"

Dryness

Chapter 15: When Skin Gets Sick

Chapter 17: "It Hurts"

Painful Sex

Chapter 10: Yeast Infections

Chapter 15: When Skin Gets Sick

Chapter 17: "It Hurts"

Chapter 18: Sexual Healing

Yeast Infections

Separating the Truths from
the Popular Beliefs

Yeast. It's the first thing most women think of when they experience V symptoms. Got an itch? Buy a tube of cream. If only it were that simple every time.

Yeast infections are harder to diagnose and self-treat than women have been led to believe. Though yeast infections are the most familiar V condition, they're not the commonest. (That distinction goes to bacterial vaginosis.) The hallmark irritation and discharge that lead many women to think "yeast infection" unfortunately characterize many other conditions as well. Grabbing a tube of OTC antifungal cream at your local drugstore won't do you any good or could even make things worse—if yeast isn't the problem. Consider these examples:

▼ Anne experiences vulvovaginal irritation, checks herself, and finds thick white vaginal discharge, so she concludes that she has a yeast infection. She goes to the drugstore and purchases an OTC yeast cream. It doesn't work. Why? She doesn't realize it, but the irritation is from exercising in thong underwear, and the suspicious discharge is actually normal.

▼ Sonya decides her inflammation and discharge stem from a yeast infection. When OTC cream does not help her, she sees me, and I diagnose the sexually transmitted disease chlamydia.

▼ Beth, who's pregnant, thinks she has yeast. Sure enough, I find that her discharge sticks to the side walls of the vagina and covers the cervix, suggesting yeast. But when I examine some secretions under the microscope, I discover she has bacterial vaginosis.

▼ Marina complains of having yeast symptoms all the time. In addition to a constantly itchy sensation, sex hurts. Though she's tried many yeast creams, they never clear up the symptoms. Turns out she doesn't have yeast; it's vulvodynia.

I don't mean to suggest that every time you think you have a yeast infection, it's probably something else. Yeast infections do happen, and often. But folklore about yeast has outpaced hard medical facts, leading to way too much assumed knowledge (which is often, as you'll see, incorrect or inconclusive). Take the following folk wisdoms, for example: *Yeast causes a cottage-cheese-like discharge with intense itching. Too many sweets cause yeast. To prevent yeast you should eat yogurt and wear white cotton underwear.* All these statements have come to be accepted as fact. However, some are only partially true; others have little or no scientific research to support them.

Misconceptions about yeast swirl through the medical community too. One study suggests that as many as 50 percent of cases of yeast may be misdiagnosed by practicing physicians.[1] Yeast infections are regarded by many clinicians as boring. They consider itching a trivial complaint not worth serious investigation. Many clinicians still believe that they can make the diagnosis without any special testing or even seeing the patient. Even when an earnest effort is made, yeast can elude diagnosis if a woman is seen at a time when she's not having symptoms or after she has used antiyeast medication. Failing to recognize the complexity of a yeast infection may lead to undertreatment and recurrence, or to the conclusion that something more serious is going on. Perhaps most damaging is the attitude that we clinicians already know everything about this grand pest. Far from it! Most clinicians are not familiar, for example, with new information that yeast is not a single condition but a spectrum of disease, ranging from the isolated episode to unrelenting recurrence.

While yeast can indeed be a simple problem, it's also often complex, showing up in many different ways. There are some women who never have a

NOTE

The name's the same

The fancy term for a yeast infection is vulvovaginal candidiasis (VVC). It was once called thrush—the name still used for a yeast infection in the mouth—and monilia.

yeast infection, or experience only one or two during their lives. Other women experience yeast only during a certain part of the menstrual cycle *(cyclical candidiasis)* but not at any other time. Still others have one infection after another and are unable to clear up the problem. Don't forget that many V problems can feel exactly like yeast: itchy skin diseases (Chapter 15), other kinds of vaginitis (Chapters 11, 12, 13), allergies (Chapter 14), and above all, that great masquerader, vulvodynia (Chapter 17). And if it isn't yeast in the first place, no yeast therapy is going to clear up the problem.

So where does this leave you when you suspect a yeast infection—besides miserable, that is? Before I chart the steps you should take, some background about yeast is in order. I know you're probably desperate for a remedy, but first we need to make sure that you're heading toward the right kind of remedy.

What is yeast?

When doctors say "yeast," we usually mean a fungus named *Candida albicans.* Yeast is not limited to the V zone. It's common on the skin and can be found in the gastrointestinal tract anywhere from the mouth

FOR IMMEDIATE RELIEF

While you're waiting to have a diagnosis confirmed, the following natural and over-the-counter remedies can help you deal with itching and burning.

▼ Sit in comfortably warm water in the tub or a plastic sitz bath container that fits under your toilet seat (available at the drugstore).

▼ Go without underwear as much as possible; when not, wear the loosest clothes you have.

▼ Use ice. Put crushed ice, frozen peas, or frozen corn in a small plastic zip-closure bag with a soft cloth around it. This molds well to V anatomy. At night keep by the bed a plastic dishwashing detergent bottle that you have cleaned, filled with water, and frozen; if you awaken with itching, put this (wrapped in a thin soft cloth) between your legs.

▼ Apply the over-the-counter preparation Vagisil.

▼ Take Benadryl or Dramamine at bedtime to help control the itching, so you can get some sleep.

▼ Ask for a prescription for a topical anesthetic, Xylocaine 5 percent ointment (gel or cream may burn).

▼ One thing *not* to do: Don't buy an over-the-counter antifungal (common trade names: Monistat, Femstat, Gyne-Lotrimin) until you have read this chapter through and decided whether you should first see your clinician. I'll explain later why these creams should not be your very first line of defense.

to the anus. Candida lives harmlessly in the vagina in as many as one in five healthy women of childbearing age without causing any symptoms.[2] Remember, all sorts of organisms normally dwell there, including such villainous-sounding bacteria as *E. coli* and group B strep. Their presence doesn't mean you have poor hygiene or are dirty. As a protective measure,

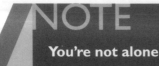

You're not alone

Most women have at least one yeast infection during their lives. The total number of cases is unknown because yeast is not a condition that has to be reported to health authorities. But in the 1980s, the number of prescriptions written to treat yeast almost doubled. An estimated $1 billion plus is spent annually on treatment in the United States.

Source: G. Cauwenbergh, Vaginal candidiasis: evolving trends in the incidence and treatment of non–*Candida albicans* infection, *Curr Probl Obstet Gynecol Fertil* 1990:8:1125–34; R. Hurley, Recurrent candida infection, *Clin Obstet Gynecol* 1981:8:209–13.

Mother Nature set us up to have bacteria—and yeast—on the skin and on every mucous membrane in the body.

Yeast gets into the vagina mainly from the neighboring intestines by way of the anal area. How does this happen? Not just from wiping yourself in the wrong direction, as women have traditionally been taught. It's just that the anus is very close to the vagina. The yeast can sprint independently from one organ to the other, or be passed along by a menstrual pad as it's worn, or be transferred during receptive oral sex, meaning that the partner's mouth contains yeast and comes into contact with the vulva, vestibule, or vagina. So you can't always actively prevent it.

Most of the time, a healthy vaginal environment and the normal immune system probably keep the harmless yeast from overgrowing and causing vaginitis. One current theory about yeast infections that keep

FIG. 33
Yeast spores and hyphae that can be seen in vaginal secretions under the microscope

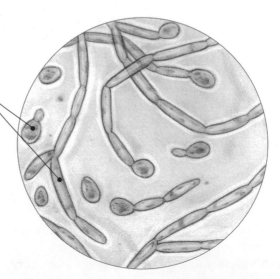

coming back is that the vaginal immune system somehow fails to police the yeast, allowing them to run amok.

Yeast lives in two different forms. It can be seen as a *spore,* a small round or oval shape, or as *hyphae,* elongated stems with the spores inside or budding on the ends. It's long been suggested that yeast can invade tissue and cause disease only in the hyphal form. Spores have been considered innocent bystanders until they are stimulated to grow into hyphae. But we now know that both forms can cause disease. Spores can be hard to see under a standard microscope, but hyphae are readily visible. So if you're complaining of itching and other symptoms and the clinician sees spores or hyphae under a microscope, it's assumed that yeast is the problem.

Like many living organisms, yeast feeds off glucose (a kind of sugar). Yeast can grow at any pH from extremely acidic (2.5) to highly alkaline (7.5), so that trying to prevent yeast infections by doing things to change the amount of acid in the vagina is not going to be helpful.[3]

To live and grow in the vagina, yeast also has to have estrogen around. *Candida albicans* has a protein on it that makes estrogen stick to it, and the cells of the vaginal lining have a protein that makes candida stick to it.[4] In addition, estrogen directly stimulates candida to switch from the yeast form that hangs out in the vagina, the spores, to the form that invades the vaginal cells and causes symptoms, the hyphae.[5] (I wish Mother Nature had hooked yeast to testosterone instead, don't you?)

The estrogen-yeast connection explains a lot. It's why young girls prior to puberty don't have yeast infections and why postmenopausal women not on hormone replacement therapy seldom do. These individuals have very low levels of estrogen in their bodies. The estrogen-yeast relationship may also explain yeast infections that occur during the second half of the menstrual cycle (cyclical candidiasis). In a 28-day cycle, with day 1 being the day menstruation begins, day 14 is the time of ovulation. Estrogen is at high levels from day 13 to day 23, then declines steadily. Yeast often flares up with the high estrogen levels after ovulation, then backs off

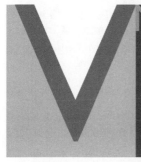

Estrogen side effect

With more women taking hormones at menopause, clinicians are seeing women in their fifties, sixties, and even seventies with their first attack of yeast.

Source: J. D. Sobel, A comprehensive strategy for managing recurrent VVC, *OBG Management,* Aug. 1998 (suppl.):14.

as menstruation begins and estrogen levels have dropped to their lowest. Finally, estrogen's link to yeast explains why women taking tamoxifen for breast cancer get recurrent yeast infections. Tamoxifen is a synthetic antiestrogen that is diverse and complex in its actions. It blocks estrogen in the breast, but it may act as an estrogen in the postmenopausal vagina.

Symptoms of a yeast infection

A yeast infection results when there's too much yeast. It overwhelms the vaginal defense system. Yeast infections are almost always (85 to 90 percent of the time) caused by *Candida albicans,* but there are more than two hundred different strains of candida. Sometimes when drugs have been used to wipe out the *Candida albicans,* different yeasts called non-albicans yeasts can increase and cause infection. The best known of these are *Candida glabrata* and *Candida tropicalis.* The yeast that makes bread rise, *Saccharomycetes cerevisiae,* can also cause vaginitis. (Though uncommon, there have been reports of tiny fragments of uncooked dough on the hands and under the nails of bakers being transferred during sexual activity.) The non-albicans yeasts are harder to treat because they require higher and longer dosing of the standard medicines used for yeast, or they do not respond at all. We don't have many alternative medications to treat non-albicans yeast.

In particular, *C. glabrata* has received attention lately because infections caused by it are on the rise. What's happening is that women are using so many OTC antifungals that although the simple *C. albicans* is getting wiped out, other, more resistant yeast forms are taking its place. (This is similar to the concern with overuse of common antibiotics.) *C. glabrata* tends to respond poorly to the main ingredient in antifungal creams (azoles) such as Monistat, Gyne-Lotrimin, or Femstat. This type of yeast is seen more frequently in diabetics. There's also a connection between *C. glabrata* and douching, and this kind of yeast is also often seen in combination with bacterial vaginosis, possibly because *C. glabrata* tolerates the alkaline pH associated with BV.[6]

No matter what the strain of yeast, severe itching and vaginal discharge are the classic complaints. Neither symptom is seen only with yeast, and neither is always associated with disease (itching has many causes, and so does discharge). But if yeast is going to give symptoms, the most frequent symptoms are vulvar itching and itching around the vaginal opening in the vestibule.

Most women expect to see a cottage-cheese-like discharge, but in fact vaginal discharge is not always present or is often minimal; even if it is profuse, it doesn't always have a telltale curdlike texture. This discharge may vary from watery to uniformly thick. Vaginal soreness, irritation, vulvar burning, pain with intercourse, and burning when the urine touches

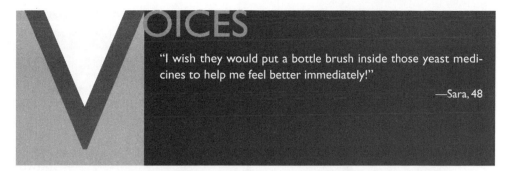

VOICES

"I wish they would put a bottle brush inside those yeast medicines to help me feel better immediately!"

—Sara, 48

the vulva are common. Odor is not a usual complaint, though candida causes a yeasty smell for some women.

An exam performed by a clinician shows redness and swelling of the labia and vulva, often with little red pimples separate from the central redness. The cervix is normal; the vagina is red and inflamed. Sometimes clumps of discharge stick to the walls, or there may be minimal secretions. Symptoms are often worse in the week preceding the menstrual period; with the menstrual flow women often experience relief.

Yeast infections produce a spectrum of symptoms. In general, the more intense the itching and redness, the greater the number of yeast organisms present. For some women secretions predominate, with profuse discharge that sticks to the vaginal wall in thick white patches or white plaques. This is sometimes called *vaginal thrush*. For other women, a more inflammatory picture emerges: minimal discharge but extensive redness over the vulva into the groin folds and down around the anus. There are also variations on both pictures.

What causes yeast?

When are you most vulnerable to a yeast infection? Let's examine each of the widely believed risk factors summarized in the box on page 198 in more detail.

THE SEX LINK

Many young women have their first yeast infection shortly after becoming sexually active. Is it just coincidence? Actually, this may occur because seminal fluid has been shown to encourage the spore form of candida to grow into the hyphal stem form.[7] The hyphal phase of candida growth has been suggested to be the more active phase for invasion of the vaginal wall by the yeast.[8] Sperm may also prevent the vaginal policemen, the white blood cells, from adequately fighting off yeast.[9]

Yeast infection is not considered a sexually transmitted disease. But there is a strong association between yeast and other STDs, such as chlamydia. So yeast is considered sexually *associated*.

In cases where the woman has repeated yeast infections, especially just

ARE YOU AT RISK?

Many long-held assumptions about the risk factors associated with yeast infections have entered the realm of common knowledge without being proven. Traditional thinking is now changing, thanks to ongoing research.

Possible Cause	Traditional Thinking	New Realizations
Sex	Yeast infections aren't an STD. Yeast is only part of the population of normal microorganisms in the vagina.	Yeast infections are sexually associated. They can be transmitted to or from partners by intercourse or oral-genital contact; they increase at onset of regular sexual activity. It is unclear if frequency of intercourse is a factor.
Diet	Sugar intake increases yeast infections. Yogurt is a good therapy.	Most studies have failed to show whether dietary excesses or deficiencies play a major role; there is only one trial reporting success in a limited number of women using yogurt.
Antibiotics	Antibiotics cause yeast infections.	Depends on type and usage. Broad-spectrum antibiotics cause more problems; length of use is also a factor.
Clothes	Tight-fitting synthetic clothing causes yeast.	The role of clothing is anecdotal and unproved.
Pregnancy	Yeast infections are more common and difficult to eradicate during pregnancy.	No one's sure. Original studies were flawed methodologically; no recent studies have been performed.
Contraception	Oral contraceptives increase risk.	The risk was greater with high-estrogen oral contraceptives (now off the market) than low-estrogen compounds. The sponge and IUD increase rates of infection. The diaphragm increases colonization but not necessarily rates of infection.

after sex, a culture of the man's ejaculate may be helpful. This can be done at home after intercourse (the man should use a condom to collect the ejaculate). Alternatively, the man can produce an ejaculate in a container. A cotton swab is dipped into the semen in the condom and then placed in yeast culture broth the woman has been given at the clinician's office. She can return the culture the next day. Culturing the penis will not give help-

COMMON QUESTIONS: Sex and yeast

Q Can I get it from oral sex?

A Yes. A number of studies have underscored a link between oral sex and yeast infection. One study using DNA matching showed that the yeast found in men's mouths was identical to the yeast in their partners' vaginas. And receptive oral sex (cunnilingus) twice or more in the previous week tripled the risk for yeast in a study where vaginal culture for yeast was part of the protocol. Yeast is a normal resident in the mouths of men who do not have symptoms; they can pass the yeast through oral-genital contact. A man's mouth can be cultured for yeast and he can be treated if positive. But we do not have good information on how long yeast is eliminated from the mouth after treatment.

Q Can I give yeast to my partner?

A Yes, though not often or with serious repercussions. There are two ways. Yeast can cause a local skin reaction (hypersensitivity, not infection) on the skin of the penis. This can cause some redness, swelling, itching, and irritation that easily clear with some antiyeast cream. It's no big deal. It doesn't mean that he's infected with yeast, and it has no long-term effects. The second way occurs when the woman actually passes the yeast to the man. Researchers have found that men can also hold yeast in the seminal vesicles. If this is the case, the man has no symptoms whatsoever but can pass the yeast back to the woman with ejaculation. This occurred in only a small number (about 15 percent) of the partners of women with recurrent yeast, however. Thirty-six percent of these partners also had oral yeast.

We do not have any information about whether one woman can give yeast to another.

Q Should I skip sexual activity while I have a yeast infection?

A While the risks to a male partner are slight, most women abstain because it just doesn't feel good. Why subject yourself to further irritation?

Q If I have lots of yeast infections, would treating my partner help?

A If he has a positive yeast culture from his ejaculate, yes. Otherwise, probably not. In most studies, partners of men who were given topical treatment did not have fewer infections. There are only two studies showing that treating male partners with oral antifungals decreased the infection rate in female patients.

Sources: J. D. Sobel, A comprehensive strategy for managing recurrent VVC, *OBG Management,* Aug. 1998 suppl.; A. M. Geiger, B. Foxman, Risk factors for vulvovaginal candidiasis: a case-control study among university students, *Epidemiol* 1996:7:182; P. Rodin, B. Kolator, Carriage of yeasts on the penis, *Br Med J* 1976:1:1123–24; J. D. Oriel, B. M. Partridge, M. J. Denny, et al., Genital yeast infections, *Br Med J* 1972:4:761–64; R. N. Thin, M. Leighton, M. J. Dixon, How often is genital yeast infection sexually transmitted? *Br Med J* 1977:2:93–94; B. J. Horowitz, S. W. Edelstein, L. Lippman, Sexual transmission of candida, *Obstet Gynecol* 1987:6:883–86; M. P. Bisschop, J. M. Merkus, H. Scheygrond, et al., Co-treatment of the male partner in vaginal candidosis: a double-blind randomized control study, *Br J Obstet Gynaecol* 1986:93:79; A. Spinillo, L. Carratta, G. Pizzoli, et al., Recurrent vaginal candidiasis: results of a cohort study of sexual transmission and intestinal reservoir, *J Reproductive Med* 1992:37:3433–47

ful information, since it is the seminal vesicles where the yeast may reside. If a man has yeast in the seminal vesicles, he will not have any symptoms but he will need oral treatment to clear the yeast.

THE DIET LINK

Various things that women eat have been accused of causing yeast infections. Unfortunately, the research is just too thin to convince me that this is a solid risk factor. Sugar has been the chief suspect because yeast, like many living things, needs glucose or other simple sugars in order to function. It breaks glucose down to carbon dioxide and alcohol in a process known as fermentation. It's the alcohol produced by this fermentation process in the vagina that produces the burning sensation women experience with yeast infection. Sugar in the human body comes in many forms. The best-known sugars are complex, meaning that the body can break them down into simple forms. (You can tell a sugar because its name has the suffix -*ose*.) We eat several complex sugars: sucrose (table sugar), lactose (found in dairy products such as milk, yogurt, cheese, and ice cream), and fructose (from fruit). These complex sugars are broken down into building blocks that the body can use, such as glucose. Different kinds of yeasts are identified in the laboratory by the sugar they ferment: *Candida albicans* works on glucose, another strain of candida ferments mannose, and so forth. There is good evidence that a type of sugar (fucose) found in vaginal cells provides an attachment area for the yeast to hook on to.[10]

The notion of a sugar-yeast link started when researchers concluded that diabetes was a predisposing factor for yeast infection.[11] This is true. We now know that diabetics are more frequently colonized by yeast than nondiabetic women—however, most diabetics do *not* have repeated yeast infections.[12] Still, sugar connections were searched for because work in the laboratory suggested that yeast was more aggressive in response to the availability of sugar.[13] Recommendations of dietary dos and don'ts mushroomed. To date, however, there is only one nutritional study on women with culture-proven yeast infections. It was done by a New England expert on yeast vaginitis. He found increased levels of three kinds of sugar (glu-

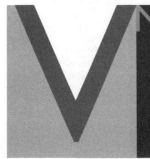

Food fads

If only you could solve yeast problems simply by reforming your diet! Unfortunately, neither a low-carbohydrate diet, a yeast-product-elimination diet, or a yogurt-rich diet has been found to cure yeast infections.

cose, arabinose, and ribose) in the urine of women with recurrent yeast infections. Dietary patterns associated with these urinary sugars were a high intake of table sugar (sucrose) or sugar-rich foods, milk (more than a quart per day), cottage cheese, yogurt, and artificial sweeteners that contain milk sugar (lactose). In that study, eliminating excessive consumption of these foods brought a dramatic reduction in the incidence and severity of yeast infections.[14] We just don't know enough, though, to make any blanket recommendations.

A diet eliminating carbohydrates and many other foods is recommended in the best-selling book *The Yeast Connection,* which has become something of a bible for women plagued by recurrent yeast infections.[15] I'm skeptical of this too, however, because the author cites one study showing a positive relationship between *Candida albicans* and baker's yeast but offers no further scientific evidence other than conversations with physicians.[16]

On the basis of such limited evidence, all I am willing to say about diet and yeast infections is that overdosing on sugar *may* be a risk factor. Ordi-

CAN YOGURT PREVENT YEAST INFECTIONS?

The recommendation that women who have yeast problems should eat yogurt is so widely held that few women realize it's not grounded in fact. This "cure" probably started as a folk remedy. In 1908, a book about the prolongation of life attributed the longevity and good health of Bulgarian peasants to their daily consumption of yogurt, which contains live lactobacilli. Since then, interest in the use of lactobacillus-containing solutions to maintain or restore the body's normal bacterial populations has waxed and waned.

It's true that several studies have reported successful treatment of yeast with use of yogurt by mouth or in the vagina. But they should be interpreted with caution: The women were included in the studies based on their own reports of yeast infection, and since no cultures were done, we can't be sure they really had yeast in the first place. Nevertheless, popular opinion latched on to the yeast-fighting power of yogurt, especially after a well-publicized 1992 study found that daily consumption of 8 ounces of yogurt containing *Lactobacillus acidophilus* decreased yeast infection. This was a really small study, though, and hasn't been replicated.

Women who eat yogurt to combat yeast infections do so because they think it will restore the good bacteria, the lactobacilli, to the vagina. While antibiotics, as we'll talk about next, do wipe out bacteria, right now *we have no evidence that women with repeated yeast infections* (that are not antibiotic-related) *don't have enough lactobacilli.* I look under the microscope all the time, and I see the spores and hyphae of yeast surrounded by tons of lactobacilli. Nevertheless, women who struggle with frequent yeast infections often eat large quantities of yogurt with the hope that the lactobacilli in it will help the problem. Or they take expensive capsules from the health food store that contain lactobacilli in the form of acidophilus.

CAN YOGURT PREVENT YEAST INFECTIONS?   cont.

Consuming lots of yogurt to sidestep yeast is a waste of time. Most of the lactobacilli-containing yogurt products currently available either do not contain the lactobacillus species advertised or contain other bacteria of questionable benefit. Also, getting lactobacilli from sources such as dairy products to stick to vaginal cells doesn't always work—adherence seems to be a unique property of human vaginal lactobacilli. Besides, yogurt contains a large amount of milk sugar (lactose), which may worsen a yeast infection. Douching with yogurt is never recommended.

L. acidophilus supplements from the health food store likewise contain a form that does not adhere to the human vagina.

The human variety of lactobacillus is now available in Europe in capsule form and is in the process of approval by the Food and Drug Administration in the United States. It may be a promising treatment for the vaginal condition associated with lack of lactobacilli, bacterial vaginosis. But its usefulness in preventing yeast infections still seems more fantasy than fact.

Sources: E. Metchnikoff, *The Prolongation of Life* (New York: G. P. Putnam's Sons, 1908); K. D. Gunston, F. Fairbrother, Treatment of vaginal discharge with yoghurt, *SA Med J* 1975:49:675–76; T. E. Will, Lactobacillus overgrowth for treatment of moniliary vulvovaginitis [letter], *Lancet* 1979:2:482; B. Sandler, Lactobacillus for vulvovaginitis, *Lancet* 1979:2:791–92; A. Friedlander, M. M. Druker, A. Schacter, *Lactobacillus acidophilus* and vitamin B complex in the treatment of vaginal infection, *Pan-minerva Med* 1986:28:51–53; E. Hilton, H. D. Isenberg, D. M. T. Alperstein, et al., Ingestion of yogurt containing *Lactobacillus acidophilus* as prophylaxis for candidal vaginitis, *Ann Int Med* 1992:116:353–57; J. D. Sobel, W. Chaim, Vaginal microbiology of women with acute recurrent vulvovaginal candidiasis, *J Con Microbiol* 1996:34:2497–99; V. L. Hughes, S. L. Hillier, Microbiologic characteristics of *Lactobacillus* products used for colonization of the vagina, *Obstet & Gynecol* 1990:75:244; S. Boris, J. E. Suarez, F. Vazquez, et al., Adherence of human vaginal lactobacilli to vaginal epithelial cells and interaction with uropathogens, *Infec and Immun* 1998:66:1985; B. J. Horowitz, S. W. Edelstein, L. Lippman, Sugar chromatography studies in recurrent candida vulvovaginitis, *J Reprod Med* 1984:29(7):441–43.

nary consumption of sweets is unlikely to trigger vaginitis. Large, well-run studies are needed to find out the truth about sugar and all the other carbohydrates before we can recommend therapies that really work.

Best advice: Eat a healthy, well-balanced diet. Make sweets a special treat. If you follow the food pyramid, you'll automatically consume a wise amount of sugar and sugar-containing foods, as well as consume dairy products in healthful moderation.

THE ANTIBIOTIC LINK

Yeast infections are often seen during or after treatment with oral antibiotics.[17] In fact, the widespread use of antibiotics is the most probable explanation for the emergence of yeast vaginitis as a widespread problem.[18] While any antibiotic can cause yeast to overgrow in the vagina, antibiotics that kill a wide variety of bacteria (called *broad-spectrum* antibiotics), such as tetracycline, are the worst offenders. The longer antibiotics are used, the more likely a yeast infection will result.[19]

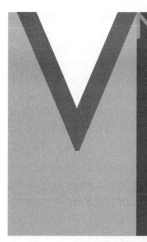

Yeast connection . . . or no connection?

Chronic exposure to *C. albicans* has been popularly blamed for causing a long litany of problems elsewhere in the body, including anxiety, depression, crying, diarrhea, premenstrual tension, hives, trouble breathing with physical exertion, headaches, abdominal pains, weak memory, poor bust development, chronic fatigue syndrome, and sexual problems. Yeast infections have also been fingered as a factor in everything from rheumatoid arthritis and Crohn's disease to schizophrenia and AIDS. The vast majority of medical practitioners, however, roundly dispute such connections, although good studies have not been done.

Why is this so? Antibiotics wipe out the normal bacteria that live in the vagina; researchers suspect that these bacteria, especially the lactobacilli, protect by providing a roadblock that prevents yeast from growing and invading the vaginal wall.

If you are a woman with a history of repeated yeast infections, look back over past prescriptions to see if a course of antibiotics started them off. If you do have yeast that seems to occur after antibiotic use, or if you have frequent yeast infections, you need to talk with your clinician about preventative measures, such as using a tube of antiyeast cream with the antibiotic. Better yet, reconsider your use of antibiotics. They are not always as necessary as believed. Many people, for example, take antibiotics before dental work because of mitral valve prolapse, a minor abnormality of one of the heart valves that can increase the chance of infection of the valve; however, the American Cardiology Society has recently indicated that antibiotics are not necessary unless an ultrasound study of the heart shows significant leaking of the mitral valve. Antibiotics are also often taken for sinusitis when conditions other than bacteria are causing the symptoms. Antibiotics are of no value to treat the common cold, since it's a virus, not a bacterial infection. Make sure you need the antibiotics in the first place.

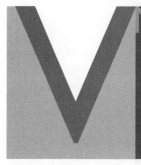

You'd probably be dead instead

Despite the long (and unproven) list of maladies that yeast infections are often blamed for, there's no medical evidence to date for such a thing as "systemic yeast." Yeast can invade the bloodstream, usually in severely immune-suppressed patients, producing massive infection that is often fatal, but this is rare.

Don't accept a prescription mutely without asking your doctor to describe the medication in detail.

THE CLOTHING LINK

Tight, poorly ventilated, and synthetic underclothing—all of which raise the temperature in the genital area and increase trapped moisture—are factors widely believed to contribute to recurrent yeast infections. Yet once again, little scientific data supports this belief. In a study of yeast infections among U.S. college women, no increased risk for yeast was found among women who wore tight clothing or noncotton underwear.[20] It's possible that contact with chemicals or allergic reactions may alter the vaginal environment and permit yeast to overgrow, but the study of college women did not identify any feminine hygiene practice as a risk factor for yeast infection. (There are other risks to this type of clothing, of course, as described in Chapter 5, "V Smarts.")

THE PREGNANCY LINK

One of the most enduring beliefs about yeast infections is that pregnant women are more susceptible to them. I'm not so sure. Some studies support this idea, having found more yeast colonization and more vaginitis, especially in the last trimester.[21] On the other hand, studies also have found that the risk of yeast infections in pregnant women does not differ from the risk in other women.[22] Many women make it through pregnancy completely yeast-free. Also, many vaginal problems in pregnancy that are attributed to yeast may be coming from other sources: bubble bath, harsh soap, hot water, thong underwear, BV, skin diseases, vulvodynia, and so on. For pregnant women, as with all women, yeast is often the only V descriptor they know to assign to *any* V condition.

Yeast infections may be harder to cure during pregnancy because high hormone levels at this time increase the starch content of vaginal cells, providing good nutrients for yeast. Estrogen also helps yeast attach better to the vaginal cell and then turn into a hypha (stem) form that can cause vaginitis.[23] Because vaginitis symptoms can be caused by things other than yeast during pregnancy, it's best not to self-treat with over-the-counter products. Check with your obstetrician or midwife first.

THE CONTRACEPTIVE LINK

Over the years reports about the relation of the birth control pill to yeast infection have varied. The older, high-estrogen pills (containing 50 or more mcg of the estrogen ingredient) thought to have promoted yeast are no longer recommended. The prevailing opinion had been that today's more common low-dose estrogen pills (20 to 35 mcg of estrogen) do not increase yeast infections.[24] Then two recent well-designed studies looking at women with *culture-proven* yeast infections showed a significantly higher

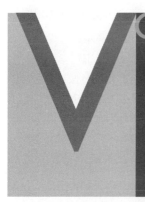

risk of yeast infections in those who use low-dose oral contraceptives.[25]

If you take oral contraceptives and have repeated episodes of yeast infection that have not responded to treatments, a "trial-of-one" therapy, in which your doctor monitors you for candida infection while on and off birth control pills, is a plan you might want to consider.[26] Be sure to use another reliable means of birth control. No one has studied the effect of discontinuing the pill for women who have repeated yeast infections.

The intrauterine device (IUD) is also associated with increased risk of yeast infections. If you have repeated proven yeast infections with an IUD, talk with your clinician about another form of birth control. The diaphragm can increase the number of yeast that live in the vagina, but it is not associated with an increased rate of infections.

OTHER LESS WELL KNOWN LINKS

Immunosuppression and Yeast

People who have to take systemic cortisone, such as those with severe asthma, rheumatoid arthritis, and many chronic diseases such as lupus and MS, are at increased risk for yeast infections. A question about the relationship of HIV to frequent recurrent yeast vaginitis has been raised, but this has been nothing more than a scare. While both men and women with HIV are susceptible to resistant oral yeast infections, no good studies have shown that women with HIV are particularly prone to recurrent vulvovaginal yeast.[27]

Genetics and Yeast

This may turn out to be one of the most important explanations for women who get one yeast infection after another. Blood group characteristics are related to a woman's susceptibility to yeast infections. Besides the common A, B, and O groups, there can be other proteins (called factors) on red blood cells with different names, such as Kell, Duffy, and Lewis. (So, for example, you can be blood type A positive and also have the Kell factor.) Women who have the Lewis factor are three to four times

Can recurring yeast impair your fertility?

There's no evidence for a connection between yeast and infertility—although there are certainly plenty of other reasons to get to the bottom of this problem.

more likely than the general female population to have recurrent yeast infections.[28] This means that up to 25 to 33 percent of patients with recurrent yeast infections are *genetically predisposed* to developing the problem, probably because along with inheriting the Lewis blood protein, they also inherited a vaginal immune system that doesn't fight off yeast the way it should. This would explain how you can be perfectly healthy, do everything right, avoid all the known risk factors, and still have yeast problems! Unfortunately, it's still only a theory; no targeted treatments exist yet.

Allergy and Yeast

Mounting evidence supports the yeast-as-allergy theory, in which yeast swamps a previously healthy immune system. Many women with recurrent vulvovaginitis have an immune system that doesn't respond during a particularly bad yeast infection.[29] Some of their white blood cells have a reduced ability to multiply and fight in response to *Candida albicans* (a condition called *reduced lymphocyte proliferative response*).[30] In response, these women also produce a compound that suppresses the immune system, prostaglandin E2.[31]

Here's how yeast allergy might work in a woman's body. During the first yeast infection, the yeast invades the top layers of the vagina and grows inside the vaginal cells. There, deep in the cells, the yeast is somewhat protected from the antiyeast cream and the immune system. Yeast proteins, called antigens, that the body recognizes as foreign are released from the cells and cause the production of antibodies, substances to fight off the foreigners. The antibodies in turn trigger the release of histamine, which not only produces itching and burning but also keeps the elements of the immune system from fighting back—white cells cannot multiply and move into the area. Thus, the vaginal defenses are paralyzed, and yeast takes over. To add insult to injury, now that the vaginal immune response is wiped out, any chemical or foreign protein coming into contact with the vagina at this point can set off an allergic reaction that causes the cells to swell and rupture, releasing the yeast inside. The whole cycle begins again. The theory of this self-perpetuating cycle, developed by Marjorie Crandall, is shown below in diagram form on page 207.[32]

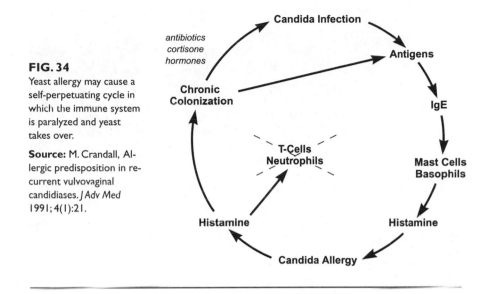

FIG. 34

Yeast allergy may cause a self-perpetuating cycle in which the immune system is paralyzed and yeast takes over.

Source: M. Crandall, Allergic predisposition in recurrent vulvovaginal candidiases. *J Adv Med* 1991;4(1):21.

If recurrent yeast infection represents an allergy, then would allergy shots against yeast work? Over the years several studies have reported success.[33] I have just finished a small pilot study on yeast-allergy shots. Five of ten women had improvement, but these numbers are too small for statistical significance. As always, we need more work.

Diagnosing a yeast infection

If you see a doctor or nurse-practitioner because you think you might have a yeast infection, you absolutely need a complete workup. Chapter 9 outlines these steps: a history, a pelvic examination, a pH test, a wet prep, and a whiff test.

A yeast infection is, in many cases, identified by performing an examination of the vaginal discharge under a microscope to detect the presence of yeast stems (hyphae). If hyphae are seen, the diagnosis is plain, and often no further testing needs to be done if the pH and whiff tests are normal. (If these tests are abnormal, there is probably a mixed infection, with trichomonas or bacterial vaginosis present as well.)

Yeast cultures are not needed in cases of uncomplicated yeast where hyphae have been seen under the microscope. There are, however, several situations that require a yeast culture:

▼ A woman has symptoms of itching, burning, and discharge, but no spores or hyphae are seen under the microscope.

▼ The clinician sees only yeast spores (not hyphae) under the microscope, suggesting infection with a non-albicans yeast that is resistant to some therapies.

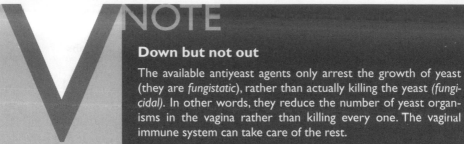

Down but not out

The available antiyeast agents only arrest the growth of yeast (they are *fungistatic*), rather than actually killing the yeast *(fungicidal)*. In other words, they reduce the number of yeast organisms in the vagina rather than killing every one. The vaginal immune system can take care of the rest.

▼ The clinician sees many white blood cells under the microscope but cannot find any yeast or trichomonads.

▼ The woman has used standard treatments for yeast and her symptoms have not improved.

▼ The clinician wishes to treat the woman with months of oral antifungal therapy for recurrent yeast.

Remember (from Chapter 9) that a yeast culture is done on a special medium called Sabouraud's medium; this is different from a vaginal culture for bacteria. Routine bacterial cultures are seldom helpful because they grow a lot of bacteria that are normally found in the vagina: strep, staph, gardnerella, and *E. coli*.

Remember too that simply looking through the vaginal speculum at the vaginal discharge to diagnose yeast is outdated and inaccurate. Be sure you find a clinician who does a complete exam and is willing to use the yeast culture on Sabouraud's medium as a backup.

There are a number of reasons why yeast may not be seen under the microscope or in a yeast culture:

▼ Microscopy is only about 40 percent accurate.

▼ A woman has been partially treated by using an antifungal cream or taking a Diflucan tablet within a few days of the visit.

▼ The checkup occurs at a time when the woman is not having symptoms.

▼ Yeast is not the cause of the problem; most vulvovaginal problems cause itching and burning.

Trying to arrange an appointment at the time of symptoms can be difficult. Many physicians work with nurse-practitioners, who may have more availability for appointments. If you have the kind of yeast that flares in a cyclic fashion, explain this in order to schedule at the right time.

Self-diagnosing a yeast infection

But wait, you're thinking. *What about those handy tubes of antiyeast cream that I can buy at the supermarket?* As you can see, yeast is a complicated problem. Without previous diagnosis in a clinical setting or a thorough education about the many faces of yeast, attempts at self-diagnosis will likely be inaccurate and will lead to ineffective self-medication. Even when a woman is completely familiar with yeast symptoms and has been treated by a clinician for a prior episode, an accurate diagnosis may still require a vaginal examination, pH determination, yeast culture, and microscopic evaluation of vaginal secretions.

Nevertheless, in 1990, the FDA approved the OTC availability of antifungal products. They're sold under brand names such as Monistat, Gyne-Lotrimin, and Femstat. Almost immediately, sales of these agents went through the roof, from nine million units per year as prescription drugs to twenty-four million units per year as OTC medications. More than $600 million in sales was recorded in 2000.[34]

Clearly, women love the convenience and sense of control that these products provide. And I'll be the first to acknowledge that a quick fix is terrific—*when it is the right one.* Unfortunately, this is often not the case. The FDA allowed OTC antifungal products based on research that is misleading when applied to the overall population of women who may self-diagnose and self-medicate. The women in the studies reviewed by the FDA were prone to yeast infections but had been carefully educated about the symptoms of other vulvovaginal conditions. Almost two-thirds of them correctly self-diagnosed yeast infections based on their symptoms, compared with four-fifths of the clinicians in the study. When the test population was limited to women who had had a prior clinical diagnosis of yeast, four-fifths were able to diagnose their problems accurately.[35] The rub: This level of knowledge is not representative of the women who are using the products now.

Other studies have shown less impressive results. One found that although the majority of women thought yeast was the cause of their symptoms, only about a quarter of them were correct. Instead, bacterial vaginosis, vulvar vestibulitis, and irritant dermatitis were their problems in almost half of those cases.[36] In another study, only 11 percent of

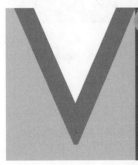

VOICES

"The first time I used a yeast cream, I was so anxious for relief that I used it in the middle of the day. What a mistake—it felt like it was running out of me all day, and I had to change my underwear and use a thick pad. After that I did it right before bed so I could be horizontal while the stuff worked!"

—April, 24

women who did not have a prior diagnosis of yeast were able to self-diagnose correctly. Of women who had previously been diagnosed with yeast, the rate of accuracy increased, but only to 34.5 percent.[37]

You can see why vulvar disease experts, including me, were aghast when the FDA approved OTC cream. Obviously it's difficult for women to figure out what's behind their vulvovaginal symptoms. As a result, over-the-counter products are being used inappropriately part of the time; women do not know about all the other conditions that may produce irritation, discharge, or itching. With self-misdiagnosis they experience prolonged discomfort or complications associated with their complaint. Millions of dollars are wasted by women trying to treat lichen sclerosus, vulvodynia, precancerous skin changes, and chlamydia with antifungal cream. Some of the complications may be serious if an STD or pelvic infection is missed, or if a urinary tract infection worsens, or if an inflammatory skin disease goes undetected. Remember, even professional medical people may find the diagnosis of yeast challenging.

So what's a woman to do when she needs help? I hope that highly accurate home tests for diagnosis will be available soon. In the meantime, women need to be educated not to rely on clinicians who diagnose over the phone, without doing an exam, or by looking through the speculum only. Women need to find a clinician who does basic simple tests: exam, pH, wet prep, and whiff test. Remember, if itching is present and yeast is not seen under the microscope, then a yeast culture on Sabouraud's medium is important.

Yes, self-treatment is faster and less expensive than making a doctor's appointment. That's why women like it. Unfortunately, it's just not the right course of action as often as most women would like it to be.

A yeast infection action plan

If you are having V symptoms that you think are an isolated or occasional yeast infection, here is an approach:

COMMON QUESTIONS: OTC yeast treatments

Q   What's the difference between the one-day, three-day, and seven-day courses of treatment?

A   We're a speed-up, faster-faster country that favors convenience and quick results. As a result, the marketing world has come up with far more choices than we need for many products—including over-the-counter antifungals. They come in suppositories, creams, and lozenges (tablets that dissolve in the vagina). There

COMMON QUESTIONS: OTC yeast treatments   cont.

has also been a major trend toward shorter treatment courses with progressively higher antifungal doses. The three-day course is a 2 percent cream, for example, while the seven-day is 1 percent. This has culminated in the one-day suppository and the prescription-only single-dose Diflucan tablet, which have enough strength to do the job in a single treatment.

It doesn't matter which you choose if you have an occasional simple, uncomplicated yeast infection. They all work beautifully. The higher doses are more convenient and less messy and may relieve symptoms a little faster. You should feel relief within two to three days, though you may not feel completely perfect for a week to ten days. Note that the one-day dosages do not mean that you will be cured in one day. (Many women fail to realize this, and complain that the medication "isn't working.") Finally, just as there are those who prefer classic Coke, there are those who prefer seven-day yeast treatments, and that's fine.

But here's the crucial caveat: The OTC options are not for you if your yeast infections are repetitive, or if you are plagued by the same symptoms again and again (in this case you may not have a yeast infection at all). But even if you have diagnosed yourself correctly, not all yeast infections are alike, especially when they are not isolated events. There are different strains that are more aggressive, different numbers of organisms at work, and involvement of different areas. There are also immune system factors to consider, as well as how long it's been since the last infection. You need a clinician to help steer your treatment.

Q How do these creams work to control yeast infections?

A They interfere with the biochemistry of the yeast's cell wall formation; without the wall the organism cannot live. No antifungal, including the new Diflucan, actually kills off all the yeast. They just reduce the numbers. For women with normal protective vaginal immune systems, this is enough to resolve an isolated yeast infection. The vaginal police clear up the rest of the culprits, and you become symptom-free again. At the other end of the spectrum are women who (we think) are probably genetically programmed to have impaired protective vaginal immune systems, so that weeks of treatment with the cream are not enough to stave off eventual recurrence. In between are women who recur because of antibiotics and a variety of other reasons.

Q Can I have intercourse during treatment?

A Intercourse is never recommended for a woman who is red, inflamed, swollen, and tender. When you are symptomatically comfortable again, it is okay. Some OTC products impair the proper functioning of latex condoms and diaphragms, so if you normally rely on one of these methods, you'll want to use backup birth control. Nor should you use contraceptive foams or jellies while being treated.

Q Can I use OTC cream while I'm pregnant?

A Sometimes they are recommended for use in pregnancy, but you should consult your clinician first and use them only under his/her care.

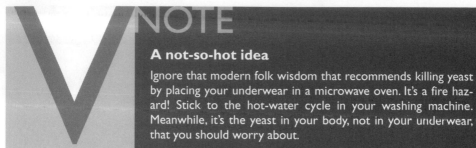

A not-so-hot idea

Ignore that modern folk wisdom that recommends killing yeast by placing your underwear in a microwave oven. It's a fire hazard! Stick to the hot-water cycle in your washing machine. Meanwhile, it's the yeast in your body, not in your underwear, that you should worry about.

1. First, don't be hasty. Don't assume all V symptoms are a yeast infection. Don't automatically purchase OTC cream for an itch. Review Chapter 7, "The Most Bothersome Symptoms," to see if anything else fits.

2. See a clinician if this is your first episode of persistent V symptoms, you are pregnant, you are 13 years old or younger, you have had more than three episodes this year, you have diabetes or HIV, or you take cortisone by mouth.

3. Choose an OTC antifungal cream for yeast if you have had prior yeast infections clearly diagnosed by a clinician and if you got prompt, total, and lasting relief from antiyeast cream. Yeast is easy to cure in most cases; symptoms that persist may not be yeast.

4. If you use an OTC product and your symptoms do not improve in three days or are not gone in seven, see a clinician. Don't bother trying another brand or strength. Choose your care provider carefully; many will merely hand out more cream. You need someone who will check for other kinds of vaginitis, do a culture for resistant yeast, and evaluate for skin diseases and vulvodynia.

Steps to controlling recurrent yeast

1. *Get confirmation.* If you think you have repeated yeast infections, it is essential to confirm this by being seen by a clinician at the time the symptoms flare to prove this is yeast. Just because you have had several episodes of yeast in the past year does not necessarily mean your current itching represents another yeast infection. You might be reacting to the ingredients in all the antiyeast creams you have used. Or maybe you are irritated from wearing a panty liner every day. You need proof that you have yeast, and you need identification of the species of yeast that you have.

2. *Reduce the risk factors.* If you have repeated yeast infections, eliminate factors that are known to contribute to yeast. Controlling blood sugar in a diabetic, eliminating antibiotics, or bringing a chronic skin condition un-

NATURAL REMEDIES

I wish I had better news about alternative approaches to V problems. Herbals have been around forever and are enjoying a high profile these days. Certainly modern medicine doesn't have all the answers. I encourage my patients to bring in anything that has helped them; I've amassed a substantial collection of products.

Unfortunately, the story that goes with them is always the same: They worked for a short period of time but that was it. "Dr. Stewart, this Yeast-Out is marvelous. It worked perfectly for three months, but today I'm itching again. What do you think the problem is?" Sometimes I find a different problem, but often the yeast is back.

At this time I don't know of any herbal that consistently works as well as the antiyeast creams and oral Diflucan. I sound like a broken record, but if these antifungals are not working for you, you may not have yeast.

I eagerly await the day when there's better research to sort out reliable remedies from useless ones. This is no small problem since many herbs are used in combination but are being studied singly. In the meantime, it breaks my heart to see women spending huge amounts of money on remedies that do not work. And because they're unregulated, there aren't any controls over what goes into the container; it may be 100 percent of the herb you want or it may be only 10 percent, with worthless fillers or possibly harmful ingredients to make up the difference. And the manufacturer is allowed to make claims about its powers that are not based on scientific study.

Here's an example of the challenges faced in finding worthwhile alternative products. At the 1999 meeting of the International Society for the Study of Vulvovaginal Disease, clinicians from all over the world who are interested in V problems were fascinated by the presentation from a Portuguese colleague who had studied the antiyeast effect of eight essential plant oils against candida. Tea tree oil had no value at all. Thyme, rose, and clove were very active against yeast, and others had intermediate effects. After the presentation, I flew across the auditorium to find out how I could use oil of thyme in Boston for my yeast patients. The answer was very clear: Undiluted essential oils are highly irritating to human tissues. The concentration of oil required hasn't been figured out, and a way to deliver the oil safely and comfortably into the vagina has to be developed. What's more, no standardization of oil quality exists—so the product itself depends on the type of thyme plant and the method of extraction. Big things need to be figured out before a doctor like me can make this promising research of any use to a patient like you.

The same situation is true of garlic, another natural substance that patients often ask me about. Its active natural ingredient inhibits the growth of some bacteria and candida in the lab. But no one knows yet if it's effective in women's vaginas and no one has developed a way of delivering the highly irritating garlic oil to the vagina.

The only natural remedy for yeast that I know works and is medically proven is boric acid. (See page 217.)

der control are examples of areas that may need work. But remember that sometimes there are no risk factors at fault; yeast may come because the vaginal police are off duty for some unknown reason.

3. *Look at your diet.* The *only* scientific nutritional study done in women

SIMPLE YEAST OR COMPLEX YEAST?

When planning a yeast treatment, I have to decide whether this is a simple case of yeast or a complicated one. Thinking about yeast in this fashion is new. Clinicians have traditionally regarded all yeast as the same, but over the years we have learned how many different forms it can take. No single treatment is suitable for all women with yeast. Simple cases of yeast need limited treatment, but complicated cases require prolonged therapy. Fortunately we have a variety of antifungal treatments to use. The following chart shows the differences between uncomplicated and complicated yeast.

	Uncomplicated	Complicated
Severity of symptoms	Mild to moderate	Moderate to severe
Frequency	Isolated, occasional, less than four per year	More than four per year
Woman's state of health	Healthy, not pregnant	Complicating factors: pregnancy, diabetes, immunocompromise, chronic skin disease, resistant yeast, recurrent yeast for many years, vulvodynia
Treatment	Any antifungal therapy will work for simple isolated yeast	Intensive regimens (avoid short courses)—these cases need longer periods of treatment and may require ongoing low-dose treatment to suppress yeast

Source: J. D. Sobel, A comprehensive strategy for managing recurrent VVC, *OBG Management,* Aug. 1998.

with proven yeast infection showed that many were drinking more than a quart of milk a day and more than a quart of sugary cola a day. That's too much! Eliminating sugar and dairy products is not realistic, but a normal balanced diet will put both of those elements under control and is recommended for every part of your health and well-being.

4. *Consider checking your partner.* This is possible by obtaining the yeast culture medium from your clinician, and by placing a cotton swab dipped in your partner's ejaculate into the culture broth (see page 198). You then bring it to the clinician for examination. Eliminate oral sex, or have your partner's mouth and throat cultured for yeast. If you have multiple partners and frequent sex, you may need to work with medication to control yeast.

5. *If all else fails, move on to suppressive medications.* If you've worked with diet and lifestyle changes and you're still having yeast—and you're sure that it's yeast—you'll need to work with suppressive medications.

SHORT-TERM TREATMENT FOR UNCOMPLICATED YEAST

Topical Medications	Formulation	Dosage Regimen
Butoconazole (Femstat)	2% cream	5 g per day for 3 days
Clotrimazole (Gyne-Lotrimin)	1% cream 100 mg vaginal tablet 100 mg vaginal tablet 500 mg vaginal tablet	5 g per day for 7 to 14 days 1 tablet per day for 7 days 2 tablets per day for 3 days 1 tablet, single dose
Miconazole (Monistat)	2% cream	5 g per day for 7 days
Monistat-1	Miconazole nitrate 1,200 mg insert with 2% cream	Use insert once, cream as desired
Monistat-3 (Packaged in 5 different combinations)	Miconazole nitrate 4% cream or 200 mg suppositories	Insert vaginally daily for three days
Monistat-7 (4 different options)	Miconazole nitrate 2% cream or 100 mg suppositories	Insert vaginally daily for seven days
Tioconazole (Monistat 1-day, formerly marketed as Monistat-1)	6.5% cream	Use insert once
Econazole	150 mg vaginal tablet	1 tablet per day for 3 days
Fenticonazole	2% cream	5 g per day for 7 days
Terconazole (Terazol)	0.4% cream 0.8% cream 80 mg vaginal suppository	5 g per day for 7 days 5 g per day for 3 days 1 suppository per day for 3 days
Nystatin	100,000 units vaginal tablet	1 tablet per day for 14 days
Oral Medications	**Formulation**	**Dosage Regimen**
Ketoconazole (Nizoral)	200 mg tablet	One tablet twice a day for 5 days
Itraconazole (Sporanox)	200 mg capsule 200 mg capsule	One capsule twice a day for 1 day One capsule daily for 3 days
Fluconazole (Diflucan)	150 mg	Single dose

Source: J. D. Sobel, S. F. Faro, R. W. Force, et al., Vulvovaginal candidiasis: epidemiologic, diagnostic, and therapeutic considerations, *Am J Obstet Gynecol* 1998: 178:203–11.

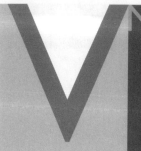

NOTE

Don't bother to try them all

It's important to recognize that all of the over-the counter and prescription azoles are virtually the same; they work only against *Candida albicans*. If one doesn't work, changing to another is like switching brands of aspirin.

Early treatment for yeast infection utilized Nystatin; while still available and still used, Nystatin has been largely overtaken by a generally more effective family of creams and suppositories, the azoles, so called because they all have a similar molecular design. The azoles include butoconazole (Femstat), clotrimazole (Gyne-Lotrimin), miconazole (Monistat-3, Monistat-7), econazole, fenticonazole, and tioconazole (Monistat-1). Recently that design was redone, producing terconazole (Terazol), reported to be more effective. Finally, in the 1980s and 1990s we started to have oral medications against yeast: ketoconazole (Nizoral), fluconazole (Diflucan), and itraconazole (Sporanox).

The azoles need high doses and extended treatment to eradicate *Candida glabrata* or other non-albicans species. These yeasts have changed themselves (mutated) so that they respond poorly to the azoles. The triazole Terazol is effective against non-albicans yeast.

Treatment for uncomplicated yeast can be either topical, by cream or suppository, or single-dose oral therapy. All of the treatments work against the standard cause of yeast infection, *Candida albicans*. Drug resistance of albicans yeast is extremely rare, with only two or three cases recorded in the world.[38] If symptoms do not improve, a yeast culture becomes vital, because the non-albicans yeast, such as *Candida glabrata* or *Candida tropicalis,* usually will not respond to the standard treatment length.

Complicated yeast

Women with complicated yeast infections need a longer course of therapy no matter how the medication is given. Conventional five- and seven-day therapy should be increased to ten to fourteen days to achieve no more symptoms and negative culture. More than one dose of oral Diflucan is needed. The initial outbreak is controlled with 150 mg of Diflucan every other day for three doses, followed by one tablet weekly for a few weeks to suppress yeast and keep it out of the picture. For women with yeast that has recurred for years, the suppression may be safely continued for up to six months. The earlier oral antifungal drugs such as ketoconazole had the risk of possible liver damage and required careful monitoring of liver function. Fortunately Diflucan, given in weekly doses, appears safe and does not require liver monitoring.

When the vulva is severely inflamed, women need special consideration. The usual creams may not be enough and may, in fact, make the burning worse. The oral medications fail to provide immediate relief. Such patients need to start oral antifungals and pursue a variety of additional remedies: sitz baths, cool compresses or ice, low-potency hydrocortisone ointment. Oral Diflucan can take three to seven days to bring complete relief.

Dealing with a resistant yeast such as *Candida glabrata* can be frustrating for both patient and clinician. Some infections can take months to respond to treatment. Studies show that most non-albicans yeast will respond to conventional therapy with azoles provided that the treatment is given an adequate length of time.[39] One to two weeks of oral and topical azole therapy—Diflucan combined with Gyne Lotrimin, for example—is the first step. If azole therapy fails, as is often the case, the next step is to use boric acid.

Boric acid is an agent that has been around since the days of the pharaohs. Little has been written about it for the treatment of yeast infections, probably because we have many effective modern antifungal agents. Yet boric acid is a very effective antifungal, particularly in the treatment of non-albicans yeast such as *C. glabrata,* where it cured about 70 percent of women in one study.[40] In another study boric acid was effective in curing 98 percent of the patients with culture-proven yeast infections that had failed to respond to the most commonly used antifungal agents.[41] Boric acid 600 mg capsules are inserted vaginally one or two times daily for fourteen days. These capsules have to be made up by a pharmacist. With this dose, systemic absorption of boric acid from

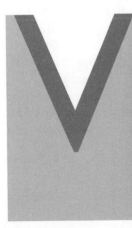

Douche not

A vinegar douche is of no value as a treatment for yeast. Making the vagina acidic will not ward off yeast, since it can grow in an acidic or an alkaline environment. Douching makes a woman feel good for a short period of time, but like mouthwash, its effects are quickly gone. Douching also carries the risk of pushing bacteria up the genital tract to cause possible infection. Nor should you douche with iodine or peroxide; these are chemicals that can cause significant contact and allergic reactions—and they're powerless against yeast.

IS THERE A YEAST HIDEOUT?

A once-popular theory that can influence treatment of recurrent yeast seems to be riding into the sunset. Some researchers have suspected that yeast may have a place in the body where it holes up its troops between attacks (called a *reservoir*). Periodically, small posses of yeast are thought to be released to wreak havoc, then retreat again. For many years, the gastrointestinal tract was pinpointed as this reservoir from which women were reinfected. This belief grew because rectal cultures from women with recurrent yeast often yielded candida. Actually, the rectal cultures were positive because the area is contaminated with yeast from vaginal discharge. The theory has also been discredited by therapy with oral Nystatin; months of this antifungal taken by mouth will not prevent yeast vaginitis.[45] Unfortunately, many clinicians are still testing and treating women based on the intestinal reservoir theory.

the vagina is minimal, but compliance is a drawback with the two-week treatment period.[42]

Boric acid has to be used as directed. It is not to be taken by mouth; the capsules must be kept out of reach of children. Its safety in pregnancy has not been studied, and so its use in pregnancy is not recommended. High dosages can lead to severe burns. It is absorbed through damaged skin and wounds but does not penetrate intact skin. When used vaginally, it stays there and does not travel through the body.[43] When boric acid fails, flucytosine (Ancobon) cream or amphotericin cream may be used for a fourteen-day regimen. These are antifungals that are not commonly used, so they have to be made up by a special compounding pharmacy.

When all else has failed against *Candida glabrata,* terbinafine (Lamisil), a new drug out for the treatment of the fungus that invades nails, is occasionally used; it may work, not because it is a great treatment for *C. glabrata* but because it is a new molecular structure that the yeast has not yet encountered.

Prolonged use of azole creams or Diflucan in daily doses over a period of weeks has an unfortunate side effect. *Candida glabrata* and other yeast can develop in a situation where all the standard albicans yeast has been eliminated by azole therapy, leaving the resistant forms to overgrow. Here is another important reason to be sure that the problem is yeast before taking these medications: Week after week of using an antifungal cream or popping a Diflucan every few days brings the risk of developing a persistent yeast infection that can take months and months of therapy to treat.

Finally, yeast-allergy shots (immunotherapy) have been used to treat difficult recurrent yeast with significant reduction in the number of relapses.[44] Weekly injections of candida extract are given for a year, with maintenance booster shots afterward. This is a therapy that is still not widely studied but has potential. You or your gynecologist would need to find an allergist to administer the injections.

▼

CHAPTER 11

BV

The Leading Cause of Vaginal Complaints

Bacterial vaginosis (BV) is the leading cause of vaginal complaints in the United States. Yet millions of women have never heard of it. How can that be? First, BV is often mistaken for a yeast infection. Second, in about half of all cases, it produces no symptoms— you might have it without even being aware of it. Or you might experience symptoms that are mild enough to ignore or "live with."

So is BV anything to be concerned about? While many physicians once believed BV was harmless, mounting evidence shows that *untreated* BV can lead to other health problems. These complications can affect your fertility or lead to premature delivery if you're pregnant. Not least, BV can be a persistent devil, recurring after treatment in up to one-third of patients. That's not to say that a single case of BV is going to torpedo your chances of having a child. But there are good reasons to not take the infection lightly.

BV is one of the best reasons I can think of for thinking twice before you follow popular habit and self-diagnose and self-treat a yeast infection. Your clinician can tell the difference. Like yeast infections, though, even persistent cases of BV can be brought under control.

What is BV?

Bacterial vaginosis is not really an infection. The term *vaginosis* is used to indicate the *lack* of any infection or inflammation. Instead, BV represents an imbalance of the bacteria that live in the vagina. The imbalance occurs

V NOTE

Important distinction

Vaginitis means vaginal infection. *Vaginosis* refers to an abnormal condition in the vagina but not a true vaginal infection.

because the vagina becomes less acidic, and without the acid it's like party time for the resident bacteria—they have an orgy and overrun the place.

BV has been reported to occur in 35 percent of women seen in clinics that treat sexually transmitted diseases, 15 to 20 percent of pregnant women, and 5 to 15 percent of women visiting gynecological clinics.[1] But since it creates no symptoms in half of all women, it's difficult to say how common it is.[2] What's more, BV is persistent—it often keeps coming back after the initial bout has been cleared up.

Signs of BV may vary considerably from one woman to the next. Typical symptoms include an unpleasant, fishy vaginal odor and excessive vaginal discharge that can vary from gray to white and from thin and watery to creamy. The discharge may stain undergarments. Women often report that the odor is bad after sexual intercourse, as semen mixes with vaginal secretions, or increased before menstruation. Mild vaginal itching or burning may sometimes be present, but BV is not a cause of vulvovaginal pain or pain with intercourse. When women have no symptoms, BV is often detected during a routine exam or during the investigation of another problem.[3]

BV has gone by several different medical names in the past. Previously referred to as "nonspecific vaginitis," this condition was first described in

IS IT YEAST OR BV?

While symptoms for these conditions can vary from woman to woman, here's a quick general comparison:

Symptom	Yeast	BV
Odor	Usually none	Strong fishy scent
Discharge	None to watery to thick curds	Thinner, gray to white
Itching	Yes	Mild, if any

1955 by Houston gynecologists Gardner and Dukes.[4] They originally named the bacterial organism most closely associated with the condition *Haemophilus vaginalis;* later the name was changed to *Corynebacterium vaginale.* Now recognized as the only member of a unique genus, it is termed *Gardnerella vaginalis* in recognition of Gardner's observation.

What causes BV?

BV is caused by a loss of the protective acid-producing bacteria known as lactobacilli. These good-guy vaginal bacteria produce the natural disinfectant hydrogen peroxide.[5] Normally, the production of hydrogen peroxide by lactobacilli combines with chlorine that is present in cervical mucus to produce a chemical defense against an overrun of certain bacteria. The combination of these substances is toxic to some of the bacteria found with BV, including gardnerella. The level of hydrogen peroxide available to combine with chlorine in the vagina may influence how susceptible a woman is to BV.[6] When the chemical conditions present when lactobacilli rule the roost disappear or are altered, there is an overgrowth of certain bacterial species. These are primarily an organism called gardnerella and bacteria requiring no oxygen (called *anaerobic*), all of which can be found in low numbers in the healthy vagina. While a lot of medical focus has been on gardnerella, it is those invaders who can do their dirty work with no oxygen around, the anaerobic bacteria, that seem to cause the worst trouble. Women who have been diagnosed with BV have been found to have up to a thousand times more anaerobic bacteria than women without the problem.

The by-products of this resulting oxygen-free bacterial factory include proteins that give a fishy odor to vaginal secretions and raise the pH of the vagina from the normal acidic range (3.5 to 4.5) to problematically high levels (above 5.0).

What triggers this loss of lactobacilli so that bacterial overgrowth leaves them outnumbered by 100 to 1? The exact reasons for this runaway multiplication are not known, but there are some clues.

The most debated risk factor is sex. It doesn't look like BV is a sexually transmitted disease such as gonorrhea, and America's expert advisors on infectious disease, the Centers for Disease Control and Prevention (CDC), do not recommend the treatment of sexual partners. Treatment of sexual partners does not reduce the risk of recurrence of BV.[7] BV is associated with sexual activity, though. Somehow, something that is put into the vagina wipes out the lactobacilli. The exact mechanism isn't yet understood. But without the neighborhood patrol of the friendly bacteria, BV holds a block party for all the less-friendly bacteria in the neighborhood— including any STDs passing through. What sexual activity increases BV? A new partner or multiple partners.[8] Male sexual contacts of women with

BV have been shown to carry similar bacteria.[9] Apparently some men have semen that kills lactobacilli and some do not.[10] Condoms can protect the vaginal lactobacilli from killer semen and prevent this kind of destruction. But condoms are of no value if semen is not harmful to lactobacilli. Currently there are no ways, other than trying a condom to see if BV improves, to see whose semen is toxic and whose isn't. BV can also be found in sexually inactive women and in lesbians.[11] It's also believed that anything introduced into the vagina, such as a sex toy or dildo, can inhibit the lactobacilli.

BV is also related to one's method of birth control. The use of an intrauterine device (IUD) has been associated with a higher rate of BV (20 percent) compared with the rate in women using other means of contraception (6 percent).[12] Women who do not use any form of birth control have also been found to have a higher rate of BV.[13] Once again, the reason for these variations is not known. Some studies report that African American women have twice the incidence of BV compared with white women, although other experts feel there is no racial variation.[14] One study suggested that the higher vaginal pH found in African American women may increase their susceptibility to BV.[15]

Routine douching for hygiene is associated with an increased risk for BV too, because douching kills off the lactobacilli.[16] Don't do it.

Why treatment is important

Even though BV is not an infection, it may lead to other health-related problems if left unchecked. For example, women with BV have an increased rate of abnormal Pap smears, usually mildly abnormal or atypical.[17] BV has been associated with infection in the tubes and ovaries (pelvic inflammatory disease), which can result in infertility.[18] It appears that the bacteria associated with BV can travel through the cervix and ascend to the tubes and ovaries. These bacteria can be found in the upper genital tract of women with acute infection of the tube (salpingitis). On top of this, BV increases a woman's chances of picking up the human immunodeficiency virus (HIV) during intercourse.

Pregnant women are at special risk. Remember that patients with BV have a hundred- to thousandfold increase in the concentration of anaerobic bacteria in the vagina. This large increase in the concentration of potentially harmful bacteria in the vagina increases the chance that, in pregnancy, the bacteria will invade the cervix and the membranes surrounding the amniotic sac cushioning the fetus and cause infection in this bag of waters. Premature rupture of the sac and preterm delivery of low-birth-weight babies have been linked to BV in several studies.[19] One study found that risk for premature rupture of the bag of waters was increased by seven times in women with BV.[20]

If you are pregnant and have BV, be sure to discuss treatment with your clinician. We're not yet sure what works to keep BV from causing prematurity, though there are some leads. For women who have a history of having had a preterm baby, early delivery or early rupture of the bag of waters can be reduced by treating BV with the antibiotic metronidazole (say "metro-NYE-dah-zoll"), trade name Flagyl, taken by mouth.[21] Unfortunately, Flagyl doesn't cut down on premature birth in women who don't have a history of this (and are therefore at low risk for premature birth), so it isn't given automatically to everyone.[22] Because some women have side effects from Flagyl, work has been done to see if another antibiotic, clindamycin, would work. It appears that clindamycin by mouth, but not vaginal clindamycin cream, reduces preterm delivery among women with BV.[23] There are currently some large studies going on to determine which pregnant women need treatment and when.

You should also discuss treatment with your clinician if you have BV and are thinking about getting pregnant or if you are planning any gynecological procedure.

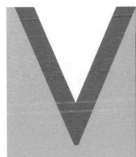

NOTE

Don't waste your money

Over-the-counter creams designed to treat yeast infections do nothing to combat BV. You need to see your clinician for treatment.

Diagnosing BV

Only a clinician can positively identify BV. You might have a strong suspicion of the problem if you have had BV in the past and are familiar with the symptoms, but you'll usually need to see a clinician for treatment. Sometimes, for patients who have been in repeatedly for BV, a clinician may give medications to try to prevent recurrences.

Clinical examination shows a normal-appearing vulva; the vagina is not inflamed and has normal ridges (rugae). To make the diagnosis of BV, the clinician needs to confirm the presence of three out of four diagnostic criteria:

1. Vaginal pH over 4.5. Yeast, in contrast, can grow at any pH. But with BV the pH is always elevated because the pH-lowering, acid-producing lactobacilli have been wiped out.

2. Clue cells (cells from the vaginal wall covered with bacteria) seen under the microscope. Clue cells are unique to BV.

3. Positive whiff test. This happens because of the smell of the proteins produced by the overgrowing bacteria. Yeast causes a negative whiff test.

4. Homogeneous white or gray-white discharge that sticks to the walls of the vagina. In contrast, the classic yeast discharge is curdier and neither grayish nor consistent. Although you can't go by the look of discharge alone, this sign helps nail the diagnosis.

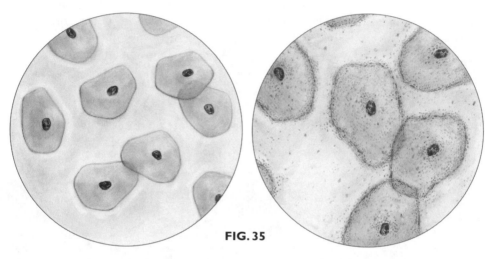

FIG. 35

Normal vaginal cells seen under the microscope.

Clue cells are vaginal cells overgrown with bacteria when a woman has bacterial vaginosis.

Doing a vaginal culture to diagnose BV is not of any value. It's worth repeating: A vaginal culture will *always* grow bacteria that can be interpreted as "infection," when in fact they live there all the time. That includes gardnerella. If your clinician merely did a vaginal culture to diagnose your problem, he or she would not actually be pinpointing the problem. A wet prep is far more useful and cost-effective and is a standard of practice.

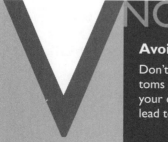

NOTE

Avoid cover-ups

Don't use a feminine spray or douche to self-treat the symptoms of BV or to make yourself smell less awful before you see your clinician. All you'll do is mask the evidence that could help lead to a proper diagnosis.

Treating BV

The good news is that the discharge and odor clear up promptly with treatment—no more BV symptoms. The bad news is that they can come back. No over-the-counter medications for BV exist; your clinician will prescribe a course of treatment, usually based on the CDC recommendations found in the box on page 226. There are two antibiotics that can be taken by mouth for seven days: metronidazole (Flagyl) and clindamycin. Both medications also come in vaginal forms, metronidazole in a gel (MetroGel) and clindamycin in a cream. All four ways of treatment are equally effective, and I use them all, depending on patients' histories and preferences. BV often returns during the month after treatment with the single-dose treatment of Flagyl, which was once very popular.[24] I don't use it as much as the other forms.

Neither Flagyl nor clindamycin is really a "cure" for BV, though. There is no cure at this time. It frequently returns and needs treatment again. Among women treated with Flagyl, 20 to 30 percent will have a recurrence in three months, and some women will have multiple recurrences.[25] It frustrates both patients and clinicians alike that there are no good answers for this problem. Restoring the balance of bacteria in the vagina so the lactobacillus is in control again is the goal. But currently in the United States we do not have a way of adding lactobacilli to the vagina and making them stay there. The most promising work being done now is with the right kind of lactobacillus to repopulate the vagina.[26] Lactobacillus treatment is available in Europe, but to date we can't import the active live bacteria into the United States.

Flagyl and clindamycin are usually well tolerated by women with BV and frequently do not cause any problems at all. Here are a few possibilities to be aware of:

▼ Allergy (itching, rash, hives, swelling, and in severe cases, shock) is possible, though not common. Any medication can cause a headache or upset stomach. Both of these antibiotics can cause yeast infections; women who are prone to yeast may need to use prevention with Diflucan tablets or yeast cream two or three times a week while taking Flagyl or clindamycin.

▼ Flagyl can cause an unpleasant metallic taste in the mouth and must not be combined with alcohol at the risk of intense nausea and vomiting. Flagyl can cause nerve damage in women who have connective tissue disease such as lupus.

▼ Clindamycin can cause diarrhea; this is more likely if it is taken by mouth. If diarrhea is severe, an overgrowth of a bacterium named *Clostridium difficile* can occur. *C. difficile* perpetuates the diarrhea until treated with another antibiotic, usually vancomycin.

TREATMENTS FOR BACTERIAL VAGINOSIS	
Standard Treatment	
Metronidazole (Flagyl)	500 mg orally twice a day for 7 days
Metronidazole gel (0.75%) (MetroGel)	5 g intravaginally twice a day for 5 days
Clindamycin	300 mg orally twice a day for 7 days
Clindamycin cream (2%)	5 g intravaginally at bedtime for 7 days
Alternative Treatment	
Metronidazole	Single 2 g dose
Low-Risk Pregnancy	
Metronidazole gel (0.75%)	5 g intravaginally twice a day for 5 days
Clindamycin	300 mg orally twice a day for 7 days
Metronidazole	250 mg orally three times a day for 7 days *or* a single 2 g dose
High-Risk Pregnancy	
Clindamycin	300 mg orally twice a day for 7 days
Metronidazole	250 mg orally three times a day for 7 days *or* a single 2 g dose

▼ A possible, but not common, side effect of MetroGel is an overgrowth of the bacterium *mobiluncus,* described in detail in Chapter 13. This glistening white, yogurtlike discharge is often mistaken for yeast, but of course yeast treatment won't fix it. Clindamycin pills for a week may get rid of it, but sometimes mobiluncus has to be treated with a week of a drug called gentamicin, given intravenously.

When BV recurs

Though most cases of BV clear up following treatment, it's notoriously persistent. One-quarter of women will experience a recurrence within four to six weeks, and up to 80 percent of women with a history of recurrent BV will have it come back again in the year following treatment. Recurrence is equally frequent whether you have taken the oral or the vaginal treatment, or whether you used Flagyl or clindamycin. BV that comes back again and again depresses patients and drives those who want to help them crazy. Prolonged cases make women feel unclean and unattractive. One hopeful thing I can tell you is that researchers have been concentrating on ways to prevent such recurrences.

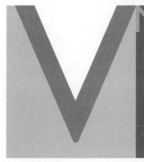

One method is to use a longer treatment period, ten to fourteen days instead of seven. You can use the vaginal form of metronidazole, MetroGel, twice weekly as a successful preventative.[27] This medication comes in a special base that works well in the vagina (carbophil) and has a low pH. Once a woman is stable on weekly dosing, she can try to stretch it to every two weeks, then every three. Sometimes women can remain free of discharge and odor by using the gel on two consecutive days each month. Flagyl given in a 2 g dose by mouth on a monthly basis is also helpful; more frequent dosing with oral Flagyl, though, isn't recommended because of side effects.[28]

During pregnancy, doctors have avoided the use of Flagyl because they worried it might harm the fetus. In 1995, a careful review of several studies found no increase in the risk of malformation from metronidazole given in the first trimester of pregnancy.[29] Nevertheless, many clinicians still prefer to use clindamycin; it must be used in the oral form, as the cream does not prevent premature labor.[30]

Treating sexual partners has no effect and is not recommended.

Another method being studied is the use of boric acid capsules. In Chapter 10, I noted that they are a great treatment for yeast. Boric acid also has a strong antibacterial action that can wipe out the hallmark overgrowth of BV. Unfortunately, for now this treatment involves sticking in a vaginal capsule (600 mg) two or three times a week. If you stop, the BV may come back.

NOTE

Vitamin V

A microbicide now being tested on women with BV is a vaginal suppository containing the protective *Lactobacillus crispatus*, which makes the vagina more acidic.

Some patients with persistent BV find the over-the-counter product Replens helpful. Replens is a vaginal acidifier containing lactic acid; it's used to moisturize the vagina. Other women tell me, however, that after a time they develop vaginal secretions that are like white cotton wool. I think this reaction comes from the chemicals in the base that Replens is made of; it's harmless and goes away when you stop using the product. Another acidifier called Aci-jel, which contains acetic acid, has not been helpful in prevention of BV, though.[31] Lactic acid is naturally found in the vagina, and acetic acid is not. A variety of other drugs that have been tried—ampicillin, doxycycline, triple sulfa cream—are not helpful.

Certainly BV is more than the nuisance condition it was formerly thought to be. But the fact that the serious risks of BV are coming to light has a silver lining: There's a certain urgency in the medical community to understand BV more fully, and to work on better diagnosis and treatment of it.

Don't be unduly alarmed if you receive this diagnosis. Yes, complications such as premature births are statistically associated with BV, but this doesn't mean that you as an individual are doomed to experience them. Also, although I've emphasized the recurrent nature of the problem, remember that BV does clear up for more women than not. What's more, even if you're stuck with recurrent BV, there are many ways, as I've discussed, to keep the annoying symptoms in check. This idea of suppressive therapy is relatively new among clinicians. If BV is a problem for you, please work to find someone who'll help you bring it under control.

▼

CHAPTER 12

Trich

The STD That Causes Vaginitis

Although it lacks the familiarity of yeast or the spotlight status of BV, trichomonas (say "TRICK-oh-MOAN-as") completes the triumvirate of the most common causes of vaginitis. Of this big three, trich has been identified the longest, so it's quite familiar to clinicians. Easily and completely treated, it's traditionally been considered a nuisance condition. In recent years, though, trich has been found to play a role in early rupture of a pregnant woman's bag of waters, preterm labor, and low birth weight, as well as the transmission of HIV, raising its profile from ho-hum bug to subject worthy of new research.[1]

Although the usual vaginitis symptoms may send you to your doctor for diagnosis, it's more likely that a routine checkup or testing for some other problem will turn up trich before you suspect a thing. Trich likes to lurk. It can hang out without causing any symptoms and is often found by happenstance.

Unlike yeast and BV, trichomonas is considered a sexually transmitted disease (STD), meaning that sexual intercourse is the only important way a woman can get it. While trich infects both sexes, most of the cases occur in young white women.[2] African Americans are frequently affected too.

What is trich?

Trichomonas is not caused by a bacterium, as is BV, or by a fungus, as with yeast infections; it is a tiny one-celled parasite called a protozoan. This is a pest with a historical pedigree: *Trichomonas vaginalis* was first reported as a

Young love

You can get trich at any age, but 16- to-35-year-olds seem most vulnerable. At peak risk: teenagers with multiple sexual partners.

cause of vaginitis in 1836 in France.[3] Because most women and virtually all men with the organisms felt no symptoms, however, it was questioned whether the protozoan could be causing disease. By 1916, a German physician proved that link, demonstrating that by eliminating the parasite one could cure the vaginitis, but little more was done to help people with this problem until 1943, when a way to grow the organism in culture was invented.[4] Once an organism can be grown in the lab, you can do all kinds of studies on the road to a cure. And indeed, researchers found in 1959 that metronidazole (Flagyl), the same medication that works against BV, kills the organism.[5] Finally there was an effective way to wipe out a trich infection— once it was detected, that is. But to this day detecting trichomonas remains a problem, as you'll see.

The trichomonas organism, called a trichomonad, is slightly larger than a white blood cell and moves rapidly because of five whiplike structures called flagellae on its edges. This vigorous motion damages cells and can cause a red appearance in the vagina.[6] Other symptoms include vaginal discharge that may vary from scant to profuse and may cause itching and odor. In addition, a woman with trich may have discom-

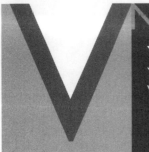

FIG. 36

Trichomonads are one-celled protozoans that swim by means of their flagellae. They are always seen with many white blood cells.

fort passing urine and mild discomfort having sexual intercourse. These symptoms may worsen after a menstrual period. The period between when trichomonads enter the vagina and when they produce disease can range from three to twenty-one days.

But different strains of trichomonas exist, and these can vary in their ability to cause disease. Up to half of women may have a mild strain that gives no symptoms. About a third of infected women develop symptoms if they receive no therapy and the infection persists untreated for six months.[7]

Trichomonas thrives in the oxygen-free environment of the vagina; it also does well in a wide acid-base range (pH 3.5 to 8.0). Trichomonas generates hydrogen, which combines with oxygen, removing oxygen from the vaginal environment. This may promote the growth of other bacteria that can live without oxygen and explains why BV is often seen with trich.[8] Because the trichomonads swim so actively, they can carry other bacteria from the vagina through the cervix and uterus and up to the tubes.[9] You can see why organisms from the vagina can cause problems far beyond the Vs.

The sexual transmission usually works like this: Because the parasite rarely causes symptoms in men, a man may not know he has it and therefore does not get any treatment. Then he infects his partner. If the woman receives treatment and the man does not, he can reinfect her. Some women can be infected for months or years, as the infection is passed back and forth between her and her sexual partner. For this reason, both sexual partners must be treated at the same time, even if they are in a monogamous relationship.

A unique feature of trich is its ability to live on in the vagina for years if it is not treated. This ability explains how a woman who has not been sexually active for some time could be found to have trich—even at an advanced age!

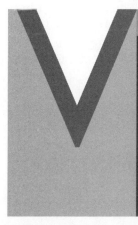

V NOTE

More ways to get it

The *Trichomonas vaginalis* protozoan has been found in hot tubs, tap water, and poorly chlorinated swimming pools. It can survive for about forty-eight hours in vaginal secretions on damp towels and clothing such as bathing suits used by infected women. Contracting trich these ways is uncommon, though, because trichomonas heavily favors living and growing in the vagina.

Source: M. F. Rein, M. Muller, *Trichomonas vaginalis*, in *Sexually transmitted diseases*, K. K. Holmes, P.-A. Mardh, P. F. Sparling, P. J. Weisner, eds. (New York: McGraw-Hill, 1984), 525–36.

Diagnosing trich

You can't diagnose yourself, since the trichomonads have to be identified under the microscope. Nor can a clinician make the diagnosis on the basis of a woman's complaints or what is seen through the speculum alone. The old medical "truisms" about trich don't necessarily hold true any more than the old saws about yeast infections do. For example, I was taught that the classic discharge associated with trichomonas is green, frothy, and foul-smelling. This is actually found in fewer than 10 percent of infected women with symptoms. The nature of the discharge depends on what

> "I've had this awful discharge for two years. It stains my underwear and causes itching and irritation. Sex hurts. My gynecologist found lots of white blood cells in the vaginal fluid and treated me for trich. I found out that's something you get by having sex. Harvey and I have been married for forty years! And anyway, the drug the doctor gave me, Flagyl, did nothing! Do I still have trich? Is it possible Harvey has been seeing someone else? Why doesn't this clear up? What's the matter with me?"
>
> —Celine, 64, who in fact never had trich; she had desquamative inflammatory vaginitis (see Chapter 13)

other bacteria are present with the trichomonas; if BV is present, there may be increased amounts of discharge and odor, though still not necessarily green and frothy. Another reported classic finding is strawberry spots, small red inflamed areas on the cervix. Fewer than 10 percent of women have these.[10] Typically, the vaginal walls are only mildly inflamed.

To accurately diagnose trich, the vaginal pH should be measured; it is always elevated, usually 6.0 to 7.0. The whiff test will be positive in three-quarters of women with trich. The wet prep, the traditional test relied on by most clinicians, will show many white blood cells, and 60 to 75 percent of the time it will also reveal the telltale trichomonads swimming around by means of their flagellae.[11]

If trichomonas isn't seen on a patient's wet prep but she has a troublesome discharge with elevated pH and many white blood cells were seen on the wet prep, culturing is the next step. A culture is the most accurate way to diagnose trichomonas. It's not routinely used, since the simpler wet prep is reliable in a large proportion of cases. Most doctors' offices do not keep the culture media on hand. The technique is expensive and takes three to seven days for results. The culture can be done using Diamond's medium, a special liquid that allows growth of the organism so that it can be seen on a wet mount. In a newer method, the clinician swirls a swab with vaginal fluid in a pouch containing soy broth. The pouch is refolded and sealed to allow the trichomonads, if they're there, to enjoy a broth meal and grow big and strong in the lab. If a culture is negative, that's up to a 95 percent assurance that you do not have trich.

Because trichomonas is so frequently symptomless, though, many women don't even know they have it. Often it's discovered as a lucky break, during routine exams or treatment for other things. Some experts suggest that a wet prep should be done on all sexually active women having a speculum examination; most primary-care clinicians don't routinely do them because of the time involved and because relatively few cases are found in low-risk

WHEN A PAP SMEAR FINDS TRICH

Trichomonads are sometimes reported on Pap smears; the diagnosis should *always* be confirmed by wet prep or culture prior to treatment, however, since some vaginal cells could look like trichomonads. The Pap could be wrong.

I got a call recently from a gynecology colleague of mine. "I'm in a really sticky situation here," he moaned. "A patient has come to me for a second opinion. Her Pap came back reporting trich, so her internist told her she had a trich infection and needed treatment. She's been monogamous for thirty years, she has no symptoms, and she's off the wall! What am I going to do?"

"Did her internist do a wet prep?" I wanted to know.

"No, he just had his nurse call her to tell her to go to the pharmacy for Flagyl. So I had her come in for an exam and a wet prep and I can't find anything—no white cells, no trich, nothing!"

So I suggested he do a culture for trichomonas, which proved negative, and everyone lived happily ever after.

populations. This could change as more is learned about trich's potential complications, such as its link to premature delivery.

In Chapter 9, I encouraged all women who have a V problem to ask for a pH analysis, a wet prep, and a whiff test. And if you are sexually active and without symptoms, it wouldn't hurt to ask for a wet prep as part of your annual exam—just ask up front so your clinician can plan on it. Remember that if you do end up with trich, it's very treatable. Though complications in pregnancy have been found in women with trich, that doesn't mean that you as an individual will necessarily have them.

Treating trich

Trich infections are treated with metronidazole (Flagyl). It works beautifully. If both partners are treated, cure rates approach 100 percent.[12] While clotrimazole (Gyne-Lotrimin) and the spermicide nonoxynol-9 help to relieve symptoms, they do not eliminate the infection and therefore are not recommended by the FDA.[13]

Both a single oral 2 g dose (four 500 mg tablets) and longer, five- and seven-day oral courses of 250 mg three times daily are effective. The FDA has also approved a 375 mg dose orally twice a day for seven days.[14] Most people prefer to take the single dose and be done with it. Trichomonas can invade the Bartholin's glands and small glands near the urethra; for this reason, topical metronidazole gel is not an appropriate treatment for trichomonas since it does not result in high enough levels of the drug in these areas.

Since infection with one STD is often associated with another STD, evaluation for multiple infections is important too.[15] Tests for gonorrhea,

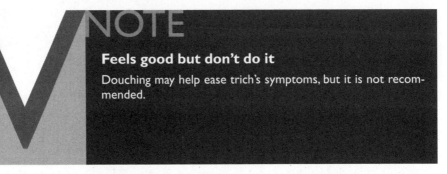

NOTE

Feels good but don't do it
Douching may help ease trich's symptoms, but it is not recommended.

chlamydia, herpes, hepatitis (hep B and C may be spread through sexual contact), and HIV may be done. Treatment is important even when there are no symptoms, in order to prevent transmission to sexual partners, to restore the vagina's normal environment, and to prevent a case of potentially harmful bacterial vaginosis.

Treating trich in pregnancy is particularly important given the infection's frequent link to BV, which can lead to preterm labor and other complications. The CDC advises a 2 g single-dose treatment for women in all trimesters of pregnancy.[16] As we noted in the chapter on BV, treatment used to be postponed until after the first trimester because of concern that metronidazole was harmful to the fetus. But there is no evidence of any such damage. Therefore, the recommendations have been changed.

Treating resistant cases

Once a woman has been treated for trich with metronidazole, the best practice would be to have her come back into the office for a follow-up wet prep to make sure the white blood cells and trichomonads are gone. Sometimes, though, they aren't gone. Or a woman reports ongoing symptoms after treatment. Then what happens?

Most of the time a woman becomes reinfected from a sexual partner with trich who was not treated, or the infection never fully goes away because she did not take the medication as directed. Other medications such as phenobarbital and phenytoin (Dilantin) can interfere with the action of metronidazole and decrease its effectiveness. A follow-up treatment with 2 g of metronidazole daily for five days is the next step. If you have taken all of the drug as directed and your partner has been treated, but you still have symptoms and/or the finding of trich on wet prep, you may have a resistant case of trich. Most strains of trichomonas fall down dead after Flagyl, but there are some strains that do not respond to mighty metronidazole. Fortunately, such resistant strains are rare.

If you took a five-day course of 2 g of metronidazole daily and still have a problem, you will need to have your physician phone the Centers for Disease Control and Prevention (CDC) in Atlanta. Experts there can give advice on the necessary drug for treatment. In the rare event of an allergy to metronidazole, consultants at the CDC can also be of help. Most of the time, however, metronidazole does the job.

▼

CHAPTER 13

Vag Itch, Continued
Lesser-Known Sources of Vaginitis

While **yeast infections, bacterial vaginosis,** and trich account for the majority of cases of vaginitis, they're not the only culprits. The following conditions cause annoying itching, discharge, and dryness too. Some, such as atrophic vaginitis, affect millions of women; others, like those caused by strep or mobiluncus, are much less common. The following descriptions won't help you diagnose and treat yourself, of course. But it's not enough to report unusual discharge or irritation and be told, "You have vaginitis." As I hope I've made clear by now, *vaginitis* is a catchall description, not the diagnosis of one certain kind of problem. It's always important to know what's *causing* your symptoms. If your clinician finds one of the following problems—or is having difficulty pinpointing the cause of your vaginitis symptoms—then you'll find these descriptions useful in understanding what you might be up against.

The estrogen-loss vaginitis: atrophic vaginitis

"What do you mean, I have vaginitis? I thought that after I went through the change I was through with all that!" Charlotte was very upset with me as I delivered the bad news. The characteristic dryness of this condition is a common problem in postmenopausal women. Estrogen cream cleared her symptoms promptly. We made an appointment to discuss the pros and cons of estrogen replacement therapy and alternatives to estrogen.

Vaginal discomfort is often the first sign of approaching menopause. As estrogen decreases in the perimenopausal period (the phase before the actual cessation of periods, which can last several years), the first indication that this is happening may be vaginal dryness and discomfort with intercourse. Long before the hot flashes and the cessation of menstrual periods, the vestibule and vagina may begin to feel like sandpaper.

Most women nowadays can look forward to decades of life after menopause, so we need to know about all the effects of estrogen and lack of it on our bodies and to make plans on how to replace or deal with the absence. As discussed in Chapter 4, without adequate amounts of estrogen in the vagina, the walls thin out and lose their elasticity. Women may complain of a discharge that is watery or sticky and yellow, while at the same time they feel "dry" regardless of whether they are sexually active. Vaginal bleeding, itching, burning, irritation, and painful intercourse may occur as well.

Menopause isn't the only cause of vaginitis caused by a loss of estrogen (atrophic vaginitis), though. It's also common in postpartum women and in women who are breast-feeding. In fact, it can be seen in any woman who doesn't have adequate estrogen. For example, atrophic vaginitis can affect athletes whose low weight and high physical activity level have shut down the central controls of the ovaries, women who have had their ovaries removed, or women whose ovaries are not working properly because of chemotherapy, radiation, or premature menopause. Some medications can also contribute to atrophic vaginitis. For example, leuprolide (Lupron) shuts down ovarian manufacture of estrogen; danocrine (Danazol) acts like a male hormone or androgen. Some low-dose contraceptives or contraceptives containing only progesterone, such as Depo-Provera and Norplant, can have similar effects.[1]

On examination, the vagina looks thin, smooth, and dry, and is light pink to white in appearance. The pH is always elevated at 6.0 to 7.0. A wet mount will show white blood cells, an absence of lactobacilli, and the presence of parabasal cells, vaginal cells that are seen when estrogen levels are low.

The treatment is estrogen added to the vagina. Adequate vaginal estrogen levels can be achieved by taking the hormones by mouth, by using estrogen cream in the vagina, or by vaginal insertion of a ring (Estring) that releases estrogen in small, steady amounts. A low-dose estrogen pill used temporarily is also available. Oral estrogen must be taken nightly; if the uterus is still present (if the woman hasn't had a hysterectomy), a progestin must be taken with the estrogen to protect the uterine lining from thickening too much under the stimulation of estrogen alone. One-half an applicator of Premarin cream or Estrace cream in the vagina at bedtime two to three times a week is usually sufficient to bring comfort. Usually, women need to continue this on an ongoing basis. The estrogen ring is

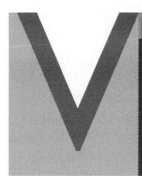

HRT may not be enough

Many people do not realize that it's possible to be taking oral estrogen in hormone replacement therapy and still have inadequate vaginal levels of the hormone. Women taking oral Premarin may still need Premarin vaginal cream or an estrogen intravaginal ring. Increasing the amount of oral estrogen may not help vaginal dryness.

placed in the vagina for a three-month period and then replaced with a new ring.

And now there are estrogens that affect different organs differently. As a woman chooses her hormone replacement, she needs to be sure that it acts in all the areas where she desires estrogen's effects. Originally we had estradiol and estrone, estrogens that worked wherever there are estrogen receptors: the breast, the bone, the uterus, and the vagina. Then along came tamoxifen. Tamoxifen has become well known for its antiestrogenic properties and its use in the treatment of breast cancer. But actually tamoxifen can do a lot of different things, depending on the hormonal status of the woman taking it.[2] In a premenopausal woman, tamoxifen thins out the vagina and it becomes atrophic. But in a postmenopausal woman, tamoxifen acts just like estrogen in the vagina, which becomes thick and elastic with an acidic pH.[3]

Unfortunately, to date there are few substitutes for vaginal estrogen. Lubricants help a little. Some herbs are helpful for hot flashes, but their contribution to vaginal comfort has to be studied. Herbs for which we still need good information include angelica, chaste berry, damiana, licorice, nettle, red clover, saw palmetto, and uva ursi. Dong quai does not produce an estrogen-like response of a thickened vaginal wall.[4] Soy products are also helpful for hot flashes and bone strength but do not cause the necessary increased thickening and elasticity of the vagina that prevent painful intercourse.[5]

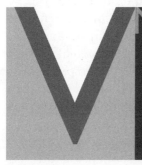

For smoother sex

Intercourse can aggravate the effects of atrophic vaginitis. Estrogen is the best therapy, but don't forget these other assists: use of a lubricant (such as vegetable oil, K-Y jelly, or a made-for-sex product such as Astroglide), lubricated condoms, and plenty of foreplay.

Strep vaginitis

Streptococcus is a problem in the general diagnosis of vulvovaginal complaints because it's always present in the vagina but doesn't always cause problems. A common situation occurs when a woman has some mild irritation, so her clinician does a routine vaginal culture, which shows strep. *This doesn't mean she has strep vaginitis;* rather, the culture has probably grown normal strep inhabitants of the vagina that are *not* responsible for the vaginal irritation. The irritation is probably coming from one of a variety of other causes.

Nevertheless, streptococci sometimes do cause vaginitis. Three kinds of streptococci (group A, group B, and group D) can, usually after use of antibiotics, cause vaginal symptoms. One cause of group D strep vaginitis, for example, is the use of clindamycin to treat bacterial vaginosis (BV).

If you have strep vaginitis, you'll experience vulvovaginal irritation and discharge. You'll have an elevated pH and a wet prep test that shows numerous white blood cells and no lactobacilli. The lactobacilli have been replaced by many small round bacteria, cocci. A culture will identify group A, group B, or group D strep in large numbers. This process is called superinfection—a good example of the balance of the friendly, protective inhabitants of the vagina being upset. An antibiotic taken to wipe out nasty bacteria also gets the healthy lactobacillus, and yeast lurking about seizes the opportunity to take over. In the case of strep vaginitis, you need the antibiotic to conquer the offending strep bacteria, but you need to fend off the yeast (with an antifungal) as well.

This infection must be treated with the antibiotic amoxicillin (500 mg three times a day) for a full ten days. A week of treatment is not enough. And you must use one of the over-the-counter antifungal creams to prevent the growth of yeast as well. A patient named Tina, for example, had BV four times in one year, treated with clindamycin cream. She came to see me when the BV didn't seem to be going away. She did indeed have discharge, and the pH was elevated. But under the microscope, where I expected to see a rioting bunch of bacteria, there were instead just a few strings of pearls—the little round streptococci lined up in chains. Her BV was gone, but strep had overgrown after she used clindamycin to handle the BV. Tina was upset over the prospect of another ten days of antibiotic and not thrilled that, on top of that, I wanted her to take the oral antifungal Diflucan to prevent yeast. She also was using boric acid to prevent the BV from recurring. So she was being given medication for three different kinds of vaginal conditions—BV, strep, and yeast. But in the long run, this was the best solution.

It is extremely important for a clinician to note the difference between strep's normal inhabitation of the vagina and actual strep vaginitis, because the unnecessary use of antibiotics won't help whatever was causing irritation in the first place, and may lead to other problems. In a case of vague vulvovaginal irritation, the discharge is unimpressive; no inflammation will be noted. There is a normal pH; the wet prep will have normal lactobacilli present and white blood cells will not be found in large numbers.

Mobiluncus vaginitis

Another bacterium that normally inhabits the vagina is a curved rod-shaped organism called mobiluncus. It comes in two forms, *Mobiluncus curtisii,* a very small organism, and *Mobiluncus mulieris,* a longer rod. Mobiluncus vaginitis, which is the overgrowth of these bacteria, does not develop out of the blue; it's always the result of using antibiotics that markedly change the bacteria of the vagina, another example of superinfection (described in the strep vaginitis section above). Mobiluncus vaginitis can strike women who have used metronidazole gel to treat bacterial vaginosis.

Symptoms include a profuse white glistening discharge, similar to the sheen and consistency of vanilla yogurt. The discharge may be foul-smelling but relatively nonirritating. Many patients (and many clinicians) mistake it for yeast.

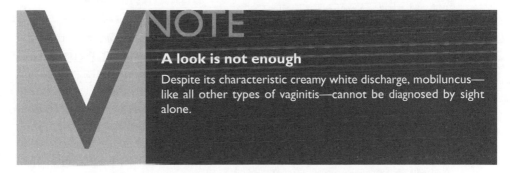

A look is not enough

Despite its characteristic creamy white discharge, mobiluncus—like all other types of vaginitis—cannot be diagnosed by sight alone.

Even with tests, mobiluncus can present a challenge to diagnose because the bacterium is difficult to see with a standard light microscope and it can't be grown in the laboratory.[6] The pH of the vagina is elevated, and a whiff test is positive. The wet prep shows clue cells like those seen in BV and many actively moving curved rods. A special microscope, the phase contrast microscope, is the best way to see the bacteria in a wet prep. With this the clinician can see that the lactobacilli are gone and in their place are many organisms that tumble across the slide rapidly. These may be attached to cells from the vaginal wall, resulting in clue cells with a different appearance.[7] The diagnosis is considered when vaginal discharge is not responding to standard therapy and the clinician suspects that something unusual is going on.

A MOBILUNCUS SUCCESS STORY

"You're telling me I need antibiotics through my veins to get rid of vaginitis?" Grace couldn't believe her ears when I told her she needed Intravenous antibiotics to get rid of her mobiluncus infection. "Can't I have some cream?" She'd had a long struggle with bacterial vaginosis and was treated with metronidazole gel on numerous occasions. The medicine worked and her symptoms would disappear for several months. Recently she had what she was sure was another recurrence, so she called her clinician and received a prescription over the phone. She used the gel for a week. It didn't work—so she got a refill and went another week. Still no help. For a third time, her clinician refilled the prescription over the phone.

By the time she was referred to me, Grace had tried MetroGel for three weeks. By now she was really uncomfortable, with discharge and mild irritation. When I checked her she had profuse discharge and an elevated pH—characteristic of BV—but under the microscope, I saw a lot of yeast as well as mobiluncus tumbling across the slide. She probably had had yeast as her original complaint, but MetroGel does nothing for yeast. And while mobiluncus is not a common problem, it can overgrow, especially after the use of MetroGel. So now she had both yeast and mobiluncus. The only way to clear up mobiluncus is with a drug that can be given only through the veins, gentamicin. With home IV gentamicin treatment for a week, combined with yeast therapy, Grace's problems cleared up. I let her know that if she has any more symptoms, she's to come in for evaluation and a new game plan.

Mobiluncus vaginitis is resistant to metronidazole but may respond to higher and longer doses.[8] It may also respond to clindamycin used orally or vaginally, but this difficult organism may require intravenous ampicillin and gentamicin for a week.

Mobiluncus vaginitis is a good example of the fact that vaginitis is often not a simple problem. Using antibiotics can lead to serious consequences, so one needs to be sure of the diagnosis before using them.

The mystery vaginitis: desquamative inflammatory vaginitis (DIV)

Sometimes women complain of profuse vaginal discharge with inflammation of the vulva and vagina. Clinicians do an examination and see vaginal inflammation intense enough to erode the vaginal wall or cause it to shed cells, or desquamate. Desquamative inflammatory vaginitis (DIV) is a cause of persistent vaginitis often accompanied by painful intercourse that can occur at any stage of reproductive life and after menopause.

Researchers don't agree on what causes this uncommon, intensely inflammatory vaginitis.[9] A leading American vulvar dermatologist, Dr. Peter Lynch, believes DIV might be a form of lichen planus (see Chapter 15), and others have suggested that some cases of DIV may have a link with LP.[10] In 1994, Dr. Jack Sobel, an infectious disease specialist, published a study of fifty-one women with desquamative inflammatory vaginitis who were successfully treated with

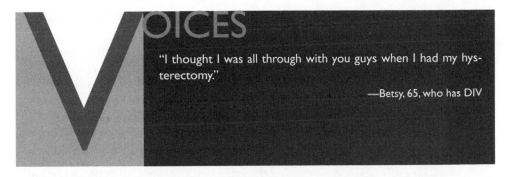

"I thought I was all through with you guys when I had my hysterectomy."

—Betsy, 65, who has DIV

vaginal 2 percent clindamycin. He believes that this unusual vaginitis is probably caused by a bacterial species not yet identified.[11] But antibiotics, the usual defense against bacteria, seem to be of little use against DIV. I have worked with both metronidazole and clindamycin without success.

Since DIV can occur in women during the reproductive years, and since it does not respond to treatment with estrogen, hormone deficiency is an unlikely cause. Infection remains a possible source, but to date no bacterial agent has been identified. It seems clear that some cases of DIV may be due to lichen planus, but more work is needed to make the association clear.

Its hallmark symptom is excessive, puslike, yellow-green discharge that may have been present for years. (Remember, not all women are familiar with what their normal discharge is like, so when there's a change, they don't readily realize it as such, and wind up enduring it for far longer than they might have if they'd reported this symptom right away.) The discharge may be bloodstained. It may be accompanied by vulvar burning, irritation, and itching. Intercourse is often uncomfortable or painful. Few women complain of odor. The vulva and vagina are reddened, and there may be red spots on the cervix. Vaginal adhesions and even scarring of the vagina may develop in cases associated with lichen planus. The pH is elevated above 4.5. The wet mount shows many white blood cells and cells shed from deep in the vaginal wall, parabasal cells. Lactobacilli are absent.

All of these findings except scarring can be seen in patients with atrophic vaginitis. Estrogen is of no value in the treatment of DIV; however, sometimes it's prescribed in order to distinguish DIV from atrophy by the lack of response to estrogen. One of my patients, Fay, 51, for example, had made many gyn visits for her vaginal discharge. It was thick, yellow, and sticky, and had ruined many pairs of underpants. She was beginning to feel pain with intercourse from irritation in the area. Several clinicians said she had atrophic vaginitis, but estrogen cream didn't help at all. Others had blamed yeast or trich. Separately, Fay needed a hysterectomy for fibroids and was told the discharge would go away after surgery. It didn't. After hearing her story, I needed only one look under a microscope to

A DIV SUCCESS STORY

Molly, age 31, came in with several problems: irritation, itching, and profuse discharge. In addition, sexual intercourse, always wonderful before, had become painful to the point that she often had to stop. On exam, she had tenderness in the vestibule all around the vaginal opening. In addition, the vagina was inflamed and tender. The pH was high, and there was a great deal of discharge. Under the microscope, there were many white blood cells that are seen with inflammation, and normal lactobacilli were nowhere to be found. Cultures for yeast and STDs were negative.

It was clear to me that Molly had DIV; with the tenderness she had in the vestibule, I thought she also had secondary vestibulodynia (Chapter 17), which was probably a result of the nerve endings in that area being triggered by all the inflammation associated with DIV.

It took some work to bring both problems under control. Molly used hydrocortisone suppositories for weeks, first nightly, then every other night. At the end of a month, she didn't look that much better, but we kept going. At the end of two months, the discharge and a lot of irritation were gone. Molly was frustrated that sex was still virtually impossible. That was the next project—conquer the pain in the vestibule after the original insult of the vaginal inflammation was gone. We kept the vaginal inflammation under control with hydrocortisone twice weekly and used one of the standard medications for the pain of vestibulodynia, nortriptyline. It took some more time—two or three months—but gradually life has improved for Molly. She maintains her hydrocortisone suppositories twice weekly and is having comfortable sex with 50 mg nortriptyline. We'll try to taper off that if she continues to be stable in another three months.

show me what was wrong: DIV. It took several months to bring the inflammation under control with cortisone, and Fay continues to use a suppository twice a week. But her discharge is now minimal and sex is comfortable again.

If the clinician is not sure of its cause, DIV tends to be difficult to treat and can recur. After much trial and error, what I've found most effective is cortisone as a cream used with an applicator or as a suppository. (I use standard rectal suppositories, which are completely safe for vaginal use. The vagina and the rectum are similar in that they're both cavities lined with mucous membrane.) Suppositories of 100 mg hydrocortisone made up by a compounding pharmacy will usually bring symptoms under control. If you're familiar with cortisone, 100 mg may sound like a lot, but hydrocortisone is the weakest of all cortisone forms. A woman uses one vaginally at bedtime every night for two weeks, then every other night for two weeks, then checks with me to see how things are going. If the inflammation is still moderate, she will need a longer stretch of the every-other-night treatment. Yes, it's a nuisance to put those things in, but they eventually do the job. If you want to have sex, you can—you just put in the suppository afterward. Once things are under control, we work to see what's necessary for maintenance. Some women need a suppository twice a week, while others can taper off eventually. Low levels of estrogen in the vagina that exist after treatment may need treatment with topical estrogen.

The discounted problem: lactobacillus overgrowth

This condition—also known as cytolytic vaginosis—is worth noting because within ten quick years it was discovered, considered an important cause of vaginal irritation, and then debunked. First described by two Boston gynecologists in 1991, this condition of discharge and itching, primarily in the second half of the menstrual cycle, along with some discomfort with intercourse, was thought to be associated with an overgrowth of lactobacilli. The story was this: A woman would have a yeast infection. She'd use yeast cream and not get better, continuing to complain of a slightly itchy discharge. The pH was normal (acidic). Under the microscope could be seen tons of normal lactobacilli. No yeast was seen, and no yeast grew in culture. To deal with what they thought was an overgrowth of lactobacilli, physicians would recommend douching with bicarbonate of soda for three weeks to try to counteract all the acid produced by the lactobacilli. Because under the microscope the cells from the vaginal wall were noted to be breaking apart (cytolysis), it was given the name cytolytic vaginosis.[12]

It now appears, however, that cytolytic vaginosis probably does not exist. Many clinicians recognize a picture of increased discharge in response to multiple vaginal treatments and suggest that this is the normal vaginal response to many therapies. If you just leave the vagina alone for a while, things will calm down. Don't douche. It's not possible to have too many lactobacilli or a vagina that's too acidic. The lactobacilli would kill themselves off if they overgrew and made too much peroxide.[13]

If you are told you have an overgrowth of lactobacillus, you need another opinion. It's possible that your vagina needs time to reequilibrate after multiple treatments. It's possible that yeast is still around but not seen on your wet prep slide. And of course there may be some other cause for your itching and discharge, which would need to be diagnosed and treated.

▼

CHAPTER 14

Could You Be Allergic?

Surprising Irritants That Trigger the Body to Attack

S **ay the word *allergy*** and most people immediately think of ragweed, dust, or cats. Who expects to be allergic to her partner's semen? Sounds more like the punch line to an off-color joke than a medical fact, doesn't it? But it's true—humans can be allergic to a vast range of substances, including semen. And the effects go well beyond sneezing and watery eyes. An allergy that causes vaginal symptoms can come from a reaction to the semen itself, or from a reaction to drugs, foods, or other proteins that come through the semen. Also, allergenic substances can also be introduced into the vagina by the fingers, by latex products, and even by the yeast that causes yeast infections (*Candida albicans*).

The whole idea of allergy connected with vaginal symptoms hasn't been well studied. Little is known about the vaginal immune system or about how the vagina reacts with the body's immune system. But what's abundantly clear is the unpleasant reaction of the women I see who experience such allergies. Fortunately, I can usually help them find some relief.

What is allergy?

Allergy occurs when something from outside the body, usually a protein, is recognized as a foreign substance (an antigen). The body then has an allergic response, manufacturing something to attack the substance and get rid of it (an antibody) or calling up special fighter cells to attack (a process called cell-mediated immunity). The antibody involved in allergic reactions is called IgE.

On a biological level, what happens is this: The foreign antigen protein reacts with the IgE antibodies that are on the surface of cells in the tissue called mast cells. This reaction leads to the release of histamine and other chemicals that cause the allergic symptoms.

What you experience as a result of this chain reaction can vary enormously. The symptoms of a semen allergy differ in type and severity. They include local symptoms of vulvar itching, burning, swelling, redness, and hives. Small blisters on the vulva may develop within hours, and a thin watery vaginal discharge may last for several days. Rarely, a woman may experience major systemic symptoms throughout her body—generalized hives, generalized itching, difficult breathing (bronchospasm), lower abdominal pain, low blood pressure, and loss of consciousness.

Allergy usually develops over time. The body must be exposed to something several times in order to develop the allergic reaction. "But, Dr. Stewart, this didn't happen the other times we made love," or "I've used that product for a long time with no problems," patients will tell me. But that is exactly how allergy develops. If you begin itching immediately after using a product for the first time, this is likely to be contact irritation, not allergy.

The woman with allergic vulvovaginitis often has a personal or family history of allergy, including food allergies.[1] She may experience mild local or systemwide symptoms over a period of months or years before showing the severe reaction known as *anaphylaxis*—difficult breathing, shock, loss of blood pressure, and loss of consciousness. The symptoms may first occur during the initial act of intercourse (really rare), after many experiences of intercourse, or following a change in circumstances, such as after a pregnancy, after gynecological surgery or the insertion of an intrauterine device (IUD), or after a vasectomy or a prostatectomy in the partner.[2] Any of these situations could either change the immunity in the vagina or alter the immune factors in semen.

Allergy to semen

It's a cruel irony that your body should attack your intimate partner (or his semen, anyway) as an enemy. A man's ejaculate contains many antigens, both in the fluid ejaculated (called the seminal plasma) and on the sperm, that can stimulate an allergic response. These symptoms (mainly itching and blisters, as described in the previous section) may begin during intercourse or immediately afterward, within fifteen minutes. They reach their greatest intensity after thirty minutes and can last for days, but usually the symptoms back down after some hours if there is no treatment.[3]

While this unusual allergy is less common than allergies to dogs or cats, more women may suffer from it than has generally been believed.[4] More than thirty cases of allergic shock (anaphylaxis) have been reported in the medical literature.[5] Most women have less dramatic symptoms, however, limited to the V zone. Often, these mild allergic reactions to semen are misdiagnosed as "nonspecific vulvovaginitis." I've seen some patients who were told they had genital herpes (but a herpes culture is negative), or who were treated unsuccessfully for years for yeast.

The problem should be suspected in a woman with a family history of allergy, a family history of vulvovaginal itching during or immediately after sex, and when symptoms improve with the use of a condom or when abstaining from sex.

When allergy to semen—a.k.a. allergic seminal vulvovaginitis—is suspected, evidence of this hypersensitivity can be confirmed by skin testing with dilute fresh seminal plasma. The allergic woman will show an immediate red, raised area of the skin (known as wheal and flare). Other evidence may be obtained by measuring IgE antibodies in the blood or by the radioallergosorbent test (RAST). With RAST, the antigen (seminal plasma) is linked to chemically treated discs that are then treated with the test subject's serum. The amount of IgE antibody that reacts with the antigen can be measured.

For some women, it's not a particular boyfriend or husband who's to blame; semen from different men can produce the same symptoms in a woman, suggesting that the allergy is broader than the individual partner. For these women, there's an allergy to some component of semen in general. And yet the problem often exists only for a short time and may disappear after several years, suggesting that natural desensitization may occur.[6]

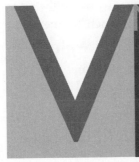

VNOTE

More than morning sickness

In 1945, a physician noted a pregnant woman who consistently experienced acute vomiting following intercourse; this was proved to be allergy-related.

Source: D. W. James, Pernicious vomiting of pregnancy due to sensitivity to semen, *West J Surg Obstet Gynecol* 1945: 53:380.

TREATING SEMEN ALLERGY

The ideal way to treat an allergy is to avoid what's causing it. When it comes to being allergic to semen, though, that means abstinence, and not too many of my patients are willing to go that route! A better option is for the male partner to use a condom—effective but, again, sometimes unacceptable. Note that some women are allergic to the latex in condoms; you may need to use a nonlatex condom to distinguish whether it's the latex or the semen that's the problem. (If conception is desired by a couple who must rely on condoms because of allergy, artificial insemination using sperm washed free of seminal plasma may be done.)

For mild cases, antihistamines taken before sexual activity can relieve vulvovaginitis reactions, although they are of no value in systemwide symptoms (such as itching elsewhere in the body, difficulty breathing, etc.)[7] Benadryl (50 mg) taken one hour before sexual intercourse works well; a nonsteroidal anti-inflammatory drug such as ibuprofen (400 mg) two hours before sexual activity and every four hours afterward on an ongoing basis may help too. Some patients also benefit from the use of an intravaginal antihistamine, 8 percent cromolyn cream.[8]

Desensitization (immunotherapy) by an allergist is an option in more serious cases. Desensitization has been used with varying results, some quite encouraging.[9] Small amounts of dilute seminal plasma are placed into the vagina over a period of several hours. The catch is that to maintain the newly gained immunity, the couple needs to have frequent intercourse, at least every other night. While for some partners this is the best prescription they've ever received from a doctor, I've also seen patients who don't want to take on this much "homework."

Other V allergies

More than the semen itself can be objectionable. Food that a man eats and drugs that he uses can show up in his ejaculate, causing an allergic response in a woman who has sex with him.

A SEMEN ALLERGY SUCCESS STORY

Cynthia had developed uncomfortable itching whenever she had intercourse. She had been with Julian for about three years, and over the past six months she noticed that every time he entered her, she immediately began to itch. With ejaculation, it got worse. Cynthia was no stranger to allergies, since she had many. "Can I possibly be allergic to my boyfriend?" she wanted to know.

She was right. I advised her to try using a condom to see if she still itched. Sure enough, when Julian wore one, Cynthia was fine. Evaluation with an allergist confirmed the diagnosis as semen allergy. Although condoms were a big help, Julian hated them, so the couple tried desensitization therapy. They understood that frequent intercourse was necessary to maintain the allergy-free state. Cynthia had an excellent response and is able to have comfortable, itch-free intercourse about three times a week to maintain her success.

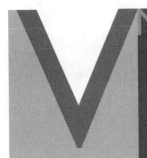

Family ties?

Researchers aren't sure if V allergies are inherited, but there is one report of four women in the same family with allergy-based vulvovaginitis.

Source: T.-W. Chang, Familial allergic seminal vulvovaginitis, *Am J Obstet Gynecol* 1976:126:442–44.

Known allergens include the tranquilizer thioridazine; a drug used in chemotherapy, vinblastine; the antibiotic penicillin; and walnuts.[10]

Allergic vaginitis may also develop when allergens such as pollen, dust, or animal hair get into the vagina by the fingers.[11] Women who have been sensitized to chemicals such as soap and spermicides can develop an allergic response to these products. Sex toys can also be culprits; though many are made from harmless plastic, they can cause symptoms if they are made of latex (see section below) or another substance to which a woman is allergic. If you're really sensitive, you might want to go so far as to find out about the materials by reading the packaging or asking the manufacturer. Stop using the item in question to see if symptoms improve.

Allergens require previous sensitization; often symptoms do not appear until several days or weeks after contact. Then, upon repeated exposures to the product, the woman develops itching, burning, redness, and swelling that last for days or up to three weeks. The pattern of breakout after the use of the product usually gives the diagnosis; avoiding the offending substance provides the cure.

Some women with recurrent yeast infections may also be allergic to the yeast *Candida albicans*.[12] See Chapter 10.

Allergy to latex

One highly allergenic material worth mentioning in more detail is latex. Latex is a substance made from the sap of a rubber tree. So many products are made from latex, you probably encounter it regularly without realizing it.

One of the most common symptoms of latex allergy is contact dermatitis, a rash that occurs on the area of the body where the latex touches the person. For example, contact dermatitis may occur on the hands of a person who wears latex gloves frequently. Or the vagina could develop contact dermatitis from condoms or the diaphragm. Another place it shows up is along the groin where the latex elastic bands of underpants touch the skin.

Latex allergy may show in other ways besides a rash. It's important to

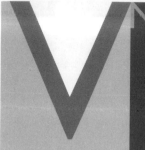

It's everywhere

Everyday products containing latex include some male condoms, diaphragms, rubber bands, dishwashing gloves, hot water bottles, shoe soles, balloons, erasers, toys, sports equipment, and medical devices such as catheters, drains, and tubing.

recognize the early milder symptoms because experts believe that the sensitivity can become more serious over time as a person is repeatedly exposed to latex. Other symptoms of latex allergy include itching, sneezing, runny nose, swelling or itching after medical or dental examinations, facial flushing, hives, shortness of breath, wheezing, rapid breathing, anxiety or confusion, feeling faint, and shock.

Specific red flags: Suspect latex allergy if you have swelling and itching after medical examinations or contact with rubber gloves. Ditto if these symptoms show up on the mouth and lips after blowing up a balloon, having a dental examination, or eating bananas, chestnuts, or avocados, which come from trees that are relatives of the rubber tree. Latex sensitivity may also show up as vaginal or rectal itching or swelling after sexual relations with a condom or diaphragm. An allergy specialist can confirm latex allergy.

Some groups face an increased risk for developing allergy to latex. Health care workers who frequently use latex gloves and touch health care products containing latex are at higher risk than average. People with medical conditions that require frequent procedures or surgery (medical or dental), as well as those who work in the manufacture of products containing latex, are also at higher risk.

Healing hands

Examination gloves in offices and hospitals were traditionally made of latex. But because of the recognition that latex allergy is more common than previously believed, in 1999 the Occupational Safety and Health Administration (OSHA) ruled that latex gloves be replaced by nonlatex synthetic gloves. Nonlatex substitutions for other products is not so easy; only the latex condom protects against STDs and viruses such as hepatitis and the AIDS virus.

Women with rubber latex allergy tend to be susceptible to certain food allergies. Well-known cross-reactive fruits include avocado, banana, chestnut, kiwi, papaya, potato, and peaches. There is also cross-reaction between latex and grass and weed pollen.[13]

Eliminating latex products is the only treatment available. That's generally easy once you know what to watch out for. Lambskin condoms (made from the intestinal lining of lambs) do not contain latex. A type of plastic called polyurethane is used to make a male condom (Avanti) and the female condom (Reality). Researchers believe that polyurethane can be highly effective against STD transmission, but more research is needed before the polyurethane condoms receive permission from the FDA to specify this protection.

THE MYSTERY ALLERGY: HIVES

Hives are itchy raised bumps caused by the release of a chemical named *histamine* from special mast cells in the body. While allergies to food, drugs, and inhaled substances often trigger hives, mast cells can also be stimulated by physical agents as well, where there is no antigen-antibody reaction involved.

Doctors are frequently unable to figure out what causes hives. The most common kind of non-allergy-related hives is dermographism, abnormal raised reddening of the skin (wheals) in response to gentle stroking. Painful intercourse (vulvodynia) is sometimes associated with dermographism.[14] Women with this will get wheals on the skin wherever it is stroked, including the vulva, and also experience vulvar swelling and itching during or after sexual intercourse. No one knows what causes this type of allergy, but antihistamines bring significant relief for this kind of problem.

▼

CHAPTER 15

When Skin Gets Sick

The Vulva Sees These
Skin Conditions Too

You've probably heard about the itchy skin conditions eczema and psoriasis—that is, in connection with other parts of the body, like hands or feet. For some reason no one expects them on the vulva; certainly many clinicians do not look there for them. Yet these skin problems, as well as a few others without such familiar household names, are some of the leading reasons behind discomfort in the vulva.

Last week, for example, Marilyn was in to see me. She'd developed intense vulvar itching, and when she did a self-exam, the area looked very red and scaly. As part of her medical history, she told me that she had psoriasis, with plaques of it on her elbows, knees, and abdomen. Her father and sister had it too. Yet Marilyn was incredulous when I diagnosed psoriasis on her labia: "You mean I have it down there? My doctor never told me that might happen!" Once she began using the same cortisone cream there that she needed for her other skin areas, the itching vanished.

Most skin diseases anywhere are very treatable, and the vulva is no exception. They don't go away completely, however; you have to learn how to manage them on an ongoing basis. Nobody likes to hear that part of the news, unfortunately. What typically happens is that my patients use a cream or ointment until their symptoms go away. Then they stop the treatment. As a result, the symptoms return, convincing the patient that something's awfully wrong. Yet this is simply the way skin diseases behave: They must be chronically managed. Think about it. If you have sensitive skin, it's always sensitive. If you have dry skin, you moisturize on an ongoing basis. If you develop a vulvar skin disease, you need to learn everything possible about it, then work actively to manage it. Once the initial problem is in control, cream once or twice a week may be all that is required.

Cheryl's problems are a good example. She had troublesome itching, with scaling and cracking of the skin of the labia, over the perineum, and even around the anus. She felt constantly irritated and uncomfortable. When intercourse started to be painful, she consulted her gynecologist. He gave her some cortisone cream that helped considerably. But Cheryl had heard bad things about cortisone and did not think she should keep using it. In addition, she was upset by the fact that the cream was just treating her symptoms and not clearing up her problem. When I diagnosed eczema, I explained that a chronic condition is one that never clears entirely. She finally relaxed after we discussed cortisone and she came to understand that it was necessary in small, infrequent doses to keep her skin disease in control.

Partly because vulvar skin conditions can be difficult to diagnose, statistics on how many women are affected don't exist. After I explain the basics about cortisone—the key treatment—this chapter maps out common skin problems, roughly in the order of how often they occur.

What to know about cortisone

Aside from careful hygiene (see box on page 262), the mainstay of treatment for vulvar skin disease is cortisone cream or ointment. Cortisone, also known as a steroid or corticosteroid, is made by the body as a natural anti-inflammatory substance. You might be fearful of using steroids because you've heard that there are many bad side effects. Cortisone is capable of thinning the skin so that it loses its suppleness and elasticity; sometimes overuse can cause striae, purple-red lines in the skin (like the ones a pregnant woman gets on her abdomen, though these are permanent). Some clinicians too worry about the side effects from powerful dosages. But I've learned that such concerns are unwarranted when cortisone is used appropriately—and the results are nothing short of miraculous. Relief of itching that has tormented for years! Scratching stopped in its tracks! Thickened skin restored to normal elasticity!

Powerful cortisone is sometimes needed to control very problematic symptoms for a short time. Then a less potent cortisone that's safe for long-term use can be substituted to keep symptoms under control. For some vulvar skin diseases, topical steroids may have to be used longer than package inserts and textbooks recommend. In twelve years of V work, I have never seen irreversible striae. (Despite the fact that vulvar experts have known from experience for almost fifteen years that ultra-potent steroids can be used safely on the vulva, the package inserts for some of them still say that this is a no-no.) Side effects do not always develop. If you work with an experienced clinician, you will be able to find a safe regimen.

Topical ointments will not work unless they are used as directed. Topical cortisone is most effective if applied in a thin film rubbed in well after a ten-minute soak in the tub. Skin adores being moisturized, and the hydrated skin will absorb the medication well. Medication must be applied regularly for the specified length of time. Once the topical has been in place for half an hour, the active ingredients will be absorbed. There is no loss of medication if you need to use the bathroom after half an hour and wipe some of the cream away.

Allergy to cortisone is extremely rare, since it's a natural body substance. Sometimes a patient will say, "Another doctor gave me a steroid cream, but it burned worse than ever!" This is caused by sensitivity to an ingredient in the cream base, especially propylene glycol. Ointments usually will avoid the problem; occasionally we need to have the corti-

STEROID SAFETY

Safe and intelligent use of steroids requires working carefully with your clinician and knowing a few basics:

▼ Carefully follow directions for use.

▼ Ask your clinician for a trusted brand name. There can be big differences in effectiveness between generic and name brand steroids.

▼ Make sure you know exactly where (labia, clitoris, vestibule, perineum, anus) to apply the cortisone. Strong steroids should not be used on the face without careful consultation with a dermatologist. So if you have a bump on the face, don't put your vulvar steroid on it without asking.

▼ Apply in a thin coating, ideally to hydrated skin for best absorption. A 30 g tube should last several months, depending on the area to be covered.

▼ Never abruptly discontinue steroid use. If the medication is stopped cold turkey, symptoms can bounce back immediately. Work with your clinician to develop a plan to taper off use gradually.

▼ Report side effects to your clinician. If itching develops after you've been doing well, the problem may be yeast. A thinning of the skin and bruising—a common side effect of cortisone use generally—are almost never seen when a topical steroid is used only for two to ten weeks, the usual duration for initial treatment.

sone made up in a neutral base by a compounding pharmacy. Chemicals in cream base can also, rarely, cause acute contact dermatitis, an immediate inflammatory reaction of the skin. A steroid commonly causes slight burning for a moment or two on initial application. Contact dermatitis produces burning that does not cease. Let your physician know if this happens.

▼ ▼ ▼

Here are some specific skin diseases, from the more common to the less common.

Eczema/dermatitis/lichen simplex chronicus (LSC)

Don't let all these ominous names confuse you. Eczema and dermatitis are the same condition. They're characterized by skin changes that disrupt the skin layers causing red patches and thin red cracks (fissures), wetness of the surface (weeping), crust formation, and yellow scale. Because the vulva is a moist area, crusts and scales are often not seen. Chronically rubbed skin thickens in a way that increases the appearance of the normal crosshatch markings. This is called *lichenification*.[1]

Vulvar eczema/dermatitis represents the most common inflammatory skin disease. It has several variations:

▼ *Endogenous eczema/atopic dermatitis* is classic eczema, usually inherited, often beginning in infancy, and, for a small number of people, persisting into adult life.

▼ *Seborrheic dermatitis/eczema* usually involves chronic inflammation in areas of sebum production: the scalp, ears, face, eyelids, chest, back, armpit, and groin. Seborrheic dermatitis is uncommon on the vulva but does occur.

▼ *Exogenous eczema* results from external factors, irritant or allergic (see definitions below) and may also be called *contact dermatitis*.

The end point for all three variations can be the same: thickened, itchy skin, called squamous hyperplasia or lichen simplex chronicus (say "LYE-ken SIM-plex CRON-eh-kus"). This skin result of scratching and rubbing is entirely different from the skin changes seen in lichen sclerosus and lichen planus, other skin diseases that have the word *lichen* in them. Confused? You're not alone. Even some physicians do not understand the differences between the lichens!

Vulvar eczema/dermatitis may occur in isolation (that is, only on the vulva) or may be part of eczematous disease elsewhere in the body. Women with eczema often go from clinician to clinician for years searching for a cure for the itching. Often they are given a cortisone cream that helps. But they're seldom told that when they stop the cream, the itching will return. When it inevitably does, they are convinced that there is something terribly wrong. There's no one-shot cure. Eczema, like most skin diseases, is chronic; it does not go away entirely, but it can be easily managed.

WHAT CAUSES ECZEMA?

The actual cause of endogenous dermatitis is not known. Exogenous dermatitis, the most common type of eczema, may be caused by an irritant *(irritant vulvitis)* or by an allergic reaction *(allergic vulvitis)*. Immediate stinging and burning upon application of a medicine or chemical to the vulva is a sign of an irritant reaction—there is direct effect on the tissues without any allergic mechanism, and itching is unusual. Allergic reactions take anywhere from forty-eight to seventy-two hours to develop (because the body needs time to figure out that this is an allergen) and usually last for about three weeks.

A big contributor to irritant vulvitis is thought to be excessive washing of the vulva. Embarrassment over itching often leads to self-medication with over-the-counter substances and household products. Even prescribed medications have potential for irritation; in one study, prescriptions were the commonest cause of allergic contact dermatitis of the vulva.[2]

THE LEADING VULVAR IRRITANTS

Here are the usual suspects that cause irritant or allergic reactions:

Irritants	Allergens
Soap, bubble bath, detergents	Benzocaine
Sanitary pads, adhesive on pads	Neomycin
Nylon underwear	Chlorhexidine in K-Y Jelly
Secretions, sweat, and urine	Ethylene diamine in neomycin
Tampon strings	Fragrances
5-FU cream, other HPV medications	Propylene glycol, preservatives
Douches, yogurt, deodorant hygiene products	Tea tree oil
Nonoxynol-9, other spermicides	Imidazole antifungals
Lubricants	Latex condoms, diaphragms
Methylated spirits	Semen
Imidazole antifungals	Disinfectants
Tea tree oil	Lanolin
Pinetarsol	Dyes
Alcohol	Nickel
Perfume, shampoo, hair conditioner, talcum powder	
Chemically treated clothing, toilet paper, water	

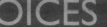

DIAGNOSING ECZEMA

The clinician needs a careful history that may reveal long-standing itching, a personal or family history of allergy and eczema, and related conditions such as asthma, rhinitis, conjunctivitis, or hives. You'll be asked specific questions about personal hygiene practices and what has been applied to the vulva—don't be shy because this information is essential. Your clinician needs to know about habitual practices—use of harsh soaps; wearing of occlusive or binding clothing such as girdles or spandex garments; daily use of panty liners—as well as any new products you've tried.

The itching may vary from mild to intolerable, interfering with sleep or activities. If mucosal areas of the vestibule are involved, there will be burning, rawness, and stinging. Symptoms are often exacerbated with menstruation and sexual intercourse.

On examination there may be mild redness in early cases or moderately extensive redness with some scaling. Cracking may be present along the labial folds. Scratches and breaks in the skin may be present, and infection with bacteria or yeast can develop on top of the affected skin. A culture of the skin surface most commonly reveals *Staphylococcus aureus, Streptococcus pyogenes,* or *Escherichia coli.*

If the condition has progressed to lichen simplex chronicus (LSC), the itching can be more intense than in any other skin disease, causing almost uncontrollable scratching and even awakening the sufferer from sleep. The skin will have become thickened and white from chronic irritation

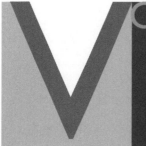

and scratching. Greatly exaggerated labial skin markings may be visible, and there may be broken hairs or loss of hair, with or without thickening of the skin.[3] Elongation of the labia, swelling, and increased or decreased pigmentation are common.

TREATING ECZEMA

LSC can be helped only if the itch-scratch cycle is ended. Sufferers have to make a great effort not to scratch. And that includes not even rubbing the area. First the itch must be brought under control with strong cortisone; then weaker cortisone may be used for maintenance. Maintenance is everything. Stopping the cortisone will result in return of the symptoms.

Modifying long-standing dressing and toilet habits is essential. The box on page 262 discusses elements of healthy vulvar hygiene. The woman also has to revise any long-standing hygiene habits that contribute to the problem (see box on page 82).

Soaks in comfortably warm water are of great help. They restore a better environment to nerve endings, lessening itching.[4] Soaking ten minutes morning and night prior to applying a topical steroid also hydrates the skin, as I have pointed out, to allow better absorption of the medication.

For simple cases of eczema, a mild to moderate topical corticosteroid ointment such as Hytone ointment 2.5 percent or Valisone ointment 0.1 percent is used in the morning and at bedtime for two to four weeks. For a little focal area a pea-sized amount (¼ inch from the tube) is usually plenty. If you need to cover both labia and the perineum, a kidney-bean-sized amount (½ inch) is necessary. When the itching is under control, application of the ointment is reduced to twice weekly.

For severe cases, a potent corticosteroid ointment, such as clobetasol or Diprolene ointment 0.05 percent, is used at bedtime for a month. Then the clinician will reevaluate. The amount used again depends on how large an area needs treating—¼ to ½ inch is usually plenty. If the itching is not well controlled, continuing the ointment may be necessary for a few more weeks, with eventual substitution of a mild cortisone twice weekly for maintenance.

In severe eczema, the skin may be so thickened that it cannot respond to creams and ointments. In these cases, injection of a cortisone called Kenalog directly under the skin may work wonders. Application of a topical anesthetic makes the injection painless.

Nighttime scratching can be controlled with a sedative antihistamine taken at bedtime, such as a small dose (10 mg) of Atarax. These drugs work against the itch-producing chemical histamine and also cause sleepiness. Antihistamines that don't make you sleepy, such as Allegra and Claritin, are of little benefit for vulvar itching. You can also use a cold pack or freeze water in an empty dishwashing detergent bottle to keep at the bedside to apply during the night.

HANDLE WITH CARE	Hygiene Help for Women with Vulvar Skin Disease

Women with skin problems are often terrified of not being clean enough and so they over-scrub, which leads to further irritation. If you have a problem, let your mantras be *gentle cleansing, avoidance of chemicals,* and *vulva-friendly clothes.* Follow the general advice found in Chapter 5, "V Smarts," and try the following substitutions:

Avoid wearing	May use
Panty hose	Stockings with a garter belt, thigh-highs, knee-highs
Synthetic underwear	Cotton underwear (always) Go without underwear when at home
Tight pants or jeans	Loose, baggy pants
Swimsuits, leotards, spandex, thongs	Loose exercise wear
Daily panty liners	Change of underwear
Do not use	**May use**
Scented soaps	Basis, Neutrogena, or Dove bar soap for bathing
Bubble bath	Tub baths morning and night, with water of a comfortable temperature
Scented detergents	Unscented detergents
Washcloths	Fingertips for washing; pat dry externally
Feminine sprays, douches, powders, or scented products	Nothing needed

Above all, remember that this condition is chronic. The treatment must continue even after the annoying symptoms go away.

Lichen sclerosus (LS)

When I diagnose patients with lichen sclerosus (say "LYE-ken sclur-O-suss"), which is a fairly common major skin disorder of the vulva, I'm quick to add that it's something we can stop in its tracks. Often women don't hear that part, because they're in shock—they hear the name and think they have something related to multiple sclerosis. (There's absolutely no connection.) An inflammatory skin disease, LS can get going anytime from childhood to old age. You may be upset to discover that science doesn't know its cause—but then again, we don't know the cause of most skin diseases. And you may be even more upset to hear that we don't have a cure. But as I said up front, most skin diseases get managed, not cured.

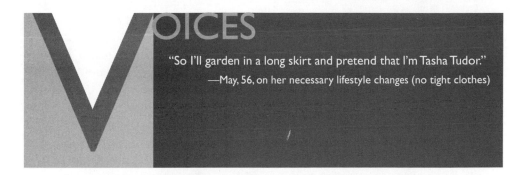

"So I'll garden in a long skirt and pretend that I'm Tasha Tudor."
—May, 56, on her necessary lifestyle changes (no tight clothes)

Too often, after receiving the diagnosis of lichen sclerosus, patients go digging in books, medical texts, or the Internet and get absolutely freaked out by scary pictures and inaccurate information. *Disregard anything written before 1995 about LS. And be careful about later material too if it wasn't written by a vulvar expert!* I'm always saddened when I hear a patient tell me, as Joanie recently did, "I saw seven doctors and they each knew it was lichen sclerosus immediately—then they each told me that there was nothing to be done." We have a marvelous and effective treatment for most cases. I follow dozens of women with this chronic skin disease that can usually be easily managed with medication and regular follow-up visits to a clinician.

LS can occur as white patches on the skin anywhere on the body. This kind of LS quickly and easily responds to topical treatment and is not a big thing. LS of the vulva may occur with these other skin patches or may exist by itself.

The most frequent sign of vulvar LS is itching. Sometimes there is burning, and intercourse can be painful, often because of cracks in the skin near the vaginal opening. However, some women have no symptoms at all.[5] The intensity of the symptoms does not correlate with the appearance of the disease clinically. The first change is a flat ivory-white area, irregular in shape with a little depression, in the middle. This may be on the labia, near the clitoris, on the perineum, or anywhere else on the vulva. There may be several white areas or they may blend together to form a

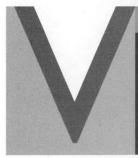

Who gets LS?

Though the disease can also affect men, it's ten times more common in women. The median age is about 50, although this condition may be seen at any age, even in kids.

larger area. Within the white areas, purple bruising and a thin, wrinkled appearance may be noted. (The thin, wrinkly skin is often compared to cigarette paper that people roll tobacco in.) The whitened areas may go on to thicken or thin out, sometimes to the point of creating an open sore (ulceration). In some cases the inflammation can cause the normal anatomy of the vulva to change, with flattening of the labia minora, fusion of the hood over the clitoris so that it is buried under the skin, and shrinkage of the skin around the vaginal opening. The whitening may extend down around the anus so that a white figure eight runs from the top of the labia, down their length, over the perineum, and around the anus. LS in the anal area may cause itching, cracking and bleeding of the skin, and discomfort with bowel movements. Women often think that they have hemorrhoids. Some women have even had surgery for anal cracking (fissures) or hemorrhoids when their problems came from LS the whole time! Involvement of the groin folds, thighs, and buttocks are common. It is generally accepted that LS does not involve the vagina.[6]

WHAT CAUSES LS?

The cause is not well understood. But it's not a disease that develops because of something that you did or did not do. It's not an infection that

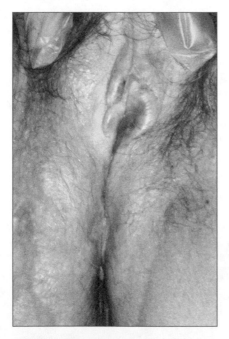

FIG. 37 **Lichen sclerosus** can cause a symmetrical white change over the entire vulva and flattened labia minora, as seen in this patient. Courtesy of Raymond H. Kaufman, M.D.

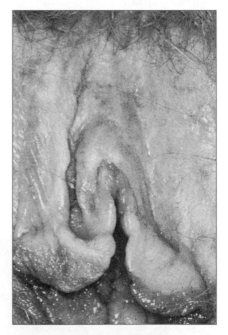

FIG. 38 **Lichen sclerosus**
Courtesy of Raymond H. Kaufman, M.D.

you got from somebody and you cannot give it to anyone else. There is a significant association between LS and some autoimmune diseases, particularly some thyroid disorders, in which the body makes antibodies that attack its own tissues.[7] But these findings do not mean that LS itself is an autoimmune disease.[8]

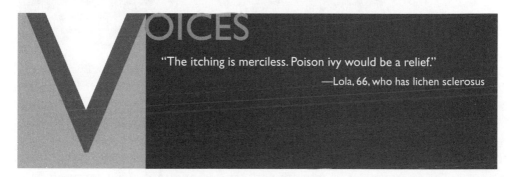

"The itching is merciless. Poison ivy would be a relief."

—Lola, 66, who has lichen sclerosus

Recently studies of how cells grow and multiply have shown that LS may be associated with some overactivity in the upper layer of the skin (keratin).[9] Researchers have also found an increase in cells that are an important part of the skin immune system and have ascertained that there is no connection between how long symptoms have been present and how the tissue appears under the microscope.[10] These findings would suggest that LS is a problem in the skin itself—a continuing inflammatory process in which activated cells of the skin immune system are involved.

It can run in families, involving both sexes, such as father (who also would have genital skin disease) and daughter, or the same sex, such as mother and daughter or two sisters. It has been seen in identical and nonidentical twins.

DIAGNOSING LS

LS is usually diagnosed by biopsy. While the diagnosis may be obvious to an experienced clinician if the typical changes of whitening and thinning are present, some of the changes of LS may overlap with other skin diseases, such as lichen planus or vitiligo. The biopsy may show either thickening or thinning of the upper layer of the skin (epithelium). Beneath the top skin layer is a zone of tissue that appears empty, with no cells in it, just fluid from swelling. Pathologists say it looks like ground glass. Special stains show the pathologist that there are no elastic fibers (which should be seen) in the tissue. Below this layer is a zone of intense inflammation characterized by a band of white blood cells that stick to the tissue like lichen on a rock. (Now you know why the name begins with the word *lichen*.)

Sometimes, especially if LS has been present for years or since childhood, the biopsy may not show definite proof of LS. In those cases a

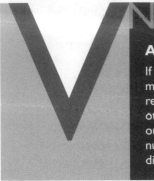

clinician has to go on his or her best judgment. This is very important! If
there are characteristic skin changes and scarring, treatment is indicated.

TREATING LS

The treatment of LS was not very satisfactory until about ten years ago,
when some British dermatologists had the courage to use and study ultra-
potent cortisone applied to the skin. Thank goodness for these women
physicians! As I have said, clinicians had always thought that this preparation was much too strong for the sensitive vulvar tissue (many still do);
they feared the vulva would be damaged, thin out, and develop striae. The
British researchers worked with thirteen women who had LS proven by
vulvar biopsy. The women were treated twice daily for three months with
a very potent steroid cream called clobetasol. The women had marked improvement in their symptoms, in the appearance of their vulvar skin, and
in the appearance of vulvar biopsy samples under the microscope.[11] On
completion of the study, the women were able to maintain their gains
successfully using less potent topical steroids. During the study, there was
only one case of allergic contact dermatitis, with no other bad side effects
despite use of this "dangerous" topical steroid for twelve straight weeks.
And long-term follow-up failed to demonstrate any bad changes in the
skin that a steroid might have caused.[12]

At the same time a study compared the efficacy of agents commonly
prescribed in the treatment of LS. Patients were treated with testosterone,
progesterone, clobetasol, or placebo (cream base without any medicine in
it). At the end of three months of therapy, the investigators concluded
that topical use of clobetasol was the safest and most effective of the
agents studied. They recommended maintenance therapy because recurrent symptoms were seen in those who ended treatment.[13] Since the original study there have been others to support it, and the ultrapotent
steroids are now the treatment of choice for LS.[14]

Treatment with clobetasol usually results in major improvement in
symptoms, and in cases where treatment is begun early, the skin may even

look normal again. So frequently we can stop LS in its tracks, eliminating itching and preventing the inflammation from progressing to alter the vulva any further. Still, women with LS need to continue the clobetasol on a twice-weekly basis or the disease will come back. A less potent steroid cream can be used in between the clobetasol doses if there is any itching.

Women who do not have any symptoms but who have evidence of LS are advised to use clobetasol for a few weeks and then continue a once- or twice-weekly program.

Vulvar specialists now know that there is no role for the use of estrogen or testosterone cream in the initial treatment of LS.[15] Testosterone, once the only available treatment for LS, has now been shown to be no better than ordinary petroleum jelly in treating LS.[16] I stress this because some physicians mistakenly continue to use estrogen and testosterone, instructing their patients that very potent cortisone is "too dangerous" to use on the vulva. Though estrogen cannot treat LS, it may be tremendously helpful in promoting healthy vaginal tissue. So estrogen cream is often combined with clobetasol treatment.

Rarely, even this wonderful clobetasol does not achieve good results. Then what? You will want to be in touch with a dermatologist who knows about the vulva. The International Society for the Study of Vulvovaginal Disease (see Resources) can give you information. Work is being done with several other medications. Derivatives of vitamin A (retinoids) given by mouth (etretinate Tegison [Roche] 25 mg daily for variable periods) have been used in difficult cases. These agents work to inhibit multiplication of the cells of the top layers of the skin and are helpful in cases of LS where there is a lot of thickening of the skin, as opposed to thinning. A recent study showed that the British form of the retinoid acitretin improved symptoms and appearance of the disease, but these progressed again when the drug was discontinued.[17] The retinoids are difficult drugs to work with because they have significant side effects and

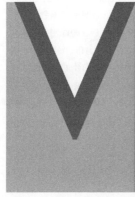

NOTE

LS and cancer

LS is not considered a precancerous condition, but there is an association of LS with skin cancer. Exactly how this connection works is unclear, but women with LS need to be checked once or twice a year to make sure that there are no nodules, thickened areas, or ulcerations that could be skin cancer. Found early, such an area can often be treated with removing the skin cancer with a little extra tissue all around. If you have LS, check yourself and have regular screenings.

I've taken care of Kerry, who is 31, for almost eight years now. She was diagnosed with LS after a long struggle with itching and irritation. A gynecologist finally noted a little white patch, did a biopsy, and found the problem. She responded beautifully to a few weeks of clobetasol and has continued to stay out of trouble with once-weekly clobetasol. When she comes in for her checkup it is hard for me to see that she has LS because all that's visible is a tiny white patch in the intralabial fold on one side. But we know it's there! Kerry ran out of her cream last year and came in a panic because the itching was back. Clobetasol clobbered her symptoms and she was on track again.

Sally, 24, found out about her LS because her sister Linda has it. When Linda was diagnosed, Sally thought, "Gee, I have itching like Linda's sometimes, but I thought it was just yeast or bath salts or something." Sally's labia minora were flattened out, and the hood had started to tighten up over the clitoris so that she couldn't pull it back. With clobetasol, the elasticity and suppleness of the hood came back. The minora are still flattened. Even though she has these skin changes, Sally has an active and enjoyable sex life without problems. Her LS stays in control with weekly clobetasol.

are known to cause birth defects, so they cannot be used in women of childbearing age. Use of the drug topically brought good results in one study group without the bad side effects.[18]

A new anti-inflammatory drug, tacrolimus (Protopic), is starting to be used, but there is no good information about its success yet.

There are some treatments you will want to avoid: laser and surgery.[19] They do not produce good results. The exception is special surgery for scarring from LS. Once the disease is under control, surgery may help to reverse the narrowing of the vaginal opening that may result from long-term progression of this condition. Before you have this done, ask about the surgeon's success rates with this kind of surgery and what will be done to keep the scarring from coming back.

Sometimes women develop pain with intercourse, and the area under the vaginal opening splits with sexual activity. The use of lubricants, estrogen cream, and clobetasol can help considerably. Sometimes minor surgery can help if this problem persists. If surgery is used to fix some of the changes brought by the inflammation of LS, it must be coupled with oral medication or aggressive use of potent steroids to prevent recurrence.[20]

Sometimes despite good relief of itching and good response of the tissues, women with LS continue to have aching, burning, and rawness as well as discomfort with intercourse. These may be occurring because of the development of abnormal nerve function leading to ongoing pain (vulvodynia). Clinicians believe that after long-term insult from the inflammation of LS, nerve fibers alter their activity and produce this pain pattern. Vulvodynia superimposed on LS can be helped with the use of medications that help vulvodynia in general, the tricyclic antidepressants and gabapentin. (See Chapter 17.)

While many patients with LS are adults, preadolescent girls are also commonly affected. Persistent scratching and/or recurrent "yeast" infections may be early indicators of childhood LS. Many cases of childhood LS spontaneously resolve by puberty, whereas others may require ongoing topical treatment.[21] We now know that the same potent steroids used for women are safe for girls.[22]

In summary, if you have LS, you have a benign but chronic skin disease. You should be screened for autoimmune conditions such as thyroid disease. You need to let other female relatives know that they might have it whether they have itching or not. You need to use strong cortisone ointment for several weeks initially and then once or twice weekly for maintenance. You need to check in at least yearly with your clinician to make sure your skin is doing well and your disease is controlled.

Psoriasis

Psoriasis is a chronic skin disease that can affect the skin almost anywhere on the body—including the vulva. Areas of dry, thickened, scaling, silvery white, and reddened skin can range from a few small spots to generalized lesions. The disease may be cyclical (coming and going) or constant with no remission.

The most common type of psoriasis, and the only one that affects the vulva, is known as plaque psoriasis. It's not common, certainly less common than LS. Between 1 and 3 percent of the U.S. population is affected by some form of psoriasis.[23] The disease is seen in all ethnic groups but is most common in people of European ancestry. Asians and Africans seem to have a lower risk. Psoriasis is not age-specific. The average age of onset is 28, but new cases are reported across the age spectrum from newborns to the eighth decade.[24]

Many different things can lead to psoriasis. Often it's genetically determined. Roughly one-third of those affected have psoriasis in their family.[25] If one parent has the disease, there is a 25 percent chance that his or her offspring will also get the disease; if both parents are carriers, the

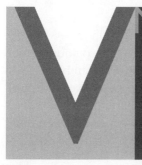

Psoriasis puzzlers

Curiously, the disease tends to go away spontaneously and to flare up without any reason. It may improve during the summer months on exposure to sunlight, or improve with weight changes and during pregnancy.

chance of passing psoriasis on to their children more than doubles.[26] Many nongenetic factors also may trigger psoriasis. For example, mechanical, ultraviolet, or chemical injury to the skin can result in Koebner's phenomenon, the development of psoriasis at the site of the injury.[27] Various infections—especially streptococcal infections, but also acute viral infections and HIV infection—can cause lesions as well.[28] Other nongenetic triggers are prescription drug use (antimalarials, lithium, beta-blockers, quinidine, withdrawal of systemic corticosteroids, and indomethacin), psychological stress, hormonal changes, obesity, alcohol, and smoking.[29]

WHAT HAPPENS

In psoriasis, normal function of the skin is altered; the cycle during which skin cells (keratinocytes) develop at the base of the epithelium and move toward the surface is speeded up. Cells divide more rapidly and move to the surface faster. Since the cells move to the surface so rapidly, they do not develop and mature properly.[30] Abnormal cells build up at the surface, making the skin thick and scaly. The number of abnormal inflammatory chemicals in the skin is increased in psoriasis.[31] Recent research suggests that special white blood cells (activated T cells) of the immune system trigger chain reactions in both the skin cells and the cascade of inflammatory chemicals that lead to the formation of the psoriatic plaque.[32]

Psoriasis starts out as round, slightly elevated bright red to reddish yellow bumps that gradually enlarge to become raised patches or plaques. These have sharp, clearly defined borders. The mons is often involved and may appear scaly. The area in between the buttocks (natal cleft) may have a crack or fissure down the middle. The lesions of psoriasis may hurt, itch, or bleed. Psoriasis does not usually affect mucosal surfaces such as the vestibule and vagina.

Psoriasis is usually diagnosed from its clinical appearance. And, of course, when lesions of psoriasis are present elsewhere on the body, diagnosis of vulvar lesions is easier. Unfortunately, many women are treated for psoriasis elsewhere on the body but the dermatologist doesn't ask—or the woman doesn't tell—about the vulvar lesions.

TREATING PSORIASIS

There are several different ways to treat psoriasis.

1. Topical corticosteroids are the mainstay of treatment for plaque psoriasis. They appear to work by constricting blood vessels to lessen blood flow and decrease redness, slowing cellular proliferation, and exerting anti-inflammatory action. A high-potency topical steroid is applied daily until the lesions are under control. The strength is then tapered and the dosage interval increased to find the lowest strength and the longest dosage interval that are still effective.

2. If the steroid applied as a topical does not help, it may work better if it is injected just under the skin of the thick plaques. An injection once or twice relieves symptoms and improves the skin.

3. Calcipotriene (Dovonex) is related to vitamin D. It decreases the severity of plaque psoriasis by promoting differentiation of the skin cells and inhibiting their proliferation. It mimics the efficacy of the midpotency steroids without their side effects.[33] The agent can be used in combination with other topical and systemic therapies.

4. In difficult cases, agents that work through the immune system can be used. The immunosuppressants cyclosporine (Neoral) and tacrolimus (Protopic) can be rapid and effective for clearing psoriasis.[34] These drugs are expensive and should be used only by clinicians with extensive experience treating with immunosuppressants.

Lichen planus (LP)

Like the other skin disorders we've discussed, lichen planus (LP) is a chronic skin disorder not limited to the vulva. In fact, it can involve the skin of body surfaces, nails, or the mucous membranes of the mouth, esophagus, conjunctiva, bladder, stomach, anus, and vagina.[35] A woman may have involvement of skin, mouth, vestibule, and vagina all at once, or she may have findings in only one area at a time. As a result, vulvar LP often escapes accurate diagnosis. If the classic rash of LP isn't present and there aren't any oral symptoms, it's easy to miss it in a patient with vulvar or vaginal symptoms. Most dentists who treat oral lichen planus do not inquire about genital symptoms, and gynecologists do not routinely examine the mouth. Lichen planus symptoms can also be confused with an-

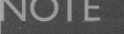

NOTE

Where does the name *lichen planus* come from?

In autoimmune disease, special white blood cells (activated T cells) are directed against cells deep in the skin (basal keratinocytes) to produce a large collection of white cells at the point where the top layer of the skin meets the deeper layer of the skin. These white cells cling to the skin layer like lichen on a rock (the cells are described as *lichenoid*). *Planus* means "square." It refers to the nonvulvar skin lesions of LP that are called purple polygonal plaques.

Source: M. M. Black, Lichen planus and lichenoid disorders, in *Textbook of Dermatology*, 5th ed., R. H. Champion, J. L. Burton, F. J. G. Ebling, eds. (Oxford: Blackwell Scientific Publications, 1992), 1675.

other skin condition, lichen sclerosus. Lichen sclerosus and lichen planus can occur together. Tricky? You can say that again!

Guess what the main symptom is? Itching! This may occur in the folds of the labia or the vestibule. Other ways LP can make itself known are by soreness of a small area in the folds or in the vestibule and by pain with intercourse. If the vagina is involved, there may be irritating yellow discharge, spotting, or bleeding from time to time and after intercourse.

Vulvar LP is relatively rare. Looking at her practice over a three-year period, a dermatologist reported that less than 10 percent of the women who came in with vulvar problems had LP.[36] However, half of all women with LP elsewhere on the body also have it on the vulva.[37] Although chronic, the condition tends to come and go in episodes that may last from weeks to years, making it difficult to decide if a particular treatment regimen is effective. Disease of the mucous membranes, especially in the vagina and vestibule, are among the most persistent; the vaginal form of LP may be the same thing as desquamative inflammatory vaginitis (DIV) (see Chapter 13).

"WHY ME?"

The cause of lichen planus is unknown, but clinicians do not think it comes from anything you did or did not do. It's not an infection that you can catch, nor can you give it to your partner. Doctors suspect that LP is an autoimmune disease where one makes antibodies against one's own skin and mucous membranes. The disease is associated with some well-known autoimmune conditions such as whitening of the skin (vitiligo), hair loss (alopecia), inflammatory bowel disease (ulcerative colitis), and a neuromuscular disorder (myasthenia gravis).[38]

A number of drugs can cause or are associated with the symptoms of lichen planus; discontinuing these drugs if one is taking them may improve symptoms remarkably. These include nonsteroidal anti-inflammatory drugs (NSAIDs), chloroquine, dapsone, furosemide, gold salts, hydroquinone, mercury compounds, methyldopa, para-amino salicylic acid, Azulfidine, penicillamine, the phenothiazines, propranolol, spironolactone, streptomycin, tetracycline, the thiazide diuretics, tolbutamide, and triprolidine.

DIAGNOSING LP

While several forms of LP may affect the vulva, the most significant is *erosive LP*, glassy, bright red areas (erosions) where the surface is worn off by inflammation; these erosions often have a white border called Wickham's striae.[39] Erosive LP is seen on the labia minora and in the vestibule; there can be separate small erosions or large erosions involving most of the vestibule. The inflammation can also scar and change the basic structures of the vulva: The labia minora can flatten or disappear, the clitoral glans can become buried under a "stuck" clitoral hood that won't retract, or the vaginal opening can narrow.

Unlike the condition called lichen sclerosus, where disease is limited to the vulva, LP usually affects the vagina as well.[40] In fact, the vagina becomes so inflamed that it bleeds on touch, with speculum insertion or with intercourse. Areas of inflammation may be small with increased vaginal discharge, or the entire vagina may be involved, massively inflamed and raw. In severe cases scarring and adhesions can lead to narrowing or closing off of the vagina.[41] The Pap smear may be abnormal (atypical) if the cervix is affected.[42] Involvement of the anus is also seen, with painful bowel movements that are sometimes mistakenly thought to be the result of hemorrhoids.

A kind of erosive LP involving the vulva, vestibule, vagina, and mouth is called *vulvo-vaginal-gingival syndrome* (VVG). It is particularly resistant to treatment.[43] Although all four areas can be affected at once, the lesions may not always occur at the same time. White lacy patches may be found in the inner cheek or on the gums, with red eroded areas of the gums near the teeth. Similar white lacy areas of painful, red, eroded areas, small or large, may be seen in the vestibule. The vagina may also have red eroded areas, particularly on either side of the cervix, or the entire vagina may appear inflamed and raw. Vaginal discharge may appear bloody or may be yellow or yellow-green. Patients complain of vulvar pain, particularly burning, rawness, and itching. Sexual intercourse may be painful. A profuse and irritating sticky yellow or yellow-green discharge may be seen. Women do not usually complain of mouth or skin symptoms, but characteristic findings are present if examination is performed.

Biopsy is the standard way to diagnose skin diseases, but unfortunately even when LP is present the biopsy may not prove it. The clinician must then rely on his or her judgment, based on the signs and symptoms that are present.

TREATING LP

Accept that the disease is chronic and will not go away; treatment will be ongoing even after your symptoms improve. Good vulvar care is essential: minimizing any irritants, using soothing soaks and cold packs, wearing loose clothes. Soaking in sitz baths, use of protective barrier creams, and topical anesthetics can improve comfort. Your clinician will review the medications you take and may advise discontinuing drugs known to promote lichenoid reactions.

Consultation with dermatologists who manage LP on a regular basis may prove helpful. Consult the International Society for the Study of Vulvovaginal Disease (see Resources).

LP is not well known in the medical community. I recently gave one of my standard talks to a group of nurse-practitioners and showed my slides of LP in the mouth, the vulva, and the vagina. After the lecture a nurse-practitioner came to tell me that she had followed a woman with these features for years. Would I see her?

Indeed, Aline's gums were inflamed and raw, and the vestibule was eroded with the classic finding of LP. The vagina was so badly scarred that it was just a dimple. I was near tears when I finished her exam.

Aline's disease had started with irritating vaginal discharge and painful intercourse. Clinicians had worked hard to help her, but no one knew what the problem was. Soon the vagina started to scar shut. She had had laser surgery to open the vagina on two different occasions by professors of gynecology at large teaching hospitals. She was never given a diagnosis or any follow-up treatment. So LP continued its inflammatory course, and the vagina scarred up again.

I gave Aline clobetasol gel for her mouth and ointment for the vulva. Those areas responded nicely. To reopen the vagina, I started her with a teeny little dilator half an hour a day in combination with more cortisone ointment. With time and hard work with dilators graduating in size, she's made nice progress, so that now she has a vagina that admits two fingers to a depth of about two inches. I hope that with continued dilators and cortisone, we can keep it open.

Treatment is based on cortisone therapy in the form of creams, ointments, or suppositories. As with other skin disorders, potent cortisone preparations are often required initially, then can be tapered to less potent preparations upon improvement. But the intense inflammation of LP can require ongoing use of strong cortisone. Getting the cortisone into the vagina can be a challenge. Suppositories that slide out easily can be refrigerated and inserted when cold and very firm. Some patients find cream introduced with an applicator easier to work with.

If the vagina starts to narrow, adhesions can be treated with cortisone and the use of a cylindrical plastic device called a dilator. Therapy begins with the smallest dilator that will fit. It is coated with cortisone ointment and inserted for a few minutes at a time, working up to half an hour three times a day and eventually to wearing it overnight with snug underpants to keep it in place. The size of the dilator is gradually increased.

While estrogen alone cannot help LP, in a postmenopausal woman it is a helpful addition to therapy to prevent the thinning that comes without the hormone support.

Yeast infections are a common side effect of the cortisone; your clinician will recommend the most appropriate treatment.

Severe LP that is not responding to the topical cortisone can be treated with cortisone injected under the skin, or oral cortisone for a short time. Immunosuppressant drugs are also used in severe cases.

Sometimes, even after the skin problem is well controlled, burning and itching can persist. These symptoms suggest a superimposed pain syndrome called vulvodynia. This is treated with a tricyclic antidepressant used for its painkilling properties. Amitriptyline (Elavil) or desipramine (Norpramin), 10 mg at bedtime, increased by 10 mg every five days until the symptoms are controlled, is the treatment of choice. The usual dose is 20 to 100 mg. Relief of this problem takes weeks to achieve; the side effects of dry mouth and constipation are common.

Skin cancer of the vulva associated with lichen planus has been reported, but this is really rare.[44] As with lichen sclerosus, it makes sense to have the skin checked once or twice a year to make sure that the skin disease is in control and no suspicious changes are occurring.

Hidradenitis suppurativa (HS)

This skin disease is the rarest in this chapter, affecting about one in three hundred people.[45] Like some of the others, it hasn't been well diagnosed or treated in the past. But if the right treatment is given early, we can prevent it from becoming extensive.

Hidradenitis suppurativa (say "HID-ra-den-EYE-tis SUP-pur-ah-TEE-va") (HS) results from blockage of hair follicles and inflammation of sweat glands.[46] After the plugging occurs, bacteria invade the sweat gland system via the hair follicles, become trapped beneath the plugs, and multiply rapidly in the nourishing environment of sweat. The glands subsequently split open and spread the infection to adjacent glands, further extending the tissue destruction and skin damage. Chronic infection and draining abscesses lead to scarring of the affected sites.

HS may occur in very limited form with one or two bumps. But more widespread and unchecked HS can reach advanced stages with great misery for those involved. Yet it now appears that the disease may be curbed in its early stages, sparing its victims later massive surgery to remove the affected tissue. This is tricky, since HS starts off subtly. Early symptoms include itching, redness, and excessive wetness in the involved area.[47] As the hair follicle becomes blocked, a firm, pea-sized nodule or cyst, similar to the zits of acne, forms. While the nodule of acne is on top of the skin, HS nodules are in part underneath, leading experts to call HS "acne inversa." This nodule can rupture spontaneously and discharge puslike material. As the area heals, it becomes thick and hard, and new nodules develop adjacent to the original ones. Some nodules rupture spontaneously under the skin surface, leading to formation of a little tunnel (called a sinus tract) deep within the tissue under the skin; other nodules remain as hard inflammatory masses. The result of all this is nodules in varying states of discharging pus, thick cords under the skin from the tunnel formation, scar pits on the skin, and deposits of dark brown pigmentation.

DETECTING HS EARLY

Early diagnosis of HS is essential, since most cases can be effectively treated when caught early, sparing you a great deal of pain. Signs that suggest early HS include:

▼ Recurrent deep boils for more than six months in places where the skin flexes and is rich in sweat glands

▼ Onset after puberty

▼ Poor response to conventional antibiotics

▼ Strong tendency toward relapse and recurrence

▼ Zits in sweat-gland-bearing skin

▼ No bacteria that cause disease grown from routine cultures of pus from boils

▼ Personal or family history of acne or pilonidal sinuses

▼ Worsening of boils premenstrually in women

One roadblock to early diagnosis is that a patient sees different physicians in different locations and no one puts together a total picture of HS. This is really important! Few processes produce recurrent abscesses and sinus tract formation with a characteristic distribution in the skin that is rich in sweat glands—the armpits, groin, and perineum.

If you are having recurrent boils that leave pits and scars and thickened cords under the skin, find a good general surgeon or a knowledgeable gynecologist or dermatologist and ask about HS.

Source: P. S. Mortimer, Hidradenitis suppurativa—diagnostic criteria, in *Acne and Related Disorders*, 1st ed., R. Marks, G. Plewig, eds. (London: Martin Dunitz Ltd., 1989), 359.

These nodules develop in the groin in women who have the problem. It's also possible to find them on the perineum and around the anus. HS may not be limited to the V zone and can occur under the arms or under the breasts.

The disease may be mild, with just a few lesions from time to time. Or it can be severe, with new lesions continually developing, leaving nodules and tracts under the skin and causing chronic, widespread, deep infection.

Physicians still don't understand the role of bacterial infection in HS. Despite the fact that bacteria seem to play a part in this disease, antibiotics alone will not cure it.[48]

Although blockage of hair follicles may be the main event leading to disease, there may be some other factors that influence whether you get HS. A relationship has been proposed between sex hormones and HS, for example.[49] HS is seldom seen before puberty, and childhood cases have been associated with puberty that comes earlier than it should (precocious puberty).[50] Women often report that the disease is worse just before their menstrual periods. However, pregnancy and menstruation do not consistently make the disease better or worse, and new HS has been reported in postmenopausal women.[51] Excessive amounts of male hormones such as testosterone and the adrenal hormone DHEA have been suggested as a causal factor in women, but the role is not yet clear.

HS has been associated with other glandular disorders, such as diabetes, excessive production of cortisone from the adrenal glands (Cushing's disease), and excess growth hormone (acromegaly).[52] It also appears to run in families.[53]

TREATING HS

Antibiotics, drugs to act against male hormones (antiandrogens), and retinoids (Accutane) seem successful in early cases. Advanced cases respond only to surgical removal of a block of affected tissue. Some details about each:

▼ *Antibiotics:* Topical clindamycin (2 percent lotion) applied twice daily to the skin over a three-month period and systemic therapy with tetracycline appear to be of value early in the course of disease to prevent the formation of pustules and abscesses.[54] Once the disease has progressed, antibiotics alone are not enough; combinations of antiandrogens, retinoids, and sugery are necessary.[55] Clindamycin also appears to prevent new lesions after existing disease has been cleared with isotretinoin and removal of sinus tracts (see "Retinoids" below).[56] Relapse is almost inevitable after withdrawal of medication.[57] Time for my familiar refrain: Skin diseases require ongoing management. They do not go away completely.

▼ *Antiandrogens:* Treatment with antiandrogens (drugs that block the action of male hormones present in small amounts in women) has produced mixed results in women with HS. A double-blind, controlled, crossover trial comparing estrogen plus a drug called cyproterone acetate showed some promising results, but the drug is not approved for use in the United States.[58] But we do have a drug named spironolactone that works against male hormones and can be used for HS treatment.

▼ *Retinoids:* Treatment with isotretinoin (Accutane) at the earliest stages of HS may correct the follicular abnormality that is at the root of this chronic disease.[59] As an example, in one trial of this therapy in sixty-eight patients, the condition completely cleared during initial therapy in sixteen cases, and eleven maintained their improvement during the follow-up period.[60] Accutane does not work if there are thick tracts under the skin.[61]

▼ *Cyclosporine:* Administration of cyclosporine, a drug that suppresses the immune system, has produced moderate improvement in a few case reports.[62] No large trials have been done, though.

Surgery has been an important treatment of HS in the past, but only because traditionally this disease was allowed to advance until it involved large areas of tissue. To avoid the knife entirely, follow the steps in the box on early detection of HS. If you have existing sinus tracts under the skin, the only way to get rid of them is surgically; then prevent formation of new ones.

▾ ▾ ▾

So here we are at the end of the scary skin section. Isn't it amazing how many problems can involve the Vs and cause itching? Isn't it astounding how many causes of itching there are besides yeast? But what great news that we know more than ever about these chronic skin woes and can fix them up!

▼

CHAPTER 16

V Bumps and Color Changes

Should You Be Alarmed? Usually Not

There's something uniquely unnerving about finding a bump of any size anywhere on your body. Why should your vulva be any different? Most women tell me that the first time they find a bump, they immediately think cancer. Yet vulvar cancer is really rare, while bumps on the vulva are really common. We get bumps because the vulva is covered with skin. And skin contains nerves, blood vessels, sweat glands, and other glands. Underneath, there's muscle and fat. With so many structures involved, no wonder dozens of different kinds of harmless bumps can show up on the vulva!

Another common moment of panic comes when, using a mirror to look because you sense an irritation, you see a red or white color on your vulva, or perhaps a darkened area. Sometimes what looks reddish to the layman's eye is actually an ulcer, an open sore where the top layer of skin has worn away. More often, a clinician first notices these discolorations during a pelvic exam, either as part of a regular checkup or for an unrelated condition. That's because the same cancer-conscious women who scan the moles on their arms or backs for the slightest change skip wholesale over the skin of the vulva.

Like a bump, a discoloration or an ulcer may be completely harmless, but in each case you need to find out what's causing this change in the appearance of your skin. Given the vast range of possibilities, trying to diagnose a change by yourself can be next to impossible. Bumps can either be fluid-filled sacs (cysts) or solid tissue. They may be caused by bacteria or viruses, or can be a precancerous growth or skin cancer. Reddish, whitish, or dark patches have varied causes too.

The following overview of the possibilities can help you to frame questions for your clinician or to know what tests to expect or request.[1] This is a mixed collection of all the things that are not covered in other chapters, so it includes a broad variety of bumps caused by bacteria, viruses, and changes in various structures. Don't let all the fancy names scare you.

Different conditions may look similar on the vulva; often (though not always), removing the bump is the only way to know what it is. Harmless, noncancerous (benign) conditions could certainly be left alone, yet removal is the only way to tell that they are benign.

How can you tell if something's not just a pimple? That's a good question. You can't tell very easily. The vulva does not get the same kind of acne you get on your face. The vulva does get folliculitis (pimples around a hair), discussed below with red discolorations. Also common are blocked oil ducts, inclusion cysts (discussed with common small bumps). It's a good idea to check out a new bump that stays more than a couple of days.

Bottom line: Should you detect any kind of skin change, whether a bump, discoloration, or ulcer, don't delay in finding out what the problem is.

Common small bumps

Small bumps of the vulva are those of half an inch or less. Many of these never grow any bigger than this small size. Others can grow to be large but usually cause symptoms early on. Small bumps may vary in color, but it is usually the fact that there is a bump that brings them to attention. Here's a catalog of small bumps, showing what structure they come from.

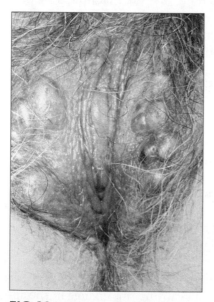

FIG. 39 Inclusion cysts, the most common small growths of the vulva, do not go away once they form but do not require any treatment.

BUMPS FROM INFOLDING OF SKIN OR BLOCKAGE OF OIL DUCTS (EPIDERMAL INCLUSION CYSTS)

These cysts are the most common small growths of the vulva. Inclusion cysts that occur in the vagina are related to trauma. Fragments of epithelium, the top layer of skin, are buried (included) beneath the skin or mucous membrane during the repair of a tear after vaginal delivery or during the repair of the small incision to enlarge the vaginal opening for delivery (episiotomy). These islands of epithelium grow and make secretions, forming a little cyst. When these cysts occur on the vulva, usually on the labia, they come from oil glands (sebaceous glands) that have become blocked. Inclusion cysts vary from several millimeters to the size of a walnut and are often multiple, smooth, and yellow-white in color. Their contents resemble thick pus but in fact are oil gland secretions (sebum), and there is no infection. Inclusion cysts do not go away once they form, but they do not require any treatment. They can be removed under local anesthesia if they are annoying.

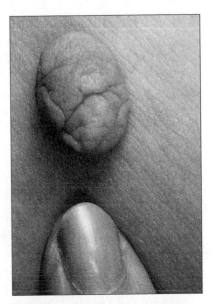

FIG. 40 **Acrochordons**, often referred to as skin tags, are soft, plump structures that do not turn cancerous and do not require treatment.

Courtesy of Raymond H. Kaufman, M.D.

BUMPS FROM SKIN AND UNDERLYING CONNECTIVE TISSUE (ACROCHORDONS)

An acrochordon is a soft, flesh-colored, wrinkled, raised growth with no hair on it. You may know it as a skin tag. It often appears on a stalk or stem (called a pedicle). Its size varies from very small (less than ⅛ inch) to about ½ inch. Skin tags are found on the vulva or the inner thigh or near the anus. They don't turn cancerous and don't need treatment. Some are removed for cosmetic reasons or if they become irritated by rubbing from clothes or activity.

BUMPS FROM THE COVERINGS OF NERVE FIBERS (NEUROFIBROMAS)

This very common bump arises from the sheath that covers a nerve fiber, but no one knows why it shows up. It appears as a small, fleshy, flabby, pinkish tan, plump mass; it seldom reaches a large size. It causes no problems and no treatment is necessary for small isolated growths.

BUMPS FROM BLOOD VESSELS (HEMANGIOMAS, ANGIOKERATOMAS, PYOGENIC GRANULOMAS)

This growth represents a malformation of blood vessels rather than a true bump. Hemangiomas on the vulva are common, and there are several types, ranging from a bright red mark (strawberry hemangioma) to purple clusters extending up into the vagina (cavernous hemangioma). The senile hemangioma (cherry hemangioma) is composed of very small

bright red or dark blue clusters. All of these are usually symptom-free unless they are injured, in which case bleeding may follow. No treatment is
usually necessary.

Another form of hemangioma is the angiokeratoma. This blood vessel
growth often appears in multiples, with a deep purple color. Because this
can be confused with a mole or melanoma or even a wart, removing the
whole area gives both diagnosis and treatment.

Still another kind of growth is the pyogenic granuloma. Pyogenic granulomas are made up of many tiny blood vessels (capillaries), often arising
on the labia during pregnancy. They aren't like varicose veins, though, in
which the walls of big veins balloon out from the extra pressure of the
pregnancy. Clinicians are not sure why tiny little capillary blood vessels
cluster to form a pyogenic granuloma. Similar blood vessels can develop
on the gums. These may become smaller after delivery but often stay or
come back. They frequently cause some bleeding and may develop infection, draining pus. They have a beefy red or purple color, and may feel
very firm and tender. Biopsy may be necessary to make the diagnosis;
treatment can be delayed until after the pregnancy, but removing the area
is necessary to prevent recurrence.

BUMPS CAUSED BY VIRUSES (WARTS AND MOLLUSCUM)

Warts (condylomas) are pesky, contagious small growths covered in
Chapter 21.

Molluscum contagiosum is a viral outbreak with a big name that in
schoolchildren affects the skin of the trunk, face, and arms. In adults the
outbreak is on the genitalia and is sexually transmitted, not by intercourse
but by close person-to-person contact. The virus may be spread by infected clothes or bedlinen (fomites). Molluscum produces no symptoms,
but appears as small translucent or waxy dome-shaped bumps that may
have a tiny depression (umbilication) in the center. Sometimes these are
called water warts. They may disappear spontaneously in a few months,
but may last for years. When they are present, they can be passed on to
another person.

Because molluscum is sexually tranmitted, clinicians always look for
other STDs when it is present. Treatment is achieved by freezing (cryotherapy) or removing with a small needle (curettage). Molluscum can also be
treated with the medicine used against warts, imiquimod (Aldara). There
are no known long-lasting problems with molluscum.

Less common small bumps

The following small growths are seen less often.

BUMPS CAUSED BY PRECANCEROUS SKIN CHANGES

See Chapters 21 and 22.

BUMPS FROM STRUCTURES USED IN FETAL DEVELOPMENT (GARTNER'S DUCT CYSTS)

Cysts can form in structures that are used temporarily in the embryo as it develops and then are replaced by more highly developed systems. In the vagina, Gartner's duct cysts form from tubules left as the kidneys develop. These cysts usually create no symptoms; in fact, a clinician tends to find them coincidentally during an exam, rather than because a patient has complained about them. If the cyst is large enough to interfere with intercourse, it is removed; often the cyst causes no trouble at all.

BUMPS FROM THE DUCTS OF GLANDS IN THE VESTIBULE (VESTIBULAR CYSTS)

If there is blockage of the duct of one of the many small glands that make a mucous secretion to lubricate the vestibule, a cyst can form. Most of these cysts are small, asymptomatic, and benign, requiring no treatment. If a cyst becomes large, interferes with intercourse or movement, or causes the patient concern, it can be removed. If the cyst is just drained, it will almost always form again.

BUMPS FROM SWEAT GLANDS (SYRINGOMAS)

A growth from a sweat gland, syringoma, may be seen on any part of the body, especially the eyelids. On the vulva, they look like many skin-colored papules, often coming together to make a short ridge. They can be hard to see if covered by labial hair. These are not always itchy, but they can be. Some women notice a rough surface of the vulvar skin, or a single bump, but most have no symptoms. Biopsy is the only sure method of diagnosis. No treatment is usually necessary, but a syringoma may be removed if it is causing problems.

BUMPS FROM SPECIAL GLANDS (HIDRADENOMA)

The hidradenoma is a growth found on the vulva of adult Caucasian women. It is usually a single growth, probably arising from a gland similar to a sweat gland called the mammarylike anogenital gland (MLG).[2] These are located on the vulva, in the depression between the labia (intralabial folds), or on the perineum around the anus (the anogenital area). The hidradenoma has a reddish color and can develop a little ulceration on the surface. Though it is noncancerous, bleeding or infection is possible. Because diagnosis may not be clear just by looking, removal will be both diagnosis and treatment.

BUMPS FROM THE HAIR SHAFT (PILONIDAL CYSTS)

It's not supposed to be there, but sometimes a shaft of hair is found near the clitoris. (Hair shafts don't always read the textbooks!) A cyst filled with hair and oil develops in a sleeve of tissue covering the hair. Pilonidal cysts

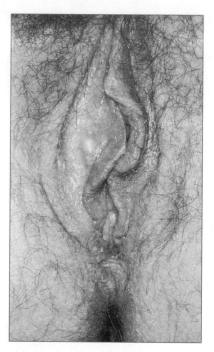

FIG. 41 **Hidradenoma** is a growth found on the vulva of Caucasian women, probably arising from a gland similar to a sweat gland.

are most often found next to the clitoris and may make tunnels that run beneath the skin for some distance. They cause pain and swelling in the region of the clitoris and can become infected and drain pus. In the stage of acute abscess, a pilonidal cyst needs to be drained surgically as a temporary measure. But to keep the cyst from coming back, the physician needs to remove the entire cyst and any tunneling it has made under the neighboring skin. This can be done only when there is no active infection.

Really rare small bumps

Although most women are not likely to encounter these problems, they're important to include in a roundup.

BUMPS FROM TISSUE LINING THE UTERUS (ENDOMETRIOSIS)

Glands and the surrounding tissue from the lining of the uterus (endometrium) may be transferred to the vulva after a procedure where the uterine lining has been scraped (curettage). Most cases have occurred in the site of a previous incision to enlarge the vaginal opening for delivery (episiotomy) after uterine curettage for bleeding after the delivery. This kind of endometriosis is usually not related to pelvic endometriosis. These bluish cystic nodules will often enlarge with the menstrual period, since the tissue responds to estrogen. They are removed for diagnosis and for treatment of discomfort.

V NOTE

Breast tissue in the vulva

Very rarely, special glands in the vulva called mammarylike glands (MLG) can enlarge during pregnancy or shortly afterward to make bumps that have milk inside them. If the bumps persist after pregnancy, they can be removed.

BUMPS FROM SWEAT GLAND DUCTS (FOX-FORDYCE DISEASE)

This is a disease of the sweat gland openings that affects women ages 20 to 50; it may affect the vulva or the armpits or both. The ducts become plugged with skin surface covering (keratin); the ducts then expand, the glands enlarge, and many little fluid-filled sacs (vesicles) result. Secretions leaking out into the skin are thought to cause the intense itching associated with this disease. Topical drugs used to treat acne, such as Retin-A and benzoyl peroxide, may be helpful for this problem. Estrogen applied to the skin is also helpful.

Common large bumps

The following conditions are harder to ignore.

BUMPS FROM THE DUCT OF THE BARTHOLIN'S GLAND (BARTHOLIN'S DUCT CYSTS AND ABSCESSES)

The cysts that probably cause women the most vulvar problems are Bartholin's duct cysts. Bartholin's glands, as you'll remember, are responsible for helping to lubricate the vagina. If a blockage occurs near the opening of the main duct into the vestibule, mucus builds up and the duct swells. If infection occurs, the contents turn into pus and a Bartholin's duct abscess has formed. The cause of obstruction is unknown; a combination of a narrow duct at birth and production of especially thick mucus might account for many cysts. The size of the cyst depends on how much mucus builds up. Since secretions from the Bartholin's gland are part of sexual activity, the size of the cyst is influenced by sexual stimulation. During sexual activity the cyst can enlarge rapidly, while cysts may stay the same size or even shrink in women with diminished sexual activity.

A Bartholin's duct cyst forms a single nontender swelling at the base of the labium, varying from the size of a grape to cysts bigger than an orange. Most women with a small Bartholin's duct cyst have no symptoms other than the swelling, although minor discomfort on sexual intercourse may be experienced. If the cyst becomes enlarged or infected, it may cause discomfort or difficulty walking. Small cysts producing no symptoms can be left alone; cysts that are large enough to cause discomfort, that become infected, or that keep coming back need to be treated. An abscess is a very tender, red swelling that causes severe vulvar pain.

Removal of the entire Bartholin's gland is seldom necessary and is usually *not* recommended. If, however, removal of the gland is really necessary—for example, a woman who is on drugs to suppress the immune system so that she will not reject a kidney transplant is developing a Bartholin's duct abscess every month—the procedure should be done by a surgeon with extensive experience, since most gynecologists have never removed a Bartholin's gland. Such surgery can lead to heavy bleeding and formation of painful scar tissue.

Simply draining the cyst or abscess may result in only temporary improvement, with return of the cyst after a short time. There are two ways to preserve the function of the gland and prevent reformation of a cyst or abscess: marsupialization and use of a Word catheter. With marsupialization, the clinician opens and drains the cyst, then sews the walls of the duct open so that a new opening is formed to allow drainage. To use the Word catheter, the clinician opens and drains the cyst, then inserts a tiny inflatable bulb-tipped catheter to stay in place for two or three weeks so that a new opening is established. Both these procedures can usually be done under local anesthesia in the office.

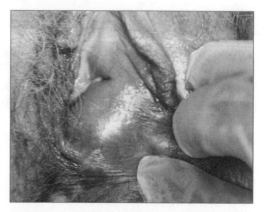

FIG. 42   A **Bartholin's duct cyst** forms when a blockage occurs and mucus builds up in the duct.

Courtesy of Raymond H. Kaufman, M.D.

LARGE BUMPS FROM FATTY TISSUE (LIPOMAS)

This growth is composed of fat cells. A lipoma is soft and smooth, sometimes on a stem, or pedicle. It can become very large, but produces symptoms only when it becomes large enough to produce sensations of heaviness or cause ulceration of the skin on top of it. It needs to be removed only if it is enlarging and causing symptoms.

LARGE BUMPS FROM FIBROUS CONNECTIVE TISSUE (FIBROMAS)

A fibroma is a firm, smooth mass on a pedicle; sometimes it appears as a small, firm nodule just under the skin. A fibroma is made up of bundles of fibrous tissue. It also can become as large as a fist. It needs removal if it is large or causes discomfort.

Uncommon large bumps

These are uncommon because women usually notice and do something about them when they're small.

LARGE BUMPS CAUSED BY BLEEDING FROM A BROKEN BLOOD VESSEL (HEMATOMA)

The vulva has a rich network of blood vessels. When injured, these vessels bleed, resulting in a blood clot, or hematoma. Most hematomas come from falls against a sharp object or from straddle injuries involving bikes, horses, or amusement park rides. Injury at the time of intercourse and being kicked cause others. A hematoma can also develop as a postoperative complication after any surgical procedure performed on the vulva.

Seeing a clinician for evaluation and follow-up after an injury is important. Hematomas always need careful evaluation and observation because they can continue to enlarge. Small hematomas are usually self-limited; an ice pack and pressure dressing will often stop expansion of the bleeding. After twenty-four hours, warm wet packs or baths will promote circulation and encourage resorption of the blood. If the mass continues to enlarge, however, surgical treatment (incision and drainage) may be necessary. Hematomas can also become infected if a surface wound occurred at the time of the injury.

LARGE BUMPS CAUSED BY INFECTION (LYMPHOGRANULOMA VENEREUM)

Lymphogranuloma venereum (LGV) is one of the classic sexually transmitted diseases caused by *Chlamydia trachomatis*. The disease is common in tropical and subtropical climates. Though it used to be a rare finding in the United States, it's on the rise thanks to increased travel and sexual contact.

The disease begins with fever and a generally uncomfortable feeling of malaise. These symptoms are accompanied by the development of a bump (papule), which becomes a painless vulvovaginal ulcer after one to four weeks. This stage often goes unnoticed. About one month later, lymph nodes in the groin, in the pelvis, or near the rectum become inflamed (adenitis). Inflamed, tender lymph nodes on one side lead clinicians to suspect LGV. The enlarged lymph nodes may mat together, forming a ridge that looks like a second fold of skin in the groin (a groove sign). But when the lymph nodes near the rectum or in the pelvis are involved, few signs are present.

Because LGV is an STD, clinicians always check for other STDs. LGV must be treated with antibiotics, usually tetracycline; sometimes the enlarged glands need to be opened and drained.

LARGE BUMPS FROM A LOOP OF BOWEL (HERNIAS)

Loops of bowel pushing through a weak place in the abdominal wall (hernias) can present as vulvar masses and be mistaken for large cysts or growths. The mass may be in the labia or in the groin. Hernias may produce no symptoms, but some give a sensation of heaviness. Generally the clinician can push the hernia back up into the abdomen (reduce the hernia); doing so makes the diagnosis. Surgical repair is usually indicated.

LARGE BUMPS FROM MUSCLE (FIBROIDS)

Fibroid growths are very common in the uterus but rare on the vulva. A fibroid is made of smooth muscle and is solitary and firm, but it is capable of enlarging, sometimes very rapidly. Because of its rapid growth, a fibroid (the official medical term is *leiomyoma*) of the vulva is usually removed.

LARGE VERSIONS OF SMALL BUMPS

Some of the growths that are usually small may occur in a large form. They may be confused with other conditions until a biopsy confirms their identity. Acrochordons, or skin tags, for example, may (rarely) enlarge to considerable size. Epidermal cysts occasionally reach diameters greater than half an inch. Neurofibromas may also reach a large size. Large growths are usually removed in order to confirm a diagnosis and because they cause discomfort.

Conditions with a red color

Normal skin gets its flesh tone in part from the redness of blood cells flowing through the superficial blood vessels. Abnormal redness results when these vessels are easier to see. They are easier to see when there are a lot of them, when they are enlarged (vasodilatation), when they fill up with blood (engorge), and when the layer of skin on top of them is very thin. Vasodilatation is part of the local immune and inflammatory response and accounts for the redness of conditions such as yeast infections, allergic reactions, folliculitis, and vestibulitis. Psoriasis, Paget's disease, and reactive vulvitis are red because of the decreased number of cell layers between the surface and the blood vessels.

Red conditions usually cause symptoms. Many cause itching; some result in soreness or pain. Because the surface blood vessels are so fragile, some lead to bleeding. It is always important to figure out what is causing a red condition.

Red conditions covered in other chapters are yeast (Chapter 10); eczema, psoriasis, and lichen planus (Chapter 15); vulvar vestibulitis (Chapter 17); and precancerous changes and Paget's disease (Chapter 22). The following sections describe some others.

REDNESS FROM INFECTED HAIR FOLLICLES (FOLLICULITIS)

Blockage and infection of the hair follicle will cause a raised red bump (papule) around the hair. The papule may develop pus in it (pustule). These pustules are usually small; they open and drain spontaneously. Large pustules may need to be drained surgically. Antibiotics may be needed to treat severe, recurrent folliculitis.

Folliculitis is common. It may occur in relationship to hair removal practices, such as shaving. Folliculitis can often be prevented by washing with an antibacterial soap (Dial, Lever 2000, pHisoHex). Please see Chapter 5 regarding hair removal.

REDNESS FROM FUNGI
(RINGWORM OF THE GROIN, *TINEA CRURIS*)

Infection of the groin and upper thighs by fungi (different from the yeast, *Candida albicans*) that thrive in the skin results in a red, usually symmetric area with clear-cut margins and raised edges. Heat and humiditiy often allow fungi to be transferred to the area by hands or inert items such as a bath towel. Genital-to-genital contact with someone who has tinea is another way to pick it up. Tinea is most common in women who wear tight, occlusive underwear, particularly during warm weather.[3] The skin between the vagina and rectum (perineum), the anal area, and the crack between the buttocks may be involved. Often the feet are infected. Itching is common; obesity, sweat, friction, and heat make the problem worse. Diagnosis is made by taking skin scrapings to view under the microscope. Treatment comes from topical application of clotrimazole (Gyne-Lotrimin) or miconazole (Monistat-7) for seven days.

REDNESS FROM BACTERIAL INFECTION (ERYTHRASMA)

This is an uncommon problem, but it can look just like candida and *Tinea cruris*. Erythrasma does not usually cause symptoms, but makes symmetric red patches in the groin or on the labia. It is caused by the bacterium *Corynebacterium minutissimum*. It is diagnosed with a special light, the Wood's lamp, which makes the bacteria appear fluorescent orange in color. Treatment with antibacterial soap and erythromycin by mouth will clear up most cases.

Conditions with a white color

A white appearance comes from three factors, which may act together or separately: the amount of a skin protein named keratin, the loss of special cells containing colored pigment (melanocytes), and a lack of blood vessels (avascularity). Vitiligo and albinism, two conditions characterized by a lack of pigment in the skin and described below, result from problems with melanocytes. Thickened, itchy skin (squamous cell hyperplasia) results from all three of these factors. If radiation is given for pelvic tumors, it destroys the melanocytes as well as blood vessels in the skin, leading to a pale, white appearance with loss of hair.

A white condition covered in another chapter is lichen sclerosus (Chapter 15).

WHITENESS RESULTING FROM LOSS OF PIGMENT
(DEPIGMENTATION DISORDERS)

Conditions that can cause a loss of pigment in the vulva include vitiligo, albinism (piebaldism), and loss of normal skin color after repeated inflammation (postinflammatory hypopigmentation, or leukoderma).

Vitiligo is an inherited condition resulting from the loss of pigment-carrying cells (melanocytes) from the skin. The melanocytes associated with pigmented hairs are among the last to be affected, so one may see black hairs growing from a whitened patch of skin. Any area of the body may be involved, including the vulva. The edges of the whitened areas may be scalloped with milky white depressions in the pigmented, darker skin. There may be other family members with the condition. Sometimes people with vitiligo have other autoimmune conditions such as thyroid disease or underactive adrenal glands (Addison's disease).

Partial albinism (piebaldism) is also an inherited condition. From infancy onward, patches of nonpigmented skin and hair are seen on the forearms and forehead. Small patches may be seen on one labium. Partial albinism is different from vitiligo in appearance because the hair in albinism loses pigment and is as white as the skin. Albinism has no clinical significance and does not need treatment.

Postinflammatory hypopigmentation (leukoderma) describes lack of color seen in areas affected by inflammation, injury, or ulceration. It may be temporary, with growth of new melanocytes into the area, or permanent. Leukoderma differs from vitiligo and albinism because the skin surface in the white area is thin, there is a history of previous inflammation, a familial history is lacking, and other body areas are not affected.

WHITENESS FROM INFLAMMATION (INTERTRIGO)

Intertrigo means "between the three corners." An inflammatory problem, it's found in the groin folds, underneath the abdominal fold (panniculus), and under the breasts. With constant moisture present on the skin between the folds, the superficial surfaces become white. Debris from skin cells that are shed, oil gland secretions, bacteria, and sometimes yeast form an accumulation of white, yellow, or gray matter on top of the reddish, shiny skin fold.

Minimizing moisture is essential. Women with intertrigo need loose cotton clothes, especially underwear. Washing with antibacterial soap is important. Dry the area well and apply a thin dusting of Zeasorb powder, which can be obtained over the counter at drugstores. If yeast is also a problem, Lotrimin powder is prescribed. Strips of plain cotton cloth (tear an old bedsheet into strips) may be placed under the folds to help with the moisture.

WHITENESS FROM SKIN REACTION TO RADIATION

Contemporary equipment allows the radiotherapist to give pelvic irradiation with little effect on the overlying skin. But some women have skin changes from older equipment used some years ago. Radiation changes result in loss of hair and pigment as well as blood vessels so that the skin appears pale and hairless. Unfortunately, there is no treatment to repair radiation damage.

Common dark discolorations

Melanocytes are specialized cells found deep in the skin layer that produce pigment. The amount of pigment in your skin is racially and genetically determined. Look at your hand, first palm down and then palm up, and you can probably see that the amount of pigment also varies in regions of the body. Vulvar skin is generally darker than other skin because of an increased number of melanocytes.

Any stimulus that leads to more melanocytes, such as inflammation, infection, or trauma, may result in a dark discoloration. There are also dark discolorations that come if an injury has left a blood clot (hematoma). The clot is gradually absorbed by the body but leaves some pigmented material from the red blood cells behind. Much less likely would be precancerous changes or a melanoma.

To diagnose a dark discoloration, a clinician needs to take a biopsy; no one can absolutely identify the source by inspection alone. A general rule in gynecology is that any dark area on the vulva, even if you think it's been there forever, ought to be biopsied. Most likely you'll be told it's one of the harmless dark discolorations below.

DARK DISCOLORATION FROM PIGMENT CELLS IN THE SKIN (LENTIGO)

The most common vulvar dark discoloration is the lentigo. It comes from localized excess production of melanin pigment from melanocytes. A lentigo looks much like a freckle. There are often more than one; they are flat, vary in size from a tiny dot to half an inch, and are usually a shade of brown. Lentigo may be found on the labia majora or minora or in the vestibule. They produce no symptoms. A lentigo needs to be biopsied or removed because, rarely, it can be an early form of melanoma.

DARK DISCOLORATION ARISING FROM SPECIAL CELLS IN THE SKIN (NEVUS)

A nevus—more commonly known as a mole—is a growth from the cells in the skin that contain color or pigment. Moles vary in color from light tan

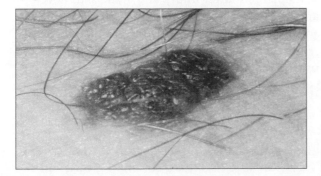

FIG. 43 A **nevus**, or mole, is a slightly raised pigmented lesion. Because of the small chance of melanoma, any dark lesion on the vulva should be biopsied or removed.

to dark brown or black. They do not produce symptoms. Normally they're perfectly harmless, yet moles are significant because they can develop into a cancer called malignant melanoma, which is a rare but very serious kind of cancer. Certain types of moles carry a greater risk for the development of melanoma, but figuring this out by appearance is not possible, even for experts. Doctors recommend that pigmented moles be removed when found on the vulva.

DISCOLORATIONS CAUSED BY INSECTS (PUBIC LICE, CRABS)

Pubic lice, or crabs, are usually confined to the hair-bearing areas of the genitalia, but sometimes they can be seen in armpit or eyelash hair. Crabs are different from the head and body lice that are usually confined to those areas. While sexual contact is a frequent means of the spread of pubic lice from one person to another, bedlinen, upholstery, and clothing can also serve as sources of infection. Lice are almost transparent gray in color, but they can be seen because they contain dark pigment from the digestion of blood that they feed on. To the naked eye, the louse looks like a tiny rusty spot on the skin surface near the base of the hair shaft. Louse eggs (nits) are olive-shaped, pale gray specks on the hair shafts.

Itching of the mons or upper labia is the most common complaint. Because lice are sexually transmitted, other STDs must be checked for when lice are found. One or two applications of Kwell (lindane) as a cream or lotion after a shower are effective (though Kwell should not be used in pregnancy). All clothing and bedlinen should be washed as part of the treatment program. It's important to know that egg cases may remain attached to the hairs for a week or two after treatment, but their presence does not mean treatment failure.

DARK DISCOLORATION AFTER INJURY (REACTIVE HYPERPIGMENTATION)

Skin can react to chronic inflammation, persistent low-grade irritation, or injury with the development of extra pigment. (Clinicians don't understand why some skin loses pigment after injury and some skin develops extra pigment.) This darkening can be seen in skin that constantly chafes, as in diabetics with chronic fungal infection in the thighs. The pigmentation is totally flat. Once the diagnosis is made, no treatment is necessary, but the pigmentation usually remains.

Rare dark discolorations

DARK DISCOLORATIONS ARISING FROM SKIN (SEBORRHEIC KERATOSIS)

A seborrheic keratosis is a slightly raised, uneven growth that may be small or reach several inches in size. It is not a common growth on the vulva, but it's sometimes seen in postmenopausal women. The cause is unknown. There may be a single growth or a cluster. Often dark brown and greasy in appearance, it looks as if it has been stuck on the skin surface and could be peeled off like a sticker. It does not become cancerous and requires no treatment unless it enlarges to cause discomfort.

DISCOLORATIONS ARISING FROM SPECIAL CELLS IN THE SKIN (MELANOMAS)

Melanomas are rare tumors, but 10 percent of vulvar cancers are melanomas. The tumor can appear in several different fashions: A flat freckle (lentigo maligna) is extremely rare on the vulva; the superficial spreading melanoma is the most common type found on the vulva; the nodular melanoma is a raised tumor with an irregular surface.

Vulvar melanomas may occur at any age but are most frequent after age 50 and are almost always seen only in Caucasian women. Since the outcome is directly related to the depth of the melanoma in the skin, it is *essential* to find the problem early. For this reason, all dark growths on the vulva need to be biopsied. If melanoma is diagnosed, it is treated surgically.

Ulcers

A final category of skin disorders seen in the vulvovaginal area is the ulcer. An ulcer occurs when part of the top layer of the skin is destroyed. It appears as a raw, reddish depression in the skin that may have some sticky clear or yellow material on it. Because the surface skin is gone, ulcers often bleed easily. Some start as a blister that pops, leaving the ulcer.

Ulcers come from a huge number of problems. An ulcer similar to a canker sore is a common problem. Most other vulvar ulcers aren't that common. Skin diseases, medications, inflammatory bowel disease, and autoimmune diseases can all cause ulcers on the vulva. Pressure sores or bedsores in immobilized women can appear as deep vulvar ulcers. An inflammation of blood vessels (Behcet disease) is a rare cause of ulcers.

Some ulcers are the result of infection by bacteria or viruses. Herpes, syphilis, chancroid, granuloma inguinale, lymphogranuloma venereum (LGV), and HIV are all sexually transmitted diseases that can cause ulcers at some point in their course. STDs are always considered when a woman has an ulcer on the vulva.

Cancers also can cause ulcerations on the surface. If there is an open sore on the vulva, it is essential to see a clinician and find out what it is. Ulcerative conditions covered in other chapters include herpes (Chapter 20) and hidradenitis suppurativa (Chapter 15).

It's important to understand that vulvar ulcers are hard to figure out. A physician can't just look at them and say what they are. Since vulvar ulcers are sometimes part of diseases in other parts of the body, your clinician needs to know if you have symptoms anywhere else. Often some initial tests—cultures and blood work—are necessary. Antibiotics may be given just in case there is an STD. Then, based on the test results and whether the ulcer is clearing up, other tests, and perhaps a biopsy, may be necessary.

ULCERS OF UNCLEAR ORIGIN (CANKER SORES, APHTHOUS ULCERS)

Canker sores (aphthous ulcers) are usually mild but recurring ulcers of the mouth. Sometimes these can occur in what's called the major form of aphthous ulcers, with more severe mouth ulcers associated with recurrent vulvar ulcers. These usually involve the labia minora or vestibule. This problem often gets started in adolescence; there may be a family history. There are no other disease symptoms that go with it. The cause of aphthae is unknown. Aphthae of the mouth or vulva can be helped with prescription topicals such as clobetasol (Temovate) or fluocinonide (Lidex)—gel for the mouth, ointment for the vulva—dabbed on the ulcers several times a day until they start to disappear.

ULCERS CAUSED BY INFECTION WITH BACTERIA OR VIRUSES

These include the following sexually transmitted diseases.

Syphilis

Ulcerations of the vulva may be seen in the first (primary) and later (secondary) stages of syphilis. The first ulcer, called a chancre, is usually single, hard, and painless, but sometimes many ulcers, infected by bacteria, develop that are soft and painful. The primary chancre appears about three weeks after infection and heals spontaneously after one to six weeks. At this time a blood test for syphilis will usually come back positive. Lymph nodes in the groin will be swollen.

Three to six weeks after the development of the chancre, syphilis goes into its secondary stage. This is systemic disease, as the infecting organism spreads. On the vulva ulcerations are soft white papules or patches. Eventually these open up to form an ulcer that contains large numbers of the infecting organism, *Treponema pallidum*. If untreated, syphilis may progress to a third stage involving the central nervous system and the aorta.

Syphilis is easily treated with two doses of penicillin a week apart. A search for other STDs must also be done.

Granuloma Inguinale (GI)

This STD is not common in the United States, though it's seen more frequently in tropical countries. It is caused by *Calymmatobacterium granulomatis*. The disease sometimes begins with superficial ulcerations, or sometimes starts with a painless reddish nodule. The ulcers have irregular edges and a bright red base. The groin lymph nodes may be swollen. The ulcerations may form scars. GI is treated with tetracycline.

Chancroid

Chancroid is a sexually transmitted disease caused by a bacterium called *Haemophilus ducreyi*. As with GI, it is a disease of the tropics but has been seen in the United States. It begins with raised bumps of the vulva on or between the labia. The bumps become pimples, then tender ulcers. They may be present for weeks or months before they become bothersome. Swollen groin nodes develop. Chancroid is treated with erythromycin.

Acquired Immune Deficiency Syndrome (AIDS)

Vulvar disease may be the first complaint of AIDS, which is a consequence of infection of white blood cells with the human immunodeficiency virus (HIV), resulting in failure of the immune system. The ulcers created are frequently multiple and may involve the perianal, vulvar, and vaginal surfaces. They are frequently painful and may become infected. The diagnosis is made by excluding other causes of ulcerations. Zidovudine may be effective in controlling the ulcers; systemic cortisone is also helpful.

ULCERS CAUSED BY INFLAMMATORY BOWEL DISEASE (CROHN'S DISEASE)

Crohn's disease causes ulceration of the vulva and perineum in up to 30 percent of women who have this problem.[4] Sometimes these ulcers are the first symptom the patient experiences, and may develop years before the bowel problems start. Actually, swelling may be the first sign, followed by cracking of the skin (fissures) and then ulcers. At other times, the vulvar ulcers are caused by connections to the diseased bowel. Mouth ulcers are sometimes seen as well. Treating the bowel disease will treat the vulvar problems, although surgical removal of the diseased bowel and the vulvar area may be required.

ULCERS CAUSED BY MEDICATIONS (STEVENS-JOHNSON SYNDROME)

This rare problem involves the mucosa of the mouth, eye, and vulva, with sudden inflammation and ulceration accompanied by fever and general discomfort. The vulva has painful shallow ulcers and blisters on all parts of the labia and surrounding skin. Any drug can cause a reaction like this, but antibiotics and laxatives are the most frequent offenders.

ULCERS CAUSED BY AUTOIMMUNE DISEASE IN THE SKIN (PEMPHIGUS AND PEMPHIGOID)

These are very rare diseases of middle and old age that cause blistering of the skin and mucous membranes; they are not common on the vulva, but this may be the area where they are first seen. Biopsy makes the diagnosis;

cortisone is the standard treatment. It is essential that a dermatologist be involved with the case of a woman with pemphigus.

ULCERS CAUSED BY BLOOD VESSEL INFLAMMATION (BEHCET DISEASE)

Behcet disease is very rare but because it's on the list of vulvar ulcers it is often considered when someone has an ulceration of the vulva. It is a disease that involves other body systems besides the vulva, and without signs of inflammation in other areas, Behcet disease is probably not the diagnosis.

Ulcerations of the mouth and genitals, along with inflammation of the eyes, are seen in Behcet disease; other symptoms include arthritis, inflammation of the veins (thrombophlebitis), acne, inflammatory bowel disease, and neurological symptoms. The symptoms come and go and sometimes do not occur all at the same time. The ulcers on the vulva are painful and leave some skin changes or scarring after they heal. The disease is caused by inflammation of blood vessels (vasculitis), but the cause of the inflammation is unknown.

Usually a biopsy is necessary to make the diagnosis. The vulvar ulcers are managed with cortisone; topical Xylocaine helps with the tenderness. Systemic cortisone or other drugs are sometimes necessary for severe disease. A rheumatologist usually manages the nonvulvar problems.

▼ ▼ ▼

Whew! We've been through the whole collection of garden-variety V bumps and color changes as well as most of the weirdos. If there's one message this litany should underscore, it's that you need to make vulvar self-exams a part of your life. Get acquainted with your Vs, and little changes are much less likely to sneak up on you.

▼

CHAPTER 17

"It Hurts"

New Insights into the V Pain Syndrome Vulvodynia

For a vulvovaginal specialist like me, this chapter is one of the most exciting in this book. For someone who suffers from V pain, I hope it may provide an "Aha!" moment—or at least be a source of answers and empathy. A great deal is finally being learned about a long-ignored, long-mysterious group of vulvar symptoms. Chronic stinging, irritation, pain, rawness, burning, or painful intercourse has been a problem for women and those who care for them for centuries. The first written records of painful intercourse were in Egyptian papyri and the Talmud.[1] Medical textbooks of the 1800s contained accurate descriptions.[2]

Not until 1983, though, did we have a name for this large group of vulvar symptoms: *vulvodynia*.[3] And it's taken almost another twenty years for this term to start creeping into public awareness. As one of the characters on the TV series *Sex and the City* said when her friend's diagnosis entered the plot line, "Vulvo-*what*-ia?" (Surely a TV first!) Vulvodynia is extremely new turf even for most physicians. Studies funded by the National Institutes of Health (NIH) only began in August 2000. I'm working with Dr. Bernie Harlow from Brigham and Women's Hospital in Boston on one of the NIH grants. Finally we're going to learn about this problem, which plagues so many women!

There is still some overlap of terms used, but the following quick summary (based on new categorizations from the International Society for the Study of Vulvovaginal Disease in 1999) can help you keep them straight:

▼ *Vulvodynia (VVD)* (say "VUL-vo-DIN-nee-ah"): spontaneous, generalized pain in the vulvar area. There may or may not be pain with intercourse, which is called *dyspareunia* (say "dis-par-OON-ee-ah"). You may also hear *vulvodynia* used as the overall term for any kind of vulvar pain, including the following conditions.

▼ *Vestibulodynia (VBD)* (say "vess-TIB-u-lo-DIN-ee-ah"): pain on touch in the vestibule. It almost always causes painful intercourse. Also called *vulvar vestibulitis* or just *vestibulitis,* it's a specific kind of vulvodynia localized in the vestibule.

▼ *Clitorodynia* (say "KLIT-or-oh-DIN-ee-ah"): another localized form of vulvodynia with pain in or around the clitoris.

For years, the *only* term used to describe pain with intercourse—and a diagnosis still inaccurately handed out—was *vaginismus* (say "VAAH-gin-IZ-muss"). This means that the muscles around the vaginal opening clench up like a brick wall. Vaginismus is a legitimate condition that may develop because of VBD. With repeated pain on touch and pain with intercourse, the muscles go into spasm. Not every woman with VBD has vaginismus, though. Or vaginismus may occur as a result of sexual trauma or abuse, and not be related to vulvodynia. (See Chapter 18 for more on vaginismus.)

I suspect that vulvodynia affects many more women than most doctors have traditionally believed, probably because for so long this problem was not recognized as a specific syndrome. According to one survey, at least two hundred thousand women in the United States have significant vulvar discomfort that greatly reduces their quality of life.[4] But the actual numbers of vulvodynia are probably higher, and rising.[5] A gynecologist in private practice in Oregon, Dr. Martha Goetsch, reported that 15 percent of all patients seen in her general gynecological private practice fulfilled the definition of VBD.[6] In a week of my own specialty practice, I see ten to fifteen new patients for VBD. In a month I see more than a hundred patients, new and established, with vulvar pain.

Clinicians consider VBD and VVD chronic pain conditions. Although the exact cause of vulvar pain hasn't yet been confirmed, one of the leading theories concerns a glitch in the central nervous system. Nerve endings don't work well and messages get all mixed up, so that touching hurts or burning is present for no good reason. What follows is a theory about how a woman can develop this pain.

Pain theory

Vulvar pain is complicated to diagnose because there are virtually no physical signs of disease. Women complain of severe pain and/or inability to be touched, but when the physician does an examination, nothing looks unusual other than some redness. How can there be nothing to see when the pain is so bad?

Over the years, as clinicians struggled to understand, some flashes of insight began to occur. As we wondered why touching the vestibule should hurt, we realized that our colleagues who study the nervous system (neurologists) had specific terms to describe what women with vulvodynia were experiencing. When a touch that should be pleasant causes pain, this is called *allodynia*. When something that normally causes a small amount of pain causes excessive pain, this is *hyperalgesia*. Allodynia and hyperalgesia are features of vulvodynia and vestibulodynia. And then clinicians realized that women with terrible burning of the vulva but no findings on physical examination were like surgical amputees with phantom limb pain. The leg and the insult causing the amputation were long gone; there was no abnormality to be seen, but the burning pain (hyperalgesia) persisted. Even a bedsheet over the stump caused pain (allodynia), just the way underwear can set off vulvodynia.

From these experiences in other areas of medicine, a theory then developed that VVD and VBD are primarily pain disorders that come from abnormal pain circuits set up in the central nervous system. VVD and VBD may be two different kinds of pain disorders. VVD may involve pain from nerve injury. VBD may involve pain from nerve inflammation.

I believe that VBD is a form of inflammatory pain. The nerve is not injured but is so continuously bombarded by inflammation that signal changes occur in the spinal cord to keep the pain going.

Here's how the inflammatory pain theory may work. The vulva, and especially the vestibule, are rich in special nerve endings called C fibers. These guys respond to pain or any disagreeable sensation and carry this message through the spinal cord to the brain and back again to the vulva. The vulva also has A fibers, which respond to light touch.

Chronic irritation triggers the C fibers. The list of possible causes includes just about any V aggravation imaginable: yeast infections, skin inflammation from an irritant (contact dermatitis) or an allergic response, mechanical irritation from chronic unlubricated and undesired

VOICES

"I had absolutely no idea that it wasn't supposed to hurt there."
—Donna, 28, when I showed her the vestibule and the painful places

intercourse or from constant stretching of the nerve when a joint is out of line, chemicals such as treatments for warts or HPV, or a natural chemical in the urine called oxalate. This theory appeals to clinicians because there are so many individualized triggers, which helps explain why women with so many different histories wind up with the same pain. We'll discuss the possible triggers in detail below.

The irritation causes the release in the tissue of various inflammatory chemicals that affect the C fibers: prostaglandins, histamines, and others. If the irritation continues, prolonged firing of the nerve fibers alters nerve centers in the spinal cord. These nerve centers then mix up signals coming from light-touch nerve fibers in the vulva (those A fibers) and tell the central nervous system that usually pleasurable light touch is painful. The result is painful intercourse and the pain with touch that are classic symptoms for VBD.

If the irritation continues, the chronic stimulation may eventually result in the creation of a new, spontaneous signal that travels from the spinal cord to the vulva, creating a burning pain even without any touch at all.

This theory is the first reasonable explanation of the mystery of vulvar pain. With this explanation, we can view VBD as a disruption of the normal neurological response to a variety of chronic irritations that occur on the vulva.[7]

Scientific support is starting to accumulate. Two studies have shown that tissue removed from women with VBD has an increased number of nerve fibers that are coarse and thickened, suggesting chronic inflammation.[8] These nerve fibers are C fibers, responsive to pain and irritation. Elevated levels of two inflammatory chemicals have been found in specimens from women having surgery for VBD.[9] In the ducts of glands in the vestibule are special nerve fibers that make a highly inflammatory chemical, substance P.[10]

Recently researchers looking for changes in genes that regulate the extent of inflammation found that women with VBD possess a form of a gene (IL-IRA 2,2) that makes inflammation more prolonged and more severe.[11] This finding suggests that women with this form of the gene have a greater susceptibility to developing a prolonged inflammatory response that could lead to the malfunctioning pain circuits described in the pain theory.

On the other hand, VVD may occur when a nerve is actually injured (neuropathy). The nerve continues to send pain signals even after the injury has gone. Neuropathic pain is seen when a nerve or a nerve root near the spinal cord is injured, stretched, or pinched. Neuropathic pain can be tricky because the original nerve injury may be insignificant or not apparent. The pudendal nerve, which supplies the vulva, is formed from several nerve roots in the lumbosacral spine. It could be pinched by any abnor-

---

ASK YOURSELF   Clues to Vestibulodynia

Have you ever said the following? Such statements can help a clinician diagnose VBD.

"I have never been able to use a tampon; it hurts."

"The doctor needs to use the smallest speculum."

"Sex is painful; my doctor says I need to relax more."

"I always have yeast; the creams don't work."

"I had a baby months ago but the episiotomy stitches still hurt."

"I am very small down there, and it's just too tight."

"Sex has been painful since menopause, and even with estrogen cream I am not comfortable."

Source: M. F. Goetsch, Vulvar vestibulitis, Contemporary Ob/Gyn Oct. 1999:56.

---

mality in the spinal area—a ruptured disc or a bone spur from arthritis, for example. The pudendal nerve then travels a long way from the spine through the pelvis to get to the vulva. In its course over ligaments and muscles it can easily be pulled or pinched if joints are rotated and out of alignment. We'll discuss this more in the VVD section below.

With these pain theories in mind, let's look at the two different kinds of vulvar pain, vestibulodynia and vulvodynia.

Vestibulodynia (VBD)

Of the various V pain conditions, vestibulodynia seems the most common. I see five cases of VBD for every one of vulvodynia. Women with VBD have irritation, pain, or discomfort that is specific to the vestibule, the area between the thin inner lips (labia minora) of the vulva. Women may be aware of some constant discomfort in the vestibule. The irritation often makes them (and their clinicians) think that they have frequent yeast or bacterial infections that do not clear with standard treatment. Their main complaint, however, is the pain that occurs with any kind of touch in the vestibule. Putting in a tampon hurts; women with VBD often say they were never able to use a tampon comfortably and have always relied on pads. It hurts when a clinician inserts the speculum for a vaginal examination. These are women for whom sex has never been comfortable or for whom sex was once comfortable but then became miserable. Penetration during intercourse causes such pain that women have to stop, limit their sexual activity, or avoid sex altogether. Tight clothes, washing during a bath or shower, or wiping after using the toilet can cause pain. Some sports activities, such as biking, may cause great misery.

Although the woman with VBD may have some degree of spontaneous burning, her major pain occurs only with attempts to enter the vagina. The pain that comes with intercourse is called introital or super-ficial dyspareunia, to distinguish it from deep dyspareunia in the pelvis that is usually associated with endometriosis or chronic pelvic inflam-matory disease. (This is also mentioned in the next chapter, on sex and pain.) A rating of the discomfort associated with intercourse was de-signed to define the severity of the condition. Level I dyspareunia causes discomfort but does not prevent sexual intercourse. Level II dyspareunia sometimes prevents sexual intercourse. Level III completely prevents sexual intercourse.[12]

VBD seems to come in two forms. Primary VBD occurs in women who have had pain on touch from their first sexual experience or attempt to use a tampon. Secondary VBD is seen in women who, prior to developing a problem, had months or years of comfortable touch, sex, and/or tam-pon use.

POSSIBLE CAUSES OF INFLAMMATORY PAIN IN VBD

The pain theory explains the pain of VBD, but what sets this off? One of the problems with the pain theory is that women with primary VBD—that is, who have pain with their first attempt to use a tampon or have sex—often deny any history of trauma or irritation that could have led to abnormal pain circuitry. These women, however, tend to have other pain problems, such as constipation, diarrhea and abdominal cramping (irrita-ble bowel syndrome), urinary frequency, urgency and bladder pain (inter-stitial cystitis), chronic fatigue syndrome, migraine headaches, painful joints and muscles (fibromyalgia), and jaw pain (temporomandibular joint syndrome). Clinicians wonder if these women are lacking the chem-ical necessary for the manufacture of endorphins that help us deal natu-rally with pain.[13] But the actual trigger for women with primary VBD remains unclear.

For women with secondary VBD that arises after a period of comfortable intercourse, there are, as I indicated, sometimes factors that could trigger inflammatory pain. Let's look at them.

Could the cause be . . .

▼ *Persistent infection and inflammation?* Bacterial infection as a cause for the pain is not likely.[14] There is no evidence of infection in the vulvar tissues, and the vagina is normal. But VBD certainly appears to be an inflammatory process. Because the tissues look so red and irritated in many women, many clinicians try some type of cortisone, whether shots, pills, or cream. Some women report improvement, but cortisone has not brought significant reduction of the pain. Antihistamines have also been tried without much success. A recent study showed a significant increase in the number of mast cells, which release histamine, a chemical that causes inflammation.[15] But when the antihistamine cromolyn was used in a cream in the vestibule to block the release of histamine, it proved no more effective than a placebo.[16] However, the action of cromolyn against mast cells in the body is modest and short-lived, and it does not prevent histamine release from mast cells that are in mucosal tissue such as the vestibule.[17] A promising report on the success of the drug Elmiron for the painful bladder condition interstitial cystitis (discussed in Chapter 19) suggests that it reduces bladder pain because it prevents release of histamine from mast cells, the presence of which has long been noted in bladder biopsies. Mast cells are also found in biopsies from women with VBD. I have just started to use Elmiron for my patients with VBD, but it's too soon to know if this has any value.

▼ *Human papillomavirus (HPV)?* In the 1980s, a great deal of attention went to this virus as a possible cause of vestibulodynia. Since HPV caused warts on the vulva and cancer of the cervix, clinicians wondered if it could be causing pain in the nearby vestibule. Though a few studies suggested that vestibulodynia might be related to infection with HPV, many others disagreed.[18] I always look for another reason for VBD; after all, HPV is a *skin* virus, not a *nerve* virus (like herpes) that can cause pain.

▼ *Herpes?* The pain of nerve involvement from the herpes virus is well described by people who have experienced the pain of shingles. In fact, herpes is considered a cause of pain in vulvodynia, and suppression of the herpes virus is an important treatment for this kind of pain.[19] But there's no evidence that the herpes virus is found in the vestibule.[20]

▼ *Yeast?* For a long time people have thought that frequent yeast infections might be a possible cause of VBD.[21] But, as I've noted many times in these pages, yeast is not well diagnosed in the United States, and no one can say for sure that the symptoms the women had were really from yeast infections. Virtually all women with vulvar VBD have been treated many times with yeast cream without getting better. I do believe that for some women, yeast is the trigger that sets off the whole process of inflammatory pain. You can bring the yeast under control, but you still have to deal with the aftermath of the pain. Other clinicians wonder if all the chemicals in the yeast creams used by the women lead to VBD; typically these creams pool in and around structures in the vestibule in concentrations much greater than those in the vagina.[22] We need much more accuracy in diagnosing yeast before we can answer this question. If I think that yeast is in any way involved, however, I am quick to ask a woman to go on a single fluconazole tablet weekly to keep yeast out of the picture.

▼ *Chemicals or other technologies?* All the treatments and medications used to treat HPV have been looked at as causes for vestibular pain, including freezing (cryosurgery), acid, podophyllin, and laser.[23] Some researchers think a powerful cream that causes peeling of the skin, 5-fluorouracil, helps treat VBD, while others believe that it may cause the problem.[24] Clinicians have also wondered if other irritants, such as those found in products for feminine hygiene, may be the cause of the problem.[25] Since many women use feminine hygiene products but don't get VBD, however, and many women with VBD have never used them, this seems unlikely. I have seen a number of women who have had extensive treatment for HPV of the vulva with chemicals and laser. I believe that these were the triggers for their inflammatory pain.

▼ *Hormones?* Women frequently ask if there is any connection between the pain of VBD and hormone levels. We don't have good information. Only one study found a significant connection between early oral contraceptive use and the development of vulvodynia, suggesting that hormonal factors might play a role.[26] Most women report that their pain is worst just before their period comes, when estrogen is at a low point. A common feature of VBD is cracking of the skin around the vaginal opening, particularly at the back. Estrogen is well known for its ability to thicken skin, increasing its elasticity by building up collagen in the tissue. There are reports of success with topical estrogen as well as testosterone, but no large studies have been done.[27] Currently, topical estrogen treatment is part of the medical management for VBD suggested by many clinicians; it is believed to soothe, thicken the vestibular epithelium, and promote healthy nerve functioning. Estrogen can be made up in a neutral base to avoid irritation from commercial estrogen creams. I ask every woman with VBD to use a small amount of estrogen in the vestibule every night.

▼ *Oxalate?* Oxalate is a chemical widely found in many foods and in water. It's difficult to completely eliminate oxalate from the diet and still obtain all the necessary nutrients. All women have oxalates in their urine.[28] The amount varies largely based on the foods eaten approximately twelve hours before. In 1991, biochemist Dr. Clive Solomons and gynecologist Dr. M. Herzl Melmed triggered a flood of interest when they reported a single patient who had increased vulvar pain just after she had large amounts of oxalate in her urine.[29] Her clinicians thought that the microscopic sharp-edged crystals of oxalate in the urine might be irritating the covering of the vulvar vestibule. They treated her successfully with a diet low in oxalate-containing foods and with oral calcium citrate to combine with the oxalate and make it inactive. Many women with vulvar pain have since tried the diet and the citrate, with varied results.

In another study done on oxalate, researchers found no difference in the amount of oxalate in the urine between women with no pain and vulvodynia patients.[30] The women with no pain actually had a significantly higher concentration of twenty-four-hour oxalate. The study also found that taking citrate for three months improved pain no better than a sugar pill. A group from Cornell University observed that women hated the diet and lost weight on it, but it did nothing for their vulvar pain. Most women stopped the regimen after two or three months. The success rate was 14.3 percent, no better than placebo.[31] The oxalate theory continues to be widely debated. I doubt that it is a trigger. I do think that foods *highest* in oxalate may worsen VBD and I ask women to avoid these. See page 308.

▼ *A psychological cause?* It's always tempting to suggest that any problem we do not understand is a psychosomatic condition, "all in your head." One of the great challenges facing women with vulvodynia and the clinicians who care for them is the education of the world with regard to the reality of the pain.

It's been reported that women who had surgery for VBD don't differ from healthy women with respect to marital satisfaction, psychological distress, or psychological problems.[32] One exception that makes perfect sense to me: Women who have chronic pain interfering with sexual functioning have been found to have reason to be depressed.[33]

Some authors have associated vulvar pain with a history of sexual

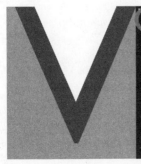

VOICES

"I've had a yeast infection that lasted eight months."

—Ashley, 22, who has VBD (this kind of mistaken self-diagnosis is typical; if the problem had been yeast, antiyeast creams and Diflucan would have cleared it up)

abuse, but others disagree.[34] Others are looking into whether the chemicals triggered by stress set off inflammation.[35]

In other words, as with all aspects of vulvodynia, we need more research. In the meantime, a psychiatric basis for vulvar pain is often diagnosed only when all other causes have been eliminated.[36] But it's a diagnosis I almost never make!

DIAGNOSING VBD

Since there are many causes of pain in the vestibule (see the box "What to Rule Out First"), it's vital to make sure that these are eliminated before the diagnosis of VBD can be made. A vulvar biopsy is not necessary on a routine basis, but it is helpful to diagnose suspected skin disorders.[37]

When other possible causes of vestibular pain have been eliminated, VBD is diagnosed by a process known as Friedrich's criteria: (1) severe pain on vestibular touch or attempted vaginal entry, (2) tenderness to swab pressure localized within the vulvar vestibule, and (3) various degrees of redness (erythema) in the vestibule with no other sign of problems. The symptoms must have been present for over six months and the tenderness moderate to severe intensity.

Women with VBD may have no visible changes in the vestibule or may have red spots. These are often hidden under little folds of the hymen and

WHAT TO RULE OUT FIRST   Other Reasons for Vulvar Irritation, Pain, or Painful Intercourse

The diagnosis of VBD or VVD is made when all other possible causes of these symptoms—infections, skin diseases, and other medical conditions—are ruled out. The following things can also result in vulvar symptoms or painful sexual intercourse. (Most are explained elsewhere in the book; see Index.)

Infections: Bartholin's gland abscess, yeast infection, herpes, human papillomavirus, molluscum contagiosum, trich

Trauma: sexual assaults, other physical injuries

Systemic disease: Behcet disease, Crohn's disease, Sjögren's syndrome, systemic lupus erythematosus

Precancerous conditions, cancer: vulvar intraepithelial neoplasia (VIN), vulvar cancer

Irritants: soaps, sprays, douches, antiseptics, suppositories, creams, the HPV treatment 5-FU, laser treatment

Skin conditions: allergic or contact dermatitis, eczema, psoriasis, hidradenitis suppurativa, lichen planus (LP), lichen sclerosus (LS), pemphigoid and pemphigus (two rare skin diseases that cause blistering)

Source: H. K. Haefner, M. D. Pearlman, Diagnosing and managing vulvodynia, *Contemporary Ob/Gyn*, Feb. 1999:110.

won't be seen unless you look carefully by gently pulling the labium out toward the side and pushing the hymen tags toward the vagina. The redness may vary from pale red to flaming red, and there may be isolated spots or widespread redness. What is red is not as important as what hurts. (See the box "The Q-tip Test" and Fig. 44.)

THE Q-TIP TEST

One of the best tests we have for diagnosing vestibulodynia is as simple as it sounds. You imagine the vestibule is the face of a clock, with 12 just above the urethra and 6 at the bottom. Touching around the vestibular "clock" with an ordinary cotton swab produces pain in one or more places. Often the most painful areas are at 6. If the Q-tip test isn't done, if a clinician just goes ahead to put a speculum in the vagina, useful information may be missed.

TREATING VBD

Since the cause of VBD is not known, and since about a third of the time any treatment, even a placebo, will create a physical change, remedies abound. They don't all work, but some may be worth trying. The first step should be stopping use of all soaps, creams, douches, fragrances, or chemicals that may come into contact with the vulva. Eliminating tight clothing and abrasive activities against the vulva (such as bicycling) is equally important. Conservative measures such as soaks in the tub, soaks in soothing solutions, topical cortisone creams, sex hormones, antibiotics, antifungals, and retinoids have

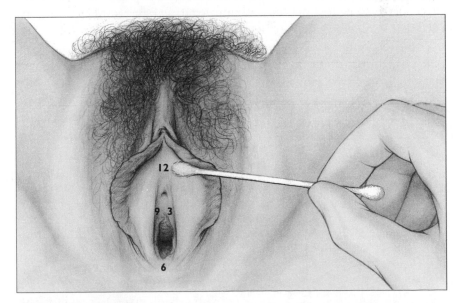

FIG. 44 The Q-tip Test
Touching around the vestibule as if touching each of the numbers around a clock face reveals tender areas often missed when the speculum is inserted without this step.

VOICES

"Eleven years ago I had a terrifying experience during a gyn exam. The gynecologist was rude, pushy, insensitive, accusatory, and intimidating. I did not have a successful Pap smear, as I felt I was being torn in two before the gynecologist could even insert the speculum. I left the office and never returned.

"Upon marriage, I had pain, pressure, and a sensation of tearing upon attempts at intercourse. Members of a new gyn team were patient, understanding, and supportive, but I still experienced pain with pelvic exam.

"Also, I have not had successful intercourse. There are many emotional issues here at present, which I feel prevent his interest, as well as mine, in pursuing a physical relationship. Counseling has been suggested, but I am not sure he is committed to what counseling will require. I feel I need to work on issues myself before I would be able to go to counseling with my husband. Too many other issues are involved.

"Successful intercourse is at times the furthest thing from my mind."

—Sarah, 28, who has vestibulodynia

not been effective in the overwhelming majority of cases.[38] Topical anesthetic agents such as 2 percent Xylocaine applied to the painful areas may help and permit the possibility of intercourse in some cases. But the anesthetic needs to be in a neutral and nonirritating base. Nonirritating topicals such as vegetable oil are also soothing and moisturizing.

What to do about sex? The vulvar golden rule: Thou shalt cause no pain. If it hurts, don't do it. Pain was invented by Mother Nature as a warning—it tells you something is wrong. It's best to take a break while you pursue your treatment. Please see Chapter 18, "Sexual Healing," about how to maintain your relationship and your sexuality in the face of pain.

Here's some information about other treatments currently in use.

Oxalate Reduction

Because oxalate is a theoretical cause of VBD, much attention has been given to reducing this chemical in the urine. But a low-oxalate diet is difficult to

HIGH-OXALATE FOODS TO AVOID

Beer, tea, cocoa, Ovaltine, beverage mixes, peanuts and peanut butter, pecans, soybean curd (tofu), all berries and berry juices, Concord grapes, citrus peel, rhubarb, tangerines, chocolate, vegetable and tomato soups, fruitcake, grits, wheat germ, black pepper, beans of all kinds, beets, celery, chard, collards, dandelion greens, eggplant, escarole, kale, leeks, mustard greens, okra, parsley, green peppers, sweet potatoes, rutabagas, spinach, summer squash, and watercress.

follow and may be nutritionally inadequate. Sometimes my patients zealously try to eliminate all oxalate but just wind up losing weight and developing a serious case of constipation. Straining with bowel movements further insults the muscles of the pelvic floor and can add to the pain. Given the limited studies that support the oxalate theory, a more reasonable approach is to eliminate foods high in oxalate (see box on page 308) and take OTC calcium citrate (200 mg of calcium combined with citrate, in two tablets three or four times a day). In theory, this regimen would prevent the formation of painful calcium oxalate crystals that might aggravate the pain. The calcium citrate may take up to six months to show any effect, though.

Tricyclic Medications

Antidepressants can help manage pain whether or not depression is present.[39] How can something that works for people who are depressed relieve pain in the genital area? Clinicians aren't completely sure. Tricyclic antidepressants improve depression by increasing levels of certain brain chemicals. Building up levels of these same chemicals is part of the way these drugs help pain. The amount necessary to treat pain is usually much lower than the amount needed to treat depression.[40]

In one study, the antidepressant amitriptyline gave relief to twenty women, ages 43 to 85, with constant vulvar or perineal discomfort.[41] Following the success of amitriptyline, other drugs in the tricyclic family were used successfully. Less clear is the effectiveness of another kind of antidepressant, the selective serotonin reuptake inhibitors (SSRIs) fluoxetine (Prozac), paroxetine (Paxil), and sertraline (Zoloft).[42] Venlafaxine (Effexor) and nefazodone (Serzone) have been reported as beneficial for a small number of patients with vulvodynia.[43]

Not all clinicians think drugs help. I do, particularly for women with secondary VBD. The medications tried have been around for many years, and much is known about their safety and side effects. Unfortunately, the gold standard study for medical research, a double-blind placebo-controlled trial, has not been performed for their use in VBD. But we use

VOICES

"I have a depressed vagina!"
—Charlotte on *Sex and the City*, on being diagnosed with vulvodynia

methods that are not well studied because they are safe and we don't know enough to have a single "best" treatment.

The tricyclic drug originally used for the treatment of vulvar pain, amitriptyline, is the best known. Its sister compounds can be equally effective. If one tricyclic doesn't work, another might. I use desipramine and nortriptyline a lot because they have the mildest side effects. (See box on page 311.)

Tricyclics are not effective when taken on an as-needed basis, but rather should be taken daily. Their effect doesn't usually kick in for several weeks, and improvement is very irregular—you'll have good periods and bad periods. I usually begin patients with a tiny dose—5 to 10 mg—and increase slowly every five to seven days to 50 mg. This allows the body to become accustomed to the medication. If there isn't any improvement with 50 mg, the dose may continue to be increased up to 150 mg if there are no troublesome side effects.

Once pain is controlled, the woman maintains that dose for two to three months before trying to taper down. Some women are able to discontinue the medication, but some need to continue for longer periods of time. *Do not discontinue this medication without first checking with your clinician.* Sudden discontinuation may cause pain to bounce back or may cause nausea and fatigue. Tapering off is necessary. Once stopped, the effects of the medication may continue for another three to seven days.

Tricyclic antidepressants are not addictive or habit-forming and may be used safely under medical supervision for long periods of time. Before taking a tricyclic, let your clinician know if you take other medications, have a chronic illness, have an allergy to any medication, are pregnant or intend to become pregnant, or are breast-feeding. While no woman wishes to take medications when she's pregnant, there is no evidence that shows that these are harmful to the baby. Ask your clinician. Alcohol and other central nervous system depressants such as barbiturates may alter the effectiveness of your medication or cause serious side effects. Before using them, talk with your clinician.

An overdose of this medication is very dangerous. Keep it out of reach of children.

A cautionary word about side effects: One of the first things that my patients do after a drug is prescribed is to read up on it in the *Physicians' Desk Reference* (PDR), available in any library and online. The PDR lists every side effect ever reported by patients. So the lists are long and the side effects may or may not be real. For example, if you develop a rash after eating a turkey sandwich for lunch one day, you might decide that the turkey sandwich caused the rash when actually the sandwich had nothing to do with it. Just because a side effect is cited in the PDR does not mean it will happen to you!

TRICYCLIC ANTIDEPRESSANTS AND THEIR SIDE EFFECTS

Generic name	Brand name	Tendency for dry mouth, constipation, flushed skin	Sedative effect	Tendency to cause a slight drop in blood pressure	Tendency to cause a slight increase in heart rate
Desipramine	Norpramin	Mild	Mild	Mild	Mild
Nortriptyline	Pamelor	Mild	Mild	Mild	Mild
Amoxapine	Asendin	Moderate	Mild	Moderate	Moderate
Maprotiline	Ludiomil	Moderate	Moderate	Moderate	Mild
Trazodone	Desyrel	Mild	Moderate	Moderate	Moderate
Imipramine	Tofranil	Moderate	Moderate	Moderate	Moderate
Doxepin	Sinequan	Moderate	Strong	Moderate	Moderate
Amitriptyline	Elavil	Strong	Strong	Moderate	Strong

Most side effects with tricyclics are usually more annoying than serious. The chief ones include the following:

▼ *Sedation.* Most tricyclics are taken at bedtime because of their sedative effect, and they bring a good night's sleep. If you are feeling tired on arising in the morning, you may eliminate this problem by moving the time you take the medication back into the evening, even to suppertime. Drowsiness is often present for only a short period of time; then it will diminish. It is very important to give the medication some time before you decide that the sedation is unacceptable.

While taking tricyclics, you may find that over-the-counter medications, especially cough or cold preparations, may cause a slight increase in the sedation effect. A decongestant called pseudoephedrine in many of these preparations may combine with the antidepressant to make your heartbeat speed up. Read labels and avoid pseudoephedrine.

▼ *Constipation and dry mouth.* Tricyclic drugs slow down the part of the nervous system that controls secretions and the activity of many internal organs. As a result, you may experience dry mouth, nose, eyes, constipation, increased perspiration, blurred vision, or a slight increase in heart rate (which is not harmful). These side effects can be effectively handled by drinking fluids, using hard candies and chewing gum, using saline nose drops and artificial tears, and adding fiber to your diet and using stool softeners such as Colace and Metamucil. (See the box "Don't Let Side Effects Stop You!")

One of the biggest problems women run into when taking tricyclics is constipation. Not only is it miserable, but also the resultant straining worsens vulvar pain. I worked with Ellen, who has VBD, for about eighteen months. Amitriptyline really helped her, and she was able to have sex. But she was so constipated, she couldn't stand the drug. So we talked about diet. I asked her if she ate breakfast. In the usual rush to get out, she didn't—she had some juice and a pastry at midmorning. "How about the rest of the day? Do you eat fruits and vegetables?" I asked.

"Oh, yes, I eat fruits and vegetables."

"Do you eat four to seven servings of fruits and vegetables a day?"

"Well, I drink lots of juice and I eat a salad every day for lunch."

Problem is that juice has no fiber in it and a salad of iceberg lettuce has almost none. I suggested that if she didn't think she could add fiber to her diet, how about taking a fiber-containing laxative such as Metamucil?

She said Metamucil didn't work.

"Are you taking it regularly every day?"

She said she'd rather drink a glass of sawdust than take that stuff every day.

I was sad to discontinue a drug that really helped. Ellen tried other medications, but none worked as well as amitriptyline for her. So she went back to it. And she really worked with her diet. She added some fruit and a bowl of raisin bran in the morning and found she actually liked eating breakfast! She packed a lunch and made a point of eating at least one apple a day, sometimes two. Her husband loved the new taco filling of black beans and corn. She tried other fiber-containing products and found one she liked better than the sawdust. Last week she reported she was ready to go off the amitriptyline because sex is now okay and she's trying to become pregnant.

▼ *Other side effects.* These may include dizziness, light-headedness, and headache (these tend to lessen within a few days); an increased appetite for sweets; weight gain; shakiness, nervousness, or restlessness; difficulty sleeping; difficulty urinating. Contact a clinician if you experience the rare symptoms of mental confusion, loss of balance, skin rash and itching, swollen tongue, difficulty swallowing, or seizures.

Antiseizure Medications

An alternative to the tricyclics are drugs classified as antiseizure medications, including carbamazepine (Tegretol) and phenytoin (Dilantin). Over the past two years, clinicians have been prescribing a new anticonvulsant drug called gabapentin (Neurontin) for nerve injury pain. I use a lot of Neurontin. Many women who come to see me have been on tricyclics, and Neurontin is a natural next step. It has fewer side effects than Tegretol and Dilantin and does not require one's blood levels to be monitored. Early studies have found that the drug is safe and gives excellent pain relief with few bad side effects, although it does not work for all patients.[44] Researchers are not sure exactly how gabapentin works to relieve pain, but believe it both blocks a doorway (the sodium channel) that needs to open so that the

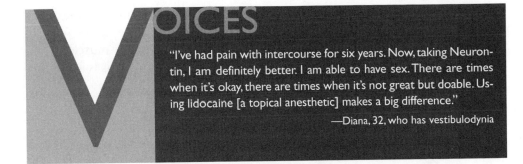

VOICES

"I've had pain with intercourse for six years. Now, taking Neurontin, I am definitely better. I am able to have sex. There are times when it's okay, there are times when it's not great but doable. Using lidocaine [a topical anesthetic] makes a big difference."

—Diana, 32, who has vestibulodynia

nerve can send a pain message and makes another nerve conduction pathway (GABAergic) work better.[45]

Women are often scared at the idea of taking a drug used to treat seizures. But nerve injury pain and seizures are similar. With pain, the injured nerve fiber discharges spontaneously, with a clocklike regularity. With seizures, the nerve also discharges spontaneously but in a disorderly and irregular fashion. Anticonvulsant drugs work to calm the nerve fibers, controlling the pain or stopping the seizure.

For seizures, Neurontin is used in doses of 900 to 1,800 mg daily. For the treatment of pain, Neurontin works over a huge range of doses. It is best to start with a small dose, such as 100 mg/day, and increase the amount slowly, adding 100 mg every five to seven days. Patients do beautifully on dosages up to 4,000 mg or more. One of the major advantages of Neurontin is that it is well handled compared with other drugs. It can, however, cause side effects. The commonest are sleepiness (which often goes away after a day or two), dizziness, less coordinated body movements (walking may feel awkward), and involuntary eye movements. Less common are facial swelling, headache, slight increase in blood pressure, loss of appetite, aching joints, and decreased white blood cell count.

Physical Therapy and Biofeedback

Women often find it unbelievable when I recommend physical therapy to the pelvic floor for vulvar pain, but it has rapidly become one of the mainstays of medical management and prevents many women from needing surgery. *But why,* women ask, *if I have pain, do I need to work on my muscles?*

In VBD, the vulvar pain causes the nearby muscles of the pelvic floor to become tense as they hold tight against the pain. Eventually the muscles go into spasm; this message goes to the spinal cord and back to the original source on the vulva, perpetuating the pain. So when a muscle goes into spasm, it can actually *maintain* the original pain even if the cause goes away. Besides having nerve fibers that are out of control, the VBD patient now has misbehaving muscles too.

The muscle involved (pubococcygeus, or PC) is the large sheaf of muscle fibers that connects the pubic bone in the front with the tailbone at the base of the spine in the back. The PC muscle fibers make up the muscles around the urethra, the rectal sphincter, and the vaginal muscles. Contractions of the PC muscle are the sensation of orgasm. This is a very important muscle for women!

If you do a study of the electrical activity that is involved in the work of the PC muscle, you find that a normal resting PC muscle shows 1 to 2 microvolts of electrical activity. In women with vulvar pain, the muscle is not only chronically tense but in spasm, showing much higher (2 to 5 microvolts) activity. Women with vulvar pain are unable to tighten or squeeze (contract) the PC muscle effectively, and they cannot sustain this tightening for more than a few seconds. A woman with a healthy PC muscle can hold the tightening up to ten seconds.

A tense muscle or a muscle in spasm causes pain. As the muscles become exhausted from working overtime in this state, they build up lactic acid, which also causes pain. This biochemical response is similar to what happens when a person overexerts athletically—like the pain of running a marathon!

With the physical therapy techniques developed by Dr. Howard Glazer, a psychologist interested in vulvar pain and muscle function, women reeducate the muscle with a simple exercise program, much like Kegel exercises for bladder control.[46] Women become reacquainted with sensation in the PC muscle through the use of biofeedback. The patient inserts a small, tamponlike device, the electomyographic sensor, into the vagina. The sensor is connected by a wire to a computer. The woman can look at the computer screen to see the electrical activity in her PC muscle.

The exercises consist of tightening the muscle and holding it for ten seconds, then relaxing it for ten seconds. This exercise is done sixty times, requiring twenty minutes. As the muscle strengthens, the chronic tension is broken, and the muscle relaxes.

Many women think they are tightening the muscle when they are not, or they are not tightening sufficiently. The biofeedback screen tells them exactly what they are or are not doing and is dramatically more effective in strengthening the pelvic floor muscles than the use of verbal instructions.

It may take two or three months to get the resting level of the muscle down to 0.5 to 1.0 microvolts. Sometimes women get worse during the first week or two, but once the resting level gets down to the desired figure, the patient begins to feel better. It may take another two to three more months of pelvic floor work for the pain to go away completely.

Other Physical Therapy

Past physical injury, scarring from surgery, trauma from childbirth, or misalignment of bones or muscles can restrict mobility, leading to pain.

For example, a fall while ice skating could cause a sacral misalignment that leads to pelvic floor tension and a burning sensation in the vulva.

The effects of chronic vulvar pain can manifest themselves throughout all body systems. Patients with vulvar pain often stand, sit, and sleep in improper positions to reduce vulvar pressure.[47] Abnormal posture develops. The inability to sit squarely often causes musculoskeletal pain in the hips, lower back, and shoulders. Gait becomes unbalanced, and body organ systems such as the bowel lose their natural action. Everything is overpowered and controlled by the relentless pain. In addition to dealing with the original pain problem, the physical therapist can identify and treat the other musculoskeletal dysfunctions that result from the chronic pain.

Besides the Glazer protocol, physical therapists have a choice of many treatment options to address physical imbalances and restore mobility. These include trigger point therapy (pressure application at the problem point), myofascial release (mobilizing soft tissue by massage), craniosacral techniques, visceral manipulation (manipulation of the abdominal organs, pelvic tendons, and muscles), postural and gait training, bony realignment, interferential electrical stimulation (application of TENS electrodes to achieve muscle relaxation), vulvar ultrasound, and the use of ice. Intravaginal treatments include therapeutic exercise, soft tissue mobilization, biofeedback, and electrical stimulation.

Not just any physical therapist can do these things. You need someone who knows about VBD and the pelvic floor. (See Resources.) It's a good idea to also ask your candidate if she is familiar with VBD and comfortable using Glazer's program of physical therapy and biofeedback.

Physical therapists also instruct women in the use of dilators. Once muscle relaxation is achieved, women learn to insert dilators in graduated sizes. *Dilator* is a confusing word that suggests opening up and making larger. But for VBD a woman uses a dilator not because she is too small but because with a dilator you control every aspect of what is happening vaginally—how fast, what angle, how quickly. We should call the device something like a Vaginal Entry Sensitization Control System! When in control of everything, you gain confidence as you learn that vaginal entry is not painful. Working with a dilator takes time and effort. You have a lot of other things that you'd rather be doing, but your hard work will usually pay off.

Interferon

When the human papillomavirus (HPV) was thought to be the cause of VBD, injections into the vestibule of a chemical that may fight off the virus, interferon, were used. Even when the viral theory started to fade, clinicians believed that the interferon could help boost the body's immune system to help fight off whatever the attacker might be. Although one of the first researchers to study this treatment reported complete relief in more than 80 percent of selected patients, the majority of investigators have had less successful results.[48] One study found surgery was more helpful than interferon.[49] The jury's still out.[50] I worked with it extensively for about five years without much success. I continue to offer it to women, since we don't have a lot of options and it has few side effects.

Psychological Treatment

Counseling for women with VBD may be valuable to treat depression that arises in response to pain and sexual difficulties. Getting rid of the pain is my foremost priority, though; no counseling will help until that is gone.

Surgery

It works—but I use it as a last resort after major medical management efforts have failed. Let me explain why. Women often want to know right away if I can simply "cut something"—sever a nerve—to relieve the pain. Severing a nerve anywhere up to the area where the nerve enters the spinal cord, or even where the nerve enters the brain, may still leave you with pain.[51] You may continue to perceive pain in the same area, because the way the brain works is to interpret an impulse from part of the nerve as an impulse from the entire nerve. This explains why cutting off nerve endings usually doesn't eliminate pain. It's also why amputees still perceive pain beyond the amputated stump (phantom limb pain): The nerve still "thinks" it is supplying the whole leg. What's more, if you cut the nerves that cause vulvodynia, you would lose bowel or bladder control. A classic operation to eliminate pelvic pain, removal of part of the nerve supply to the pelvis (presacral neurectomy), has not worked for vulvodynia, and in some cases women have become worse.[52]

For similar reasons, nerve blocks don't work. "Can't you just inject something to make the whole area numb?" I'm asked. Once again, the problem is that if you block sensation, you also block motor function and affect bladder and bowel function. And pleasure—clitoral re-

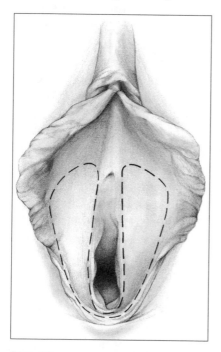

FIG. 45
The Incision for Vestibulectomy
A dotted line marks off tissue that is to be removed. The hymen is also included. Small stitches bring the area together for a satisfactory appearance afterward.

sponse—would be blocked too. In addition, nerves can become hypersensitive as a result of repeated blocks.[53] Pain clinics around the country are working with nerve blocks, but they are still in the experimental stages.

The surgery that does work, and that is in fact one of the best treatments for VBD, is the surgical removal of a section of the vestibule *(vestibulectomy)*. It was popularized by a gynecologist at Johns Hopkins, Dr. Donald

---

COMMON QUESTIONS: Vestibulectomy

Q What is a vulvar vestibulectomy?

A Vulvar vestibulectomy is a surgical procedure designed to eliminate or improve painful intercourse that comes from vestibulodynia. A strip of tissue in the vestibule between the inner lips (labia minora) is removed. (See Figure 45.) This tissue is believed to contain the hypersensitive nerve endings that cause the pain of VBD. Along the sides of the vestibule where the tissue is removed, stitches are placed. In the back, at the entrance to the vagina, a cushion of thick elastic vaginal tissue is brought forward (vaginal advancement) to provide a little padding at the point of entry for sexual intercourse.

Q Who is a candidate for vestibulectomy?

A Vestibulectomy is done only for women who have vestibulodynia. Women who have pain elsewhere on the vulva, or women who have spontaneous pain without touch, may not be appropriate candidates. Women who have urinary symptoms associated with their pain may not benefit from the surgery. Some women may want surgery as their first choice, before other management is tried, but I discourage this.

Q How successful is vestibulectomy?

A The success of the surgery depends on proper selection of the candidates and a surgeon with experience in this procedure. Women must have pain confined to the vulvar vestibule and not beyond. The procedure must remove adequate portions of the vestibule, including the painful areas. For properly selected candidates with an experienced surgeon, the initial success rate is 60 to 90 percent.

Q Does vestibulectomy interfere with sexual enjoyment?

A The procedure does not cut across or remove any areas associated with sexual pleasure.

Q Does vestibulectomy alter my appearance?

A The vestibule is narrowed from the procedure, but usually only an experienced gynecologist can tell that a woman has had the surgery.

Q Does vestibulectomy interfere with childbearing?

A There is no known relation between VBD and fertility, and vestibulectomy does not affect ability to have a normal vaginal delivery. Occasionally I will recommend cesarean delivery in a complicated situation—for example, lichen sclerosus in addition to vestibulectomy.

COMMON QUESTIONS: Vestibulectomy   cont.

Q How long does the procedure take?

A The operation is performed in an ambulatory care facility. The surgery itself lasts about an hour. Women may choose to go to sleep (general anesthesia) or to have a spinal block (regional anesthesia). The patient goes home several hours after the procedure.

Q What is the recovery from a vestibulectomy?

A It varies; most women need two to four weeks out of work and at home to recover. The surgical site is painful, especially with sitting and moving around. Vigorous physical activity must be avoided for at least two weeks. Activity at first should be limited to reading or watching TV; after five days short, easy walks are okay. A rubber ring may make sitting more comfortable.

There are a number of stitches (the kind that are absorbed into the body and do not need to be removed), and it is important to limit activity to allow healing. The suture line will feel bumpy from all the small stitches; these are absorbed in several weeks and the area smoothes out. There may be some oozing from the incision for twenty-four to forty-eight hours. Women need an ice pack applied to the vulva for twenty-four hours followed by soaks in the tub two to three times a day for seven to ten days. After each soak a small amount of anesthetic gel (Xylocaine) may be applied. Urinating may be more comfortable while warm water is poured over the vulva or while sitting in a tub of water.

Narcotic pain pills are often alternated with ibuprofen. Pain pills may cause constipation; stool softeners such as Colace will help prevent this. The antifungal drug Diflucan is usually given to keep yeast away.

Q What happens if the surgery does not eliminate the pain?

A A 60 percent success rate means that six out of ten women who have this procedure will be able to resume sexual relations with reasonable comfort; they may not be perfect, but sex will be enjoyable. Between 10 and 40 percent of surgery patients say they see no change after the surgery or continue to worsen because of the disease process of vestibulitis. There is no evidence to suggest that the surgery itself makes anyone worse.

Some women have a prompt improvement within six to eight weeks of the operation; others do not respond for up to six months. This amount of time may be necessary for the hypersensitivity to resolve and normal nerve conduction to take over again. So it may take some time to know what your result is.

Woodruff, who reported in 1981 that all eighteen patients in a study had complete relief of painful intercourse after vestibulectomy.[54] A recent major review of reports over twenty years found that 89 percent of the 646 women studied had a significant decrease in their symptoms after surgery.[55] The disappearance of painful intercourse was reported in 72 percent of 512 women; 11 percent had no response to the operation.

Because no one knows what causes VBD, the reasons for the success or failure of surgery are not well understood. That uncertainty makes it a highly debated topic. Clinicians are clear that it is useful only for women with VBD, not vulvodynia. As well as when other efforts haven't worked, I recommend surgery for women who cannot have intercourse at all. Although I recognize the controversial nature of an operation to improve nerve-related pain, if a woman is unable to have vaginal intercourse, it is difficult to withhold a procedure with a 60 percent or higher success rate.

The surgery may not help for several reasons.[56] Constant vulvar pain in addition to painful intercourse before the surgery suggests that vulvodynia is present in addition to vestibulodynia. Patients with urinary symptoms, those who often think they have a bladder infection and don't, do not respond as well to surgery. These are not reasons to avoid surgery, but the pros and cons should be considered carefully. Women who have never had comfortable sex or who have had a long stretch of sexual pain are not going to swing into satisfac-

A VBD SUCCESS STORY

Amelia, 25, had struggled with itching and burning and then painful intercourse for years. She clearly had recurrent yeast infections, but pain persisted even when these were in control. VBD was finally diagnosed and treated with vestibulectomy. But the surgery brought her only partial improvement, so she saw another expert in a large teaching hospital, who diagnosed her with the skin disease lichen sclerosus (LS) and did a revision of her surgery to take out some additional painful areas. With cortisone ointment to control the LS and topical estrogen to buff the tissues, Amelia's problems came under control.

About a year later, she moved to Boston and saw me because she was starting to have pain again. She had a rip-roaring yeast infection. Once again, even when the yeast came under control, she continued to have pain, which concerned her greatly because her wedding was coming up. It turned out that all she needed was some medication to follow up her surgery. I prescribed a tricyclic antidepressant and Neurontin to control the pain, and I sent her for some physical therapy as well. The bride was beautiful and the honeymoon went well. Finally, after a year, she has been weaned off the oral meds. She does her exercises, uses her cortisone ointment and local estrogen, and keeps yeast at bay with weekly oral medication. Though not yet completely free from discomfort, intercourse for her is comfortable and enjoyable.

tory experiences after surgery in the blink of an eye. They need considerable help with postoperative relaxation techniques and sexual counseling in order to achieve comfortable sexual intercourse.

The surgery may not help if only a small area at the back of the vaginal opening is removed. Another common problem is failure to remove the vestibule around or above the opening of the urethra; the woman may be left with focal tenderness in these areas.

Postoperative pain with intercourse may also come from a sensitive scar. This problem can be avoided by bringing a flap of vaginal tissue out onto the perineum to cover the incision line in the back (vaginal advancement). The scar will be located outside the vaginal entrance (introitus) so as to avoid painful pressure during intercourse.

Postoperative vulvar pain may be caused by the formation of a Bartholin's duct cyst. During the surgery, the ducts of the Bartholin's glands are cut, but usually the gland will form a new opening for drainage into the vagina.[57] In cases where the duct remains blocked, a Bartholin's duct cyst may develop later. If it does, women may complain of a feeling of fullness at the base of the labia majora and around the vaginal opening when sexually aroused, and a swelling at the base of the labium may be noted. If the symptoms are minimal, observation may be all that is required; a large cyst that causes significant discomfort or becomes infected will need to be drained. One clinician recommends removal of the Bartholin's glands in every case because they may be involved in the inflammatory process of VBD.[58] The removal of Bartholin's glands is not an easy operation to perform. There is the risk of increased blood loss as well as postoperative scarring and pain; this practice has not been adopted by most clinicians at this time.

Another reason for ongoing pain with intercourse after the surgery is vaginismus, or involuntary tightening of the vaginal muscles. Women are often so accustomed to experiencing pain with penetration that they automatically tighten up with any attempt at vaginal entry. (See Chapter 18.)

For women with continued pain, use of medical therapy often has benefit. One support group has had success with aloe vera cream and an estradiol cream.[59] If there is a small focal area of pain, this can often be eliminated with superficial laser therapy or possibly simple excision with local anesthesia. Postoperative interferon treatment has helped some women.[60] Repeat surgery, especially if there are sensitive areas around the urethra, may be carried out.[61] Finally, referral to a pain center is an option for women who have not had relief from any medical or surgical management.

VESTIBULODYNIA TREATMENT SUMMARY

If you have VBD, I suggest that you:

▼ Read and learn about the problem (see Resources); join a support group if you wish

▼ Eliminate any possible trigger by suppressing yeast infection, treating LS, or controlling any other source of inflammation

▼ Eliminate all possible vulvar irritants; use healthy hygiene and comfort measures (discussed in Chapter 15)

▼ Use a daily topical estrogen cream on the vestibule—about ¼ teaspoon rubbed in well

▼ Try physical therapy to the pelvic floor, with biofeedback

▼ Take a tricyclic antidepressant or gabapentin

▼ Consider interferon or surgery if medical management is not successful after three to six months

Vulvodynia (VVD)

This kind of vulvar pain is usually quite different from VBD. Women with
VBD are fine until touch in the vestibule is involved; women with vulvodynia have a burning discomfort most or all of the time. With VBD the
area involved is limited to the vestibule; vulvodynia may hurt anywhere
from the pubic bone to the anus, even down the thigh. The typical patient
with this complaint is postmenopausal (middle-aged to elderly) and not
receiving hormone replacement therapy, but I also see the problem in
younger women.[62]

Symptoms are felt over various areas supplied by the branches of the pudendal nerve; pain may occur on one side of the vulva, on both sides, or
in an asymmetric fashion. Pain may be widespread and diffuse or just in
one spot. Because the problem involves this one nerve, vulvodynia is
sometimes called *pudendal neuralgia*.

Often women find it hard to explain their symptoms to me. They speak of
a vague rawness or itching-burning sensation; they can't always even point
out exactly where it hurts. The pain may not be associated with any particular activity, though for some women it worsens with sitting or standing for
long periods of time.[63] Intercourse may hurt like a rope burn, or you may
have no problem at all sexually. Some say that light touch on the vulva
brings on the pain; even movement of their pubic hairs can lead to burning
pain.[64] Sometimes women have brief, sharp, shooting pains (paresthesia).
Some patients report burning in the mouth, and some report sciaticalike
pains over the buttock and down the back of the leg.[65] But sometimes, mys-
teriously, the burning will let up for days or weeks at a time.

Women also complain of vaginal discharge or increased vulvar secretions. When I'm having a hard time figuring out what's going on, I ask a
patient to come in during a flare. She feels terrible, with aching, burning
rawness. In addition, there is often increased normal sticky white sebum
from the vulvar glands, or increased normal vaginal secretions. I think increased secretions appear because the wacky nerve pain fibers are not reg-
ulating the glands properly. My experience has been that the medications
we use to control the pain eventually cut down on the secretions, but it
takes months.

On a physical exam, there's little to see. At most, there may be some
mild redness and a little swelling. The pelvic exam may trigger burning
discomfort. But the clinician finds no evidence of infection, no abnormal
wet mount, no pH change. If a woman complains of urinary symptoms
such as burning and frequency, urinalysis and a urine culture are done—
and these too are negative.

VOICES

What does vulvodynia feel like?

"It feels like there are knives there all the time. On good days it is little paring knives sticking me; on bad days there are butcher knives."

—Lorna, 75

"I am so embarrassed to say this, but it feels like my pubic hair is caught, or something is pulling on it."

—Bobbie, 23

"There were all these people in my house for Passover, and I was in the bathroom crying. A friend brought me some ice."

—Hadassah, 44

"The vulva and vagina feel swollen, dry, and painful—like sitting on a cactus. They are sensitive to touch and pressure. Intercourse is exquisitely painful, especially since I have major difficulty lubricating."

—Janet, 41

"This feels like it should be red and on fire when you look at it!"

—Kate, 27

Lack of physical findings is one of the key reasons women are slow to be diagnosed with vulvodynia. Most physicians, carefully trained to detect the subtlest of changes, find it difficult to believe that any problem with such marked pain leaves no visible evidence. Yet our neurologist colleagues often see patients with bad pain over the pathway of a nerve, and not much else.

CAUSES OF VULVODYNIA

Injury to the pudendal nerve is probably the root cause, and this can be caused by different things. Most of the nerve supply to the vulva comes from the pudendal nerve; its branches supply the entire area from the pubis over the labia and across the perineum to the anus.

Earlier I said that the pudendal nerve has to travel a long way from its origin in the spinal cord roots to its destination in the vulva. A disc that has popped out from between the vertebrae or a piece of vertebra thickened by arthritis could press on the nerve in the area of the spinal cord. (There's not a lot of room back there, and anything out of line can pinch a nerve.)

Other ways the nerve could be injured:

▼ *Surgical trauma.*[66] Injury to the pudendal nerve could occur during any kind of pelvic surgery performed near the course of the nerve or after a

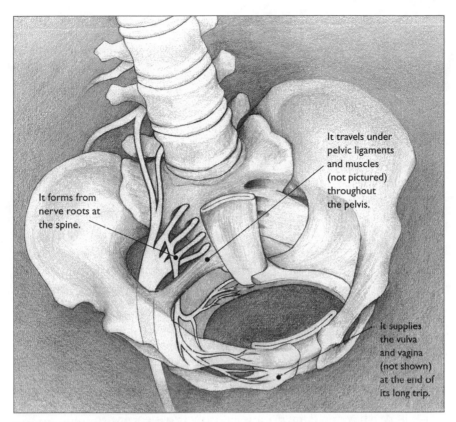

It travels under pelvic ligaments and muscles (not pictured) throughout the pelvis.

It forms from nerve roots at the spine.

It supplies the vulva and vagina (not shown) at the end of its long trip.

FIG. 46 **The Pudendal Nerve**

complication of surgery, such as a large blood clot in the pelvis. Injury to the pudendal nerve has been reported with a procedure to fix a bulge, or prolapse, of the vagina.[67] The vagina is tacked to a ligament near the base of the spine (sacrospinous ligament). Both the pudendal and sciatic nerves travel underneath the outside third of this ligament.

▼ *Orthopedic injury.* If a ruptured disc can cause vulvar pain, it seems likely that falling on the back or tailbone (coccyx) can also lead to VVD.[68] Several muscles in the pelvis can send pain signals to the vulva. The piriformis muscle runs from the front of the lower backbone (sacrum) to the hipbone (femur). It turns the hipbone outward. The pubococcygeus muscle runs from the back of the pubic bone to the coccyx. It is part of the pelvic floor that supports the pelvic organs, and also part of the anal sphincter. Another set of muscles that runs from the pelvic bone to the hip, the obturator muscles, also help turn the hip outward. Any injury to the obturators, as well as the joint that connects the backbone to the hipbone (sacroiliac joint), is commonly felt as pain in the perineum, vagina, and rectal area.[69] Sports injuries, automobile accidents,

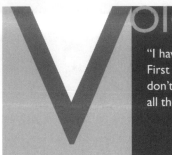

or any misalignment of these muscles or joints could lead to vulvodynia. It is not uncommon to find vulvar pain in women with problems in the hip joint, women with one leg longer than the other, and women with sacroiliac joint imbalance who pursue physical activity such as ice skating or running. Curvature of the spine (scoliosis) has the potential to cause misalignment of the hips and sacroiliac joint that can make the pudendal nerve unhappy.

▼ *Sports trauma*. Possibilities include those related to horseback riding, bicycling, or using exercise equipment in vulnerable women.[70]

▼ *Childbirth*. The pudendal nerve is stretched for long periods of time during the delivery of a baby. It appears that in women vulnerable because of their anatomy or particular delivery trauma, vulvodynia could result. We have no data, no studies, only experience with some cases.

▼ *Herpes virus*. Anyone who's had shingles knows the pain this condition can trigger. The type most commonly associated with vulvodynia is herpes simplex.[71] Another herpes virus (zoster) associated with painful skin blisters (shingles) can lead to vulvodynia if the shingles appear near the vulva. Both of these viruses damage nerves, and if they hang out in branches of the pudendal nerve, vulvodynia is the payment.

▼ *Other causes*. Vulvodynia has been seen in association with a harmless but painful growth of nerve fibers (neurofibroma) and in patients with multiple sclerosis.[72] Metabolic or connective tissue diseases, such as diabetes and Sjögren's syndrome, can sometimes involve nerves, so vulvodynia can be found with these types of problems.

DIAGNOSING VULVODYNIA

Patients and physicians alike are frustrated by trying to nail this problem. There are no clear signs, no special tests. There is no one single cause. The woman complains of the worst burning imaginable, yet on examination there is nothing to see. It's easy to understand how one might jump to a psychiatric diagnosis.

Nevertheless, a medical workup can do the job. The history comes first,

VOICES

"I tell myself I can get past the pain. It will not last. With the Elavil and what my physical therapist has taught me, I can control it."
—Ellen, 53, who has vulvodynia

to pinpoint the type of pain, its behavior, and its location. Any associated event is important—development of a vulvar blister, medical illness, recent pelvic or V surgery, childbirth, sports injuries, back surgery, slipped disc, spinal arthritis, scoliosis, or dislocated hips. Occupational or leisure-time activities that might affect the back or the pelvis count too.

A careful exam checks the mouth for lichen planus, the skin for lichen sclerosus or lichen planus, and the vulva for any skin abnormality. A vulvar biopsy may be necessary if there is a question about the skin. The exam checks for tender areas or areas of pain without tenderness to touch on the vulva. The Q-tip test tells if there is VBD, which can occur along with VVD. But there may be no findings at all on physical exam.

A culture for yeast is done, as well as cultures for herpes simplex and herpes zoster if suspicious lesions can be seen anywhere along the lower genital tract. If the clinician thinks that the pain might be caused by a chronic condition such as diabetes or lupus, tests might be done for those things. If there are extensive urinary symptoms, a consult with a urologist is important.

Studies of the spine (X rays, CAT scan, MRI) may be helpful if disc disease, arthritis, or a growth near the spine is suspected. But clinicians disagree vigorously about their benefit. A recent study suggests that routine use of MRI in the evaluation of vulvodynia is of doubtful value.[73] And, many orthopedic surgeons, neurologists, and neurosurgeons have never heard of vulvodynia. So even if I suspect that a patient's vulvar pain is related to the spine, finding a specialist on my wavelength is hard. I do order MRIs when patients have a history that suggests the spine might be involved in the pain, or if the pain just won't go away. If it's positive, I pray that I can talk one of the very few vulvodynia-friendly physicians I know into agreeing that the MRI findings might be the cause of the pain, and helping me with it. This is one of those areas in which more research is sorely needed.

TREATING VULVODYNIA

The first part of the treatment is the diagnosis. As with VBD, most women I see feel such relief after having seen a zillion clinicians without any clo-

A VULVODYNIA SUCCESS STORY

Helen came in because she had a sore bump on the inner lip of the vulva. It had come and gone a year earlier, and again six months after that. She'd seen her regular gyn; cultures for herpes had been negative both times. On the day I saw her, she had a small, smooth, tender pink bump. It certainly didn't look like the little blisters that herpes usually makes, nor anything else familiar to me. So I cultured it for herpes and did a biopsy with the hope that the lab would tell us what was going on in the skin. The culture was negative and the biopsy was not the least bit helpful.

Then Helen called to say she was starting to have pain—burning over the labium and in the labial fold. It was clear to me that whatever was going on with her skin had brought vulvodynia on top of it. I started her on a tricyclic antidepressant and got on the phone to a dermatologist colleague, Dr. Lynette Margesson. She reminded me that there are often atypical forms of familiar problems. Herpes, suggested by painful bumps recurring in the same place, does not always form classic blisters and does not always grow in culture. Sure enough, Helen had a blood test strongly positive for herpes type 2. As is often the case, her partner also had a positive blood test (please see Chapter 20); he had herpes without knowing it.

Helen had a raging case of vulvodynia by the time all this got figured out, and major depression set in. She was unable to work. But we gave the problem a full-pronged assault: She went on acyclovir for the herpes, increased her tricyclic dosage for the vulvodynia, and added Neurontin and another antidepressant. The bumps promptly disappeared, though it took weeks more to control the vulvodynia and to get her life back. But she won. A year later Helen was tapering off all medications except the acyclovir. We'll stay on that because we need to keep the virus out of the picture.

sure: "Oh, my gosh, you actually know what I'm talking about!"

Next I counsel women to eliminate any possible V irritant and use soothing V care. Get in the tub or get off your feet, in a spread-eagle position with an ice pack or a cool fan. A topical anesthetic (5 percent Xylocaine in ointment form) helps some.

The mainstay of treatment for vulvodynia is medication with the tricyclic antidepressant family or the anticonvulsant drugs described under the treatment for VBD. As with VBD, response is slow and uneven. Many women achieve good control but still have little flares that often seem unexplained. They tell me all the time that they are comfortable but that there is enough sensation in the background for them to know it's "still there." The goal of treatment with medication is to control the pain, keep it that way for several months, and then try to taper off the medication. Some women can; many cannot. A lot can get down to a low dose of 10 or 20 mg of nortriptyline, for example, but once they're off the drug, the symptoms return.

Eliminating activity that is suspected to contribute to the pain makes a huge difference. Women are often very clear about what triggers it—sitting, tight clothes, working out in the gym. Avoiding these makes good sense, although it is difficult for an athlete to give up horseback riding or bicycling.

I often have long discussions with women about whether an activity has to go. It's a painful choice to make. Sometimes the activity can be resumed at a later date, but not always.

In addition to dealing with the pain, the treatment of vulvodynia needs to focus on the suspected cause if there is one. Obvious problems are treated: yeast, herpes, skin diseases, any metabolic or connective tissue disorder. Low estrogen is treated with cream. If there are spinal problems, these need to be treated, sometimes with surgery.

I usually recommend evaluation and treatment by a physical therapist familiar with vulvodynia to detect old injuries, bony or muscle malalignments, or the high muscle tension and spasm that may be contributing to the pain.

Some women find help with alternative methods of pain relief. These include acupuncture, TENS, and topical anesthetics. Pain clinics with a multifaceted approach to pain problems are popping up everywhere, but the problem is that few have any experience with vulvodynia. Pain experts do have extensive experience with the use of narcotic painkillers that your providers may be unwilling to give you. Managed appropriately, these work well and allow you to continue your daily life. Don't worry about what you may have heard about painkillers being addictive. Among people who have no history of drug abuse and work in concert with a physician, the odds of getting hooked are very low.[74]

Nerve blocks have been tried and have a mixed track record. While they may help a lot of pain problems, I haven't had any luck with women with vulvodynia. Spinal cord stimulation is a well-recognized treatment for many intractable pain conditions.[75] It is believed that electrical stimulation by tiny wires implanted in the spinal cord can block pain sensation and bring dramatic relief. This is a procedure still in its infancy for the treatment of vulvodynia; it is done by anesthesiologists, usually associated with a pain unit. I haven't had any patients who have used this technique.

THE VULVODYNIA–INTERSTITIAL CYSTITIS LINK

A relationship between interstitial cystitis, or IC (a bladder disorder of unknown origin, marked by severe pain), vulvodynia, and vestibulodynia has been suspected for some years. The bladder and the vestibule have a lot in common:

▼ All the tissues—bladder, urethra, and vestibule—involved in IC and vestibulodynia are derived from the same tissue in the embryo during fetal development.

▼ Both bladder and vestibule are rich in C fibers, nerves that respond to pain.

▼ Patients with VBD have increased bladder irritability and variations in pressure in the urethra compared with women who have no symptoms.[76]

Because of these shared features, investigators have wondered if vestibulodynia and interstitial cystitis are the same problem affecting these special urinary and genital tissues. Several researchers have found women with both IC and VBD.[77] With better diagnosis of both IC and vestibulitis, I expect more cases to be identified.

A recent optimistic study found that more than two-thirds of women who had vulvodynia that wasn't getting better had IC. When the IC is treated, the vulvodynia pain improves.[78]

For more information about IC, see Chapter 19, "Bladder Pain."

CLITORAL PAIN (CLITORODYNIA)

Clitoral pain is, like VBD, a form of localized vulvodynia; here, the pain centers in the clitoris, with or without associated pain in the vestibule or vulva. It's the newest V pain problem to be acknowledged. Many clinicians, unfamiliar with clitorodynia, still assign any problem related to the clitoris to a sexual or psychological problem.

Diagnosis is made by the description of pain localized to the clitoral area. Women often have a hard time describing the pain, but refer to a constant aching or soreness. Sitting increases it, as does clothing, exercise, and sexual activity. Pain worsens with the engorgement of sexual stimulation, making intercourse impossible for many.

On exam, the Q-tip test is negative (meaning the vestibule is fine), but touching the clitoris produces the pain.

Many cases of clitorodynia do not have clear causes. Possible causes include skin disease such as lichen planus, lichen sclerosus that causes blistering or cracking (see Chapter 15), or pemphigus, a very rare autoimmune skin disease that causes blistering and then the loss of skin surface, sometimes causing a small tender area on the clitoris under the hood. All these can be treated with cortisone. A small tangle of nerve fibers called a neuroma can cause a painful bump on or under the hood, or small cysts can form under the hood, causing pain. These can be removed surgically. Compression of the pudendal nerve under pelvic ligaments when there is joint misalignment can produce clitoral tingling and burning. A good physical therapist can show you how to realign the joints and give you exercises to keep them that way.

More difficult to deal with is clitoral pain from trauma. I have seen injury to the clitoris from violent stimulation with a vibrator, straddle injuries from bikes and balance beams, and damage caused by parachute harnesses. Extensive or deep laser treatment and harsh chemicals can cause pain. All the drugs that help vulvodynia have potential to help clitorodynia.

▼

Sexual Healing
Help for Coping with Painful Intercourse

S exual intercourse isn't supposed to hurt, not ever. It's meant to feel wonderful—so good (and so important) that Mother Nature tied the entire future of humankind to it. Having babies simply wouldn't happen if it hinged on anything less than orgasmic delight.

Unfortunately, things don't always work the way they should. I'd like to talk to Mother Nature about that part. Each week I see dozens of women who have pain with sex—pain some of the time, pain all the time, pain so bad they have given up vaginal intercourse altogether. It's hard to say which is worse, the pain from the physical problem or the pain of being a woman unable to be sexual. These are not easy problems, but we go to work on both of them. It's music to my ears when I hear, "Dave and I had sex Saturday night. It wasn't perfect, but it was just fine!"

Many aspects of sexual relations can go awry. In addition to painful intercourse, the other most common kinds of dysfunction for women are lack of desire, inability to become aroused, and delay or absence of orgasm. In fact, as many as a third to two-thirds of women experience some type of sexual problem at some time in their lives.[1] Most of these are the province of sex therapists and psychologists. I approach the physical problems. Problems with orgasm can be physical, but women rarely see me because they are anorgasmic. Pain during sex, though, is something I help women with all the time.

Painful intercourse is called *dyspareunia* (say "dis-par-OON-ee-ah"). When it involves the vulva, vestibule, or vagina, it's *superficial dyspareunia*.

There's another kind of sex pain known as *deep dyspareunia,* which originates up in the pelvis and lower abdomen. Deep dyspareunia may come
from a variety of conditions that affect the pelvic organs, such as pelvic
inflammatory disease (PID) from chronic infection, endometriosis, or
large uterine fibroids. Your regular gynecologist can help with deep dyspareunia. Superficial dyspareunia is a V problem.

Causes of painful sex

Let's just recap the many possibilities. Yeast infections (Chapter 10) will
certainly interfere with pleasure, especially if the yeast has set up permanent housekeeping. But—alert, alert, big *V Book* message—before you
blame recurrent yeast, you must have a clinician make sure it can be seen
under the microscope or proven by a culture. It could be another problem.
Trichomonas (Chapter 12) and other vaginitis (Chapter 13) could be to
blame. Urinary tract infection (Chapter 19) will do it too.

Occasionally the problem boils down to technique. As I explained in
Chapter 6, direct clitoral stimulation or touching that's too intense may
be painful to some women. Telling a partner what feels good solves that
one. If a partner tries to come inside before a woman is adequately lubricated, there will certainly be pain. These things are easily fixed. You've got
to say (and keep saying) that you're not ready or wet enough, and possibly
use a good lubricant (Chapter 6).

A misperception that I run across again and again is that sex hurts if a
man is "too big" or a woman "too small." Remember, when a baby can't
make it out, a problem with the passageway of the bony pelvis is to blame,
not the vagina. So the vagina is not the problem if someone can't get in either. Many gynecologists (we have little training about sex) actually be-

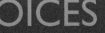
VOICES

"Woman is like a fruit, which will not yield its sweetness until
you rub it between your hands. Look at the basil plant; if you do
not rub it warm with your fingers, it will not emit any scent. Do
you not know that the amber, unless it be handled and warmed,
keeps hidden within its pores the aroma contained in it. It is the
same with woman. If you do not animate her with your toying,
intermixed with kissing, nibbling, and touching, you will not obtain from her what you are wishing: you will feel no enjoyment
when you share her couch, and you will waken in her heart neither inclination nor affection, nor love for you; all her qualities
will remain hidden."

—*The Perfumed Garden of the Cheikh Nefzaouim,*
translated by Sir Richard Burton

lieve that there are cases where the penis is too big for the woman's vagina. Impossible! Turn her on adequately and "too big" will be history.

But caution, caution, caution! When some women think they're in pain because they're too small, the actual problem is pain in the vestibule (Chapter 17). To tell a woman with this problem, vestibulodynia, that she needs only to be turned on adequately would be a terrible mistake. The pain in the vestibule has to be diagnosed and treated. Vaginismus, muscle spasm making the vaginal opening like a brick wall, may result from the pain in the vestibule, or it may be the result of sexual trauma and abuse. If pain in the vestibule is the source, it has to be fixed. Once the trauma or abuse is dealt with or the vestibular pain is fixed, this muscle spasm must also be treated with careful sexual therapy.

Sometimes dryness can be traced to hormonal changes that occur with breast-feeding, perimenopause, and menopause (Chapter 4). Women vary in the amount of estrogen their bodies make, so you may not automatically have a problem. But a vagina without estrogen is like a fish without water. Only water will do for the fish, and to date, only estrogen provides the thick, supple elasticity so important for a woman's comfort as well as sexual pleasure. As I've said, this is so easily remedied; it takes only a small amount of estrogen directly added to the vagina as cream, a tablet, or a ring insert. We do not have a shred of information to date that properly used local estrogen is a health hazard.

Older women often blame menopause for painful sex caused by other problems, especially vulvodynia (Chapter 17). But midlife is a time when V skin diseases, which can lead to vaginal pain, like to show up. Lichen planus and lichen sclerosus (Chapter 15) cause cracks, raw areas, and tightening of the skin around the clitoris or vaginal opening— which naturally can lead to pain. Lichen planus can even inflame and scar the vagina.

Finally, it's important to know what *doesn't* cause pain with intercourse. If you are given any of the following reasons for your discomfort, you need to keep looking. Bacterial vaginosis (BV, covered in Chapter 11) does *not* cause painful intercourse. Discharge, yes; odor, yes. Dyspareunia, no.

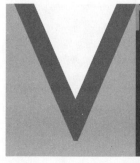

V NOTE

What do sex and vulvar self-exams have in common?

Regular checks, including regular gyn exams, can help you spot potential problems early—before they wreak havoc in your bedroom.

Neither does the human papillomavirus (HPV, Chapter 21), whether in the skin of the vulva or causing an abnormal Pap, make sex painful.

The downward spiral

Most of the causes of painful intercourse get fixed quickly. Cure or control the vaginitis, buff the vagina with a little estrogen, refine the sexual technique, and you're on your way. Of all the reasons sex hurts, ongoing pain from vulvodynia or vestibulodynia (whether new or layered on top of a skin disease) seems to shatter women's sexual confidence most.

If sex hurts, sexual desire goes out the window and the ability to have orgasm goes down the drain. Some women who have had pain beginning with their first sexual experience might be saying, "What orgasm?" As my patient Susie told me, "If intercourse is supposed to be fun, I'd rather have a root canal." With this kind of pain with sex, you must go through some stages in coming to grips with your sexuality in the face of pain.

First, you realize that something's wrong. Sex doesn't feel good and becomes more painful with the passing of time. You have to figure out how to tell your partner. You try to handle things on your own. Use a lubricant, change positions. No luck. *Maybe it will just go away,* you hope. You wait. It doesn't. You try abstaining for weeks, only to be disappointed that when you resume, intercourse is just as painful as ever.

If you're new to sex, you look around for reasons for this baffling pain. You rationalize: "The first time is never so good, right?" "Maybe I just need more time than most." You look for something to blame: "Gee, tampons have always hurt too, so maybe I'm just too small."

Then you try to get help. You confide in friends or family and follow their well-meant advice about spicing up your sexuality, without improvement. But many women tell me they wouldn't dream of discussing painful sex with their mothers or sisters. If they do, they find that Mom or Sis never had or heard of such a problem. Trying to be helpful, they hint at stress and the need for counseling. You scan books and magazines for references to painful sex, but they too suggest a shrink or more lubricants. Your partner can't relate.

VOICES

"You can't believe how bad this is. Ow! Don't touch here. No! Get away from there. Stop! That hurts. Oh! I don't think you'd better do that right now."

—Mattie, 46, who has vestibulodynia, describing sex with her husband

Effort to find professional help may be frustrating as well. Numerous medical visits and treatments follow. Many clinicians work really hard to help, but they have little reliable information about what to do for women with vulvar pain and sexual issues. Maybe you had the experience of screwing up your courage to go to your ob-gyn with great reluctance and embarrassment about so intimate a problem, only to be disappointed by being told to relax more or to see a psychiatrist. I hear this from patients all the time.

You struggle with battering questions. *Are these people right? Is this all in my head? Shouldn't I just get a hold on myself and move forward? Do I have some disease I can give to my partner? Did he give something to me? How will I ever find a mate?* or *How can I keep the mate I have when sex is so awful? Will I ever be able to have children?*

The realization dawns that you cannot function sexually the way you used to or always heard you were supposed to, and you must confront what is an initial problem or change in sexuality. You feel like an incomplete woman and defective sexual partner. And when sexual activity is so painful, part of you never wants to be sexual again, while the rest of you yearns for the pleasures of sexual arousal and satisfaction. *Why can't sex be pain-free? Why can't I have what I always dreamed of?* or *Why can't I get rid of this pain to get back to the old life?*

Changes in your sexual functioning start to occur. Desire droops and then rides off into the sunset. Many women don't make the connection that pain caused this. They scurry around looking for hormone tests or Viagra. My nurse-practitioner partner Diana often puts it this way: If you were a carpenter and every time you went to work you smashed your thumb with a hammer, you'd soon stop wanting to be a carpenter! And there's the emotional impact of each sexual encounter too. You try so hard to make it work, but it still hurts. Your partner tries to understand, but everybody gets frustrated and you end up in tears. With everything so unpleasant, who wouldn't shut down?

To a certain degree, the pain itself starts to build a wall between partners. It's physically painful for you and emotionally painful for both of

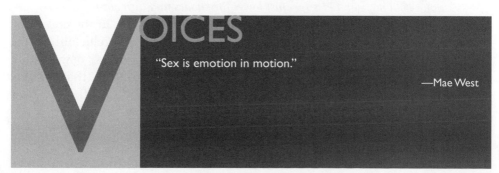

"Sex is emotion in motion."

—Mae West

you. Another change occurs. You start to become a watchdog to guard against the pain. During sex, you coil up like a cobra, ready to spring on the slightest adverse sensation. This means that you lose all sense of pleasure and become a spectator outside of your body, watching for the pain, waiting for the pain. The sensual side of sex? Not here. Spontaneity, enjoyment, and ecstasy, while a no-brainer for many, are not part of the experience for someone with ongoing painful intercourse.

The partner's pain

It's not easy for the partner of a woman who has vulvodynia either. Even though the woman is the one with the pain, it's her partner's problem too. No one wants to hurt someone he or she loves. That person wrestles with parallel questions: *But what is this? Is it all in her head? Does she have something awful?* And, in the case of a male partner, *Well, a guy needs what a guy needs. So what about me? What about my needs?* For many men, if it isn't vaginal intercourse, it isn't sex.

A lot of men have trouble understanding the degree of pain that women feel. Our society has put out a lot of misinformation that pain with sex is psychological. (Sexual difficulty for men used to be written off as psychological too. And then along came Viagra. How things change!) But you can count on this: The pain that women feel in the vestibule when nerves are not working is absolutely real and awful. Women are accustomed to give their all for others, but this is one area where the pain overwhelms.

Anger adds to the stew. You're angry at the doctors you may have seen who are unable to diagnose your problem and who tell you it will go away. Or anger at your doctor may be aimed instead at your partner. You may be angry at friends or family or employers who are clueless about what you're going through or about what it's like to have a chronic invisible illness.[2]

So for everyone involved in both sides of the relationship affected by vulvar pain, there is a great loss. And to this insult, couples often add the injury of isolation. Sex is often viewed as all or nothing. She starts to think, *If I can't have vaginal intercourse, forget it. I don't want anything. Don't touch me, don't hold me, don't kiss me. Just lower the shades and turn out the light.*

For male partners there are changes in function also. In the effort not to hurt her, he starts to monitor his physical response, reluctant to trip her hair-trigger pain. So for him as well, the sensual focus goes. Trouble with erections may follow. Or if the partner starts to think that if intercourse is not possible, any sexual stimulation is pointless—the thinking goes, *Why lead the other person on?* So next comes avoidance of any activity that might be sexually provocative, even touching and hugging. Men often respond to situations differently than women. A woman talks. A man withdraws into a cave to do nothing and say nothing. That doesn't mean he doesn't care. But it's unfortunate that he seems unavailable just when she desperately needs *not* to be allowed to lower the shades and turn out the light.

Most women are aware of their partner's needs and try to continue to function sexually. In fact, it's typical for a woman to endure significant, often severe pain in order to be a woman and meet her partner's needs. It's a feminine characteristic to make great sacrifices for others.

But sex is not about duty and meeting an imaginary standard. No one is entitled to sex. It's not a given. We have sex because both partners feel wonderful about each other and want to express this joy in bodily activity as the ultimate expression of love. It's a personal choice on the part of both. Unfortunately, not everyone sees it this way. Many men believe sex is something they are entitled to. And women, even with great pain, go on having sex because of pressure, guilt, or "duty."

It's important to remember in the middle of all this mess that it is always a woman's (or man's) right to *choose* whether or not to be sexual. That choice exists whether she or he is single or in a relationship. The choice can be temporary or permanent. It's a choice that exists whether a woman has vulvodynia or not. Choosing not to be sexual may be the right choice, but if you are in a relationship, your partner will be affected by that choice.[3] So both partners need to arrive at the decision about what to do. Professional counseling may well need to accompany this choice, which impacts a relationship and needs to be accepted by a partner. Such a choice needs to be talked out and mutually agreed upon, not just silently put into place.

VOICES

"VENIS (very erotic noninsertive sex) is sex without penetration. It involves broadening your ideas of what sex is beyond intercourse, to focus on non-goal-oriented activities. In other words, VENIS aims to turn foreplay into a home run. This may involve a whole range of activities, which may or may not lead to orgasm . . . erotic wrestling with maximum body and genital contact, massaging each other with oils or other materials, manual stimulation, light bondage with feathers or fur, mutual masturbation, erotic dancing, intercourse between breasts or buttocks, and body kissing are just some of the possibilities."

—Dr. Laura Berman, sex researcher and coauthor of *For Women Only: A Revolutionary Guide to Overcoming Sexual Dysfunction and Reclaiming Your Sex Life*

A coping plan

Refraining from sex is, of course, not the way many women go. So what do you and your partner do if you are living with the pain of vulvodynia and want to be sexual?

Before you can be sexual, you have to deal with the pain. Nothing counts, nothing works, nothing matters if it hurts. You have to find a savvy clinician to make the diagnosis and work with you on the available treatments for your painful condition outlined in the previous chapter. You don't have to give up the idea of being sexual until you are pain-free, but you do have to start by attacking the root problem.

Then you have to decide about counseling. There's nothing a counselor can do about your pain, but sometimes other issues in a relationship (perhaps born out of your condition) need to be worked on along with the pain. A lot of couples don't need counseling, however.

It's a natural reaction, as I've described, for both parties to want to quit and withdraw into their shells. You don't have to do that. Please don't do that. Why we cut ourselves off in this way is a little hard to understand, because in the rest of our lives we accept substitutes all the time. Think about it. If they're out of french fries, we'll take mashed potatoes; we don't just give up on dinner that night. If they don't have the red dress or tie, we'll take another color; we don't go without clothes. If the hotel of our choice is fully booked, we choose another; we don't cancel the trip. Yes, there is disappointment and frustration. On the other hand, this fork in the road gives us the opportunity to try something new. In fact, it's the chance to be somewhat daring and experiment a bit. Given the choice, we use it to find pleasure in a different fashion. There is a sexual menu, and you can choose other things to do. So if you're handed a lemon, make lemonade.

Pregnancy and vulvodynia

Just because you have a vulvar pain condition—even one that has you ready to give up on a normal sex life—doesn't mean that you can't have a

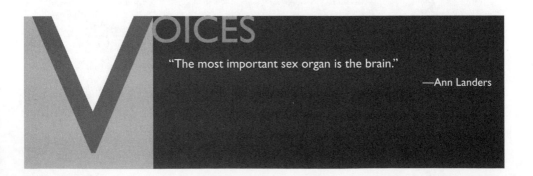

"The most important sex organ is the brain."

—Ann Landers

COMMON QUESTIONS: Vulvodynia and sex

Q **How do you find a satisfactory sexual experience despite pain that prevents vaginal intercourse?**

A Sexuality implies the totality of a being. It refers to human qualities, not just to the genitals and their functions. It includes all of the qualities—biological, psychological, emotional, cultural, social, and spiritual—that make people who they are. And people can express their sexuality in any of these areas; it doesn't have to be solely through the genitals.[4] Not having vaginal sex does not mean that a woman (or a man) is not being sexual. This is an important and liberating concept.

Q **But how about a more satisfactory genital experience?**

A Well, first you talk with each other. You tell each other how you feel. You speak of the loss, frustration, and disappointment you are feeling. You let the other person know where you're coming from. You acknowledge that all these feelings need talking about, and you agree to work on understanding where your partner is coming from. You reiterate your love and commitment to the relationship. You state your interest in exploring new avenues, your willingness to try something new.

Q **Try something new? Okay. What about anal intercourse?**

A No problem if you both want to do it. But lots of women are totally turned off by the idea. Trading something painful for something repulsive is not a good deal. And by the way, if you're going to have anal intercourse, it must be gentle and super-lubricated. Rough anal intercourse can damage the anal sphincter. Once again, if it hurts, don't do it! And vaginal entry immediately after anal sex is a total no-no.

Q **What do you mean by a new way of thinking about sex?**

A Researchers in sexual functioning tell us that there are two commonly held views of sexual activity.[5] The more common view is goal-directed, which is the same as climbing a flight of stairs. The first step is kissing; the next step is caressing; then there's vagina-penis contact, which leads to intercourse. The top step is orgasm. One or both partners has a goal in mind, and that goal is orgasm. If the sexual experience does not lead to the achievement of that goal, then the goal-directed couple or person is dissatisfied with all that has been experienced. Goal-directed sex when a woman has vulvar pain is often going to lead to dissatisfaction. That goal just isn't possible for now.

The alternative is to go after pleasure-directed sex. Think of a circle, with each form of sexual expression merging around the edge of the circle as an end in itself. These expressions might include kissing, touching, holding, and oral sex. But each of these activities is complete in itself, and each is satisfying to the couple. There is no need for any particular form of expression to lead to anything else.

So after you've talked and agreed to change the goal of vaginal sex at every encounter, you work on pleasure-directed sex.

You need to start by building the emotional ties between you. At first you do nothing physical or particularly sexual, just pleasurable: fireside talks, strolls by the river, breakfast in bed, sunsets, rain on the roof, butterflies in the garden, Beethoven, Bruce Springsteen, whipped cream, candlelight. You know what helps you feel close.

Once you're connected emotionally, you move on to a time-honored and magical means of expressing love without words—touch. Touch and caress. Focus on the sensations and feelings without the goal of sex in mind. Trade back rubs with lotion and take in the curves of your partner's glistening muscles. Shower or bathe together and enjoy the feeling of skin all lathered up. Lie side by side and trace little circles over arms and legs and back and shoulders. Enjoy the naturalness of your partner's nude body. You express your affection physically without talking. Skin-to-skin contact, whether holding hands, hugging, or genital caressing, releases important internal chemicals that promote bonding between partners and elevate mood.[6] When you're out of words, touch says it all, and you come to realize that you can have wonderful, soothing, and affirming experience without "going all the way."

Then the two of you need to find other ways to achieve sexual satisfaction if vaginal intercourse is not possible. Couples use stimulation by hand and mouth. A woman can climax by clitoral stimulation when vaginal penetration is not an option, and she can bring her partner to climax with oral or manual stimulation. Some women have such clitoral sensitivity that touch in this area is not possible, but they can enjoy vaginal sex. If a woman is unable to participate sexually at all, her partner can consider self-stimulation for gratification. This can be particularly important when finding relief from her pain is such a priority that she needs time off from focusing on her sex life.

It is also possible for a man to allow sexual urges to subside, unexpressed physically. There is no danger of bad effects from lack of sexual activity. People don't get sick or go crazy from lack of sex.

Finally, for a woman who has had pain and needs to regain her sexuality, positive thinking will move her forward. You need to think about sexual pleasure, remembering a particularly enjoyable encounter with your partner and focusing on the pleasurable sensations that went along with it. Fantasy and provocative thoughts that are meaningful to the woman also work.

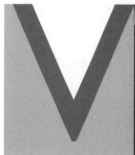

OICES

"The physical therapist taught me about Mr. Frosty. She took a condom and filled it with frozen peas and tied the end shut. It fits between the labia comfortably and really helps the stinging. Sometimes I use a cold pack or some aloe gel I've chilled in the refrigerator."

—Phoebe, 24, who has pain after intercourse

SEX PAIN AND THE SINGLE WOMAN

If you're not in a relationship when your vulvar pain first develops, it's natural to worry about how you'll share this information with future intimate partners. People with herpes struggle with this problem all the time. Not everyone you go out with has to receive this information. In our society, dating is the way that we decide whether we want to enter into a longer relationship and share our most intimate selves with another. You don't have to tell it all on the first date!

As the relationship develops and you find that trust is growing, information about your problem can be shared. The best advice is to keep it simple and straightforward. The time to talk about it is the time when you think that information about your pain problem will be important to the relationship. This is unlikely to be the first evening. As you begin considering sexual involvement or as you suspect that the other person is, the time to talk has arrived.

It makes sense to have more than one talk about vulvar pain. Your first effort might cover what you can and cannot do. If you are able to have sex but experience great soreness and burning afterward, you may need to indicate that reduced frequency is necessary for you. Or if you may not be able to participate in vaginal sex, explain that you can enjoy orgasm with manual or oral stimulation. In later conversations you can provide more details and history. As you reveal yourself, you will be receiving information in return about the other person. The response you receive will allow you to decide whether continuing with the relationship is something you want to do.

The fear of every woman with vulvar pain is that she will meet Mr. Right, find the courage to tell him her problem, and be rejected because of it. A guy who takes off because a woman has vulvar pain and cannot function in all aspects of physical sex leaves one message: He was so interested in physical sex that he couldn't see the rest of the package. Perhaps Mr. Right only seemed right on the surface. All over the world, women with vulvodynia have relationships that continue, proposals of marriage that are made, weddings that take place, and honeymoons that glow with sexual activity.

child. Many women ask me about this: "How can I get pregnant? Will my vulvodynia worsen during or after pregnancy?" We don't have good statistics about this. The general thinking, which matches my own experience, is that the effect of pregnancy on vulvar symptoms is variable. Most patients find that their symptoms are no worse, and some improve.[7] Although it can cause painful intercourse, there is no known connection between vulvodynia and the ability to conceive. Nothing about vulvodynia affects the growth of the baby or the healthiness of the pregnancy.

For some women, deciding about pregnancy and VBD or VVD is tough because they are playing beat the biological clock. You probably know that as you reach thirty, fertility starts to decline, dropping sharply at forty. This has nothing to do with vulvar pain. But you have to make a choice: Either work full-time on the VBD or VVD, or work on being pregnant. Treatment takes time and should not be cut short for pregnancy or the pain will bounce right back. No one wants to be on medications while attempting conception. On the other hand, if time is running out and you want a family, don't keep putting it off. If intercourse is too painful, go with insemination. You can work on the pain after the baby (or babies).

Becoming pregnant with vulvodynia is a challenge if a woman can engage in sexual intercourse only rarely, if at all. Knowing when you ovulate becomes important. The most popular method for finding out when ovulation occurs is the use of an ovulation kit, which can be purchased at any drugstore. A less expensive method is to record your temperature each morning before getting out of bed. This method cannot tell you that ovulation is about to occur, because once the temperature has risen, the egg has already been released. To use this technique you need to record your temperature during one menstrual cycle prior to the month of planned conception, so you can see when ovulation occurred. If you have regular cycles, there is an excellent chance that you will ovulate at the same time during the next cycle. To increase the chance of conception, you need to have sexual intercourse on the day before the temperature rise. (You'll know this only after you've mapped out several cycles.) If you do not have regular cycles, the test kits may be best. To make things easier, use a topical anesthetic prior to intercourse and liberally apply nonspermicidal lubricants. (Remember that K-Y jelly contains a chemical called chlorhexidine that can kill sperm as well as irritate the vulva; it's best to use a little common vegetable oil.)

If penetration is not possible, manual or oral stimulation of your male partner with ejaculation at the introitus may work. You can then lie on your back with your knees up; this position helps the sperm to travel up into the vagina and toward the pool of vaginal secretions near the cervix. Alternatively, the man could ejaculate into a diaphragm, which you then place over the cervix. Then there's the Thanksgiving way, placing the semen in a clean, new turkey baster and inserting it into the vagina. A turkey baster is often a little smaller than a penis, so you can minimize discomfort by controlling how you put it in, and it doesn't have to stay in as long or with as much thrust as in normal sexual intercourse. Alternately, in the clinic, the semen can be placed at the cervix and kept there with various devices such as a cap or a sponge, or the semen can be washed to remove everything except the sperm, which is then inserted into the uterus through a thin tube (catheter). Insemination in the doctor's office costs about $200 to $300 per cycle. Some but not all insurance covers this.

Many women with vulvodynia are taking tricyclic antidepressants or the drug Neurontin. As a general rule, physicians recommend coming off these drugs prior to conception. This is a precaution, since there is no evidence that these drugs cause birth defects. But the medications have not been studied in great detail in relation to pregnancy (most drugs haven't), and it is always a good policy not to be taking drugs of any kind during the first twelve weeks of a pregnancy. In cases of severe vulvodynia, some women elect to resume the tricyclics after the first trimester. To date there have been no reports of problems with this. Although they have not been considered to be as effective in controlling pain as the tricyclics, the selective serotonin reuptake inhibitors (SSRIs) such as Zoloft and Paxil are considered safe to take during pregnancy.[8] Narcotics are safe, but high doses for extended periods of time could cause the baby to have some withdrawal symptoms after birth. Topical cortisone, injections of cortisone into the vulva, or the application of creams such as estrogen or lidocaine is also safe for pregnant women.

During labor and delivery, you may want to consider epidural anesthesia since your cervix will be checked for dilatation and this could be painful. There's no reason to automatically have a cesarean delivery if you've had a vestibulectomy, although the decision must be tailored to a woman's individual story.[9] Some clinicians are wondering if vaginal delivery may improve vestibulodynia, although this is only guesswork at this point. You will want to avoid an episiotomy, if possible, since this scar can increase the pain of vulvodynia. On the other hand, if there are problems as the baby is about to be born, please listen to your clinician, who may need to do the episiotomy to achieve a safe delivery.

Vaginismus

A different kind of impediment to intercourse is the condition called vaginismus. This is the spasm of the muscles surrounding the vagina during attempted entry of the vagina. This spasm cannot be voluntarily controlled. In some women, just thinking about something (a penis, a speculum, a tampon) going into the vagina can lead to muscle spasm.[10] This muscle contraction may be strong enough to prevent penetration altogether. When a woman has vaginismus, it feels as if her partner is running into a solid wall as he attempts to enter her. Vaginismus can make vaginal examination difficult or impossible, can make sexual intercourse difficult or impossible, and leads to emotional and physical pain for both parties.

Clinicians have always thought that vaginismus was psychological in origin—a physical manifestation of a woman's fear of injury, guilt about sexuality, or dissatisfaction with her relationship.[11] Psychological factors often do play a role in vaginismus. But physical factors can lead to this problem as well. It's understandable that a woman who has been injured or abused would develop this condition, for example. Other medical problems such as endometriosis, vaginal infection, or urinary tract infection can also contribute.[12]

Also, the exquisite pain of vestibulodynia can lead to vaginismus—but they are not the same thing, even though clinicians often confuse them. Consider the case of Alexandra. She'd had pain with her first sexual experience. It had been awkward and hadn't gone very well, and she had chalked it up to youth and inexperience. But the same pain occurred again with the next encounter, and then with a third. She came across a description of vaginismus in a book and figured that was her problem. She found a helpful sexual therapist and started counseling and work with dilators. When she was able through hard work to insert a medium-sized dilator, she started using a tampon and was extremely pleased that she could tolerate a Pap smear. Her mother heard about my specialty clinic, and Alexandra came to see me while she was home on vacation from graduate school. After an exam, it was clear to me that Alexandra had not a suggestion of vaginismus. Her problem was vestibulodynia—pain specifically in the vestibule. She was gratified by the knowledge that she didn't have a "psychological" problem, since despite her time in therapy, she was clueless about what events in her life could have led to vaginismus.

Vaginismus is a real problem and an entity separate from VBD. Since vaginismus can lead to painful intercourse and painful intercourse can lead to vaginismus, sorting out which condition came first is often difficult.[13] A careful history is essential. If a pelvic examination can be done, an answer may be immediately available—the physician can see and feel the muscle spasm when a finger gently presses down on the muscles surrounding the vaginal entrance. But the exam can cause a woman to flash back to a time of abuse. Sometimes the emotional and physical pain of examination makes a medical exam impossible, and clinicians have to work based on history only.

Compare these three stories: Marie was sexually abused in childhood by her uncle and date-raped in college. When I met her, she had been unable to consummate her marriage despite extensive sexual counseling. At her first visit she did not think she could go through with the exam. We just talked. I explained how valuable the exam could be to sort out whether she had VBD or vaginismus or both. I would stop at any point if she felt she couldn't handle the situation. A few weeks later, she returned with her sister to hold her hand and give her support. She had taken antianxiety medicine as well. We agreed that the exam would not involve the speculum—only looking and a Q-tip test (used to determine pain in the vestibule and thus diagnose VBD; see the previous chapter). The test was positive—she had great pain in the vestibule. But also the muscles of her pelvic floor jumped in spasm just from the touch of the swab; she clearly also had vaginismus, reinforced by the VBD. Armed with the facts and the right therapies, Marie has made amazing progress and will soon be ready for intercourse.

Susan, who had a story similar to Marie's, had a negative Q-tip test but clear muscle spasm in the pelvic floor. No vestibulodynia. She has to deal with her sexual trauma and vaginismus, and then she too can move forward.

Renee, also with a story of extensive childhood abuse, cannot even tolerate an exam. She may have VBD and she may not, but I can't get in there to tell. For now it doesn't matter. She will work with her therapist to overcome the emotional issues, and then we can figure out if we have VBD to work on.

Treatment of vaginismus involves fixing any sources of physical pain (such as if there is vestibulodynia) and working with counseling, relaxation, and guided imagery techniques as well as dilators to help the muscles stop clenching up. Dilators are used not because the vagina is too small but as vaginal entry desensitization devices. Therapy for vaginismus, as you might imagine, takes a long time.

A word about Viagra and friends

The word *Viagra* has come to mean instant potency for men, a cure-all for what sexually ails you. While this is a distortion of how the little blue pill actually works, it's led many women, especially women with vulvodynia, to wonder, *What about a similar pill for me? Could Viagra help my low libido?*

Many different medications have been used for sexual problems, with varying and inconclusive results.[14] Among the more promising drugs are those that interact with the body chemicals nitric oxide synthase (NOS) and cyclic guanosine monophosphate (cGMP) to make the muscle-relaxing substance nitric oxide. Viagra is one of these. It prevents the breakdown of cGMP. Once there's lots of cGMP around, a lot of nitric oxide is made—allowing the blood vessels of the clitoris, labia, and vagina to relax so that blood can flow in for the engorgement we feel as sexual arousal. Other substances on the horizon are L-arginine, a precursor to nitric oxide, prostaglandin E1, phentolamine (another smooth-muscle relaxer), and apomorphine, which may be involved in the mediation of sexual desire and arousal.[15]

Can women just take men's Viagra? Rumors are flying everywhere: It works. It doesn't work. It sort of works. It's not recommended yet. In theory, if the pipelines open and blood engorges all the female genitalia, it ought to feel marvelous and totally arousing when combined with all the other elements that women need to take off. But it's still unknown how much engorgement occurs in a woman, how it compares to normal, and how long the effects last. Early reports are clear that Viagra offers significant improvement for women who experience sexual dysfunction because of antidepressant medications. That's very good news, since antidepressants interfere with desire for thousands of women. The big catch, however, is that research into this is still in its infancy. Popping

THE CLITORIS'S NEW BEST FRIEND?

In 2000, the U.S. Food and Drug Administration approved a new prescription treatment for female sexual dysfunction, the clitoral therapy device called Eros. A little plastic cylinder fits over the clitoris, and the hand-held, battery-powered bulb pump (like the inflator on a blood pressure cuff) creates a gentle suction that stimulates and contains blood flow in the clitoris. With blood flow, everything else follows—arousal, stimulation, lubrication, and, one hopes, orgasm.

Eros is a small device, no larger than a vibrator or other sex toy, but it is able to generate a little more focalized pressure through its cylinder than human massage can create. A small device, it's meant to be part of foreplay (though it can be used without a partner and is bound to be used by some for self-stimulation or as a couple's sex toy, regardless of sexual dysfunction).

Both Eros and Viagra (see page 343) work by stimulating blood flow. Is one better than another? Which one should a woman having trouble use? No one knows. There are no studies, reports, or other data on Eros yet. Caution is warranted, therefore. (It's also worth noting that clitoral injuries are possible even with ordinary vibrators, and this device exerts additional pressure.)

your partner's Viagra is unlikely to trigger the exact same erotic effects in you (whether you have a problem with sexual function or not) and can even be hazardous; it's never a smart idea to take someone else's prescription. Better to see a clinician about other ways to remedy a problem and to take heart in the flurry of research for women that the Viagra trend has sparked. Nor can drugs such as Viagra help women with childhood sexual abuse or significant emotional or relationship issues.

Even when it's approved for women, Viagra is probably not the way to go for women with vulvodynia. It's such a tempting idea—relief in a little blue pill. But you must deal with the pain first. Libido will follow.

Meanwhile, while science is patiently exploring the right medications to aid female sexual function, commerce is not so restrained. Dietary supplement manufacturers are having a field day packaging combinations of herbs and other compounds purported to really spice up your love life. The eye-catching labels say it all: "Better sex! More intense orgasms! Unforgettable lovemaking experiences! Bring back the honeymoon fireworks!" The names are even better: Aroused, Climaxx, Instant Sex, Love in a Jar, Libidoblast, NiAgra. Be aware that the government has no power to regulate the accuracy of these labels or determine the safety of the contents. And they may interfere with prescription drugs. Even the more seriously packaged alternative cures should be eyed skeptically. There is little scientific evidence that *Avena sativa,* damiana, ginseng, *Ginkgo biloba,* maca, muira puama, or zinc can improve libido or sexual function.[16] There is some evidence that arginine and yohimbine help some men, but information about female use is lacking.[17]

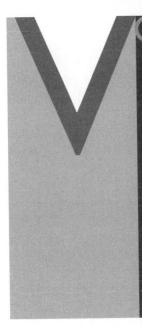

VOICES

"Sometimes I feel that this illness has brought my husband and me closer together, not only because of what we've endured together, but also because many times we are limited to just 'cuddling' and offering each other reassurance. It is still difficult for me, at times, to overcome my feelings of inadequacy as a wife and lover. I tell my support group members that sex does not make a marriage, but it sure can be an important and fun part of it.

"I think that when you have something like this to 'test' your love for each other, you realize what a good marriage you really have. I'm sure that having vulvodynia has been equally difficult for other women, and I believe for a cure to be found, we must overcome our embarrassment and let everyone know that this disease is real and that more research needs to be done.

"If we can increase public awareness, fewer women will have to suffer in silence, like so many have in the past."

—Anonymous, in *NVA News*, Spring 1995; 1(2):8.

Women need more than the next Viagra, of course. We need accurate information about social, physical, and psychological processes that influence our sexuality; sex education that illuminates differences in function and response between men and women as well as between women; services such as sexual and relationship counseling; and access to contraception and abortion.[18] These are the real developments that will empower women sexually.

CHAPTER 19

Bladder Pain

Feeling the Burn That Could Be UTI or IC

Why have I included **urinary tract** infections (UTI) and a related condition known as interstitial cystitis (IC) in a book about the Vs? They're not considered vulvovaginal problems or even gynecological problems. But symptoms associated with these bladder problems overlap with various vulvovaginal disorders. Many women see me for V symptoms that turn out to have urinary origins. Others who see me first suspected a bladder problem and have already seen a urologist, where they were frustrated that several invasive tests yielded no diagnosis. The great pretender vulvodynia (Chapter 17), for example, often feels exactly like a UTI. IC and vulvodynia can occur together. Yeast infections (Chapter 10), trichomonas (Chapter 12), herpes (Chapter 20), and assorted skin diseases (Chapter 15) can all inflame the tissue around the urinary opening (the urethra) so that urine burns on touching it. The STDs gonorrhea, chlamydia, and herpes can inflame the urethra itself, causing urethritis (say "yur-eeth-RYE-tus") with burning on irritation.

You may not be sure what the source of your problem is, except to know that something is not right "down there somewhere." The following explanations are meant to clarify what is (and what isn't) urinary trouble.

If it is a bladder problem, you're certainly not alone: Urinary tract infections are one of the most common reasons for women to seek medical care, accounting for seven million patient visits each year.[1] About one out of every five women develops UTI sometime during her life.[2]

What is a urinary tract infection (UTI)?

UTI (a.k.a. *bladder infection*) occurs when a large number of bacteria grow in the urethra (the tube that leads from the outside of the body into the bladder), in the bladder itself, in the tubes that carry urine from the kidneys to the bladder *(ureters),* or in the kidneys. Infection in the urethra *(urethritis)* generally exists along with infection of the bladder. Although these lower-tract infections can be annoying and painful, they are usually easily treated with antibiotics and clear up within days.

Symptoms include painful urination (called *dysuria*), frequent urination, and the need to go constantly or suddenly and immediately *(urgency)*. A woman with a bladder infection may also experience blood in her urine *(hematuria),* pain over the bladder, and flank (side) or back discomfort. White blood cells and bacteria in the urine may make it appear cloudy. If there is blood in the urine, it may be reddish in color.

V NOTE

Color check
Normal urine may vary in color from almost clear to dark yellow; the depth of yellow color has no relation to infection.

You can have symptoms that feel like UTI without actually having an infection. Drinking too much coffee or tea will cause frequent urination. Premenstrual syndrome, food allergies, or irritation from chemicals in bubble bath, soaps, or douche products can cause sensations similar to UTI. Vaginitis can also cause urinary symptoms—the itching and inflammation in the vestibule around the urinary opening can make urination uncomfortable, and yeast or trich can irritate the urethra or the bladder.

It's possible for a bladder infection to disappear without treatment. If you are in good health and have no history of urinary problems, you can treat yourself with fluids for twenty-four hours to see if things improve. Drink an extra quart or two of fluids on top of your usual daily consumption (a good recommendation for general health is 64 ounces of water daily) to help flush bacteria out of the bladder; 10 ounces of cranberry juice as part of the extra fluids may keep bacteria from multiplying (see box on page 356). If the symptoms persist more than twenty-four hours, or if you develop chills and fever, vomiting, or pain in the back near the kidneys, you need to see a clinician, as these symptoms suggest possible kidney infection.

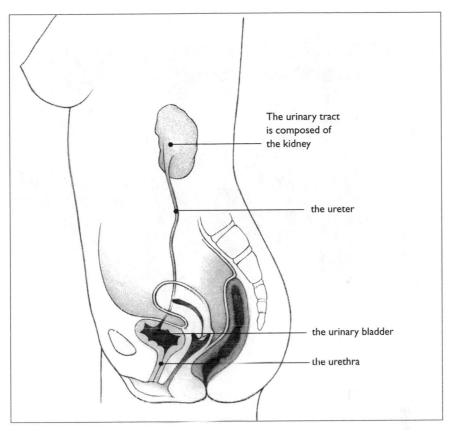

The urinary tract is composed of the kidney

the ureter

the urinary bladder

the urethra

FIG. 47 **The Urinary Tract**

WHO GETS UTI?

The way women are built predisposes them to bladder infections. The urethral opening is located very close to the anus, a common source of bacteria. Sexual activity involving the nearby vagina may also shift bacteria into the urethra. In addition, because a woman's bladder is only about an inch away from her urethra (compared to a man's, which is half a foot away), bacteria introduced into the urethra have much less distance to travel in the woman before infecting the bladder.

Most of the following categories of at-risk women are related to these hard realities of geography. Remember, it doesn't mean that if you fall into one of these categories, you will get a bladder infection. It simply means that infections are more common among these types of women. You could also get a bladder infection without a known risk factor.

▼ *Women who are sexually active.* In women who are sexually active, most bladder infections are associated with sexual intercourse.[3] Women who are susceptible to the problem develop symptoms within a short period

V NOTE

Good ideas, anyway

How fastidious you are about cleaning your genitals and the direction in which you wipe don't have anything to do with UTI. Neither do birth control pills. Nor does it matter whether you use tampons or sanitary napkins. Two recent studies reported a higher incidence of UTI in groups of college women who used tampons, but a high level of sexual activity could explain this finding.

Sources: R. Tuomala, Gynecologic infections, in *Kistner's Gynecology*, K. J. Ryan, R. S. Berkowitz, R. L. Barbieri, eds. (St. Louis: Mosby, 1996), 518; H. A. Omar, S. Aggarwal, K. C. Perkins, Tampon use in young women, *J Pediatr Adolesc Gynecol* 1998:11:143; B. Foxman, A. M. Geiger, K. Palin, et al., First-time urinary tract infection and sexual behavior, *Epidemiology* 1995:6(2):162.

of time (a few hours to a day or two) after sex. The movements of foreplay and intercourse are believed to move the bacteria hanging out around the vulva and vagina into the urethra and up to the bladder; sex briefly increases the number of bacteria in the urine up to ten times normal levels.[4]

▼ *Women who use the diaphragm.*[5] Diaphragm users, for a number of reasons, have twice the risk of UTI compared with women who do not use a diaphragm. The diaphragm may compress the urethra, making it difficult to empty the bladder completely. This can set the stage for bacteria that will invade urine that sits around in the bladder. The act of inserting the diaphragm increases colonization with bacteria that come from the intestine. The motions of foreplay and intercourse in and out of the vagina then make it easy for bacteria to move up into the bladder. The spermicide used with a diaphragm may slightly irritate the urethra, making infection more likely, and decrease the vaginal lactobacilli, especially the peroxide-producing lactobacilli that police vaginal bacteria such as *E. coli.*[6]

▼ *Women with a history of UTI.* Factors that disrupt the normal bacteria of the urogenital tract promote the further growth of harmful bacteria. The recent use of some kinds of antibiotics increases risk.[7]

▼ *Pregnant women.* The weight of the fetus on the bladder can prevent complete emptying of the bladder. Remember, urine that sits around in the bladder is an invitation for bacteria to visit. Treatment is especially important for moms-to-be in order to prevent a kidney infection from developing.

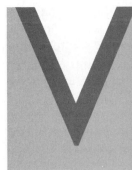

The water reminder

Try drinking a glass of water before you have sex. Odds are better that you'll need to empty your bladder afterward, which is a good idea to help flush away bacteria that have traveled where they shouldn't. Clinicians are not sure whether urinating after having sex helps prevent bladder infections—but it certainly can't hurt.

▼ *Postmenopausal women.*[8] Sagging of the bladder or uterus down into the vagina (conditions known as prolapse) may prevent proper emptying of the bladder, causing urine to remain.[9] In addition, the lack of estrogen causes dramatic changes in the bacteria of the vagina, including a loss of lactobacilli and increased colonization by *E. coli*.[10] It looks like estrogen therapy can help keep UTIs at bay after menopause. Estrogen therapy acidifies the vaginal pH and corrects the thinning of the vaginal, urethral, and bladder lining; the lactobacilli come back. One study has shown that postmenopausal women with a history of UTI had a significant reduction in infections when treated with vaginal estrogen cream.[11] Other studies suggest that oral estrogen may not be enough to buff up the urinary tract and prevent infection in postmenopausal women.[12] Further work showed that use of a vaginal estrogen ring, delivering low-dose topical estrogen, kept the majority of women free of UTI.[13]

▼ *Women with an abnormality of the structure of their urinary tract.* There could be something wrong with its shape that leaves them vulnerable to infection.

The overwhelming majority of bladder infections—more than 90 percent—are caused by two bacteria, *E. coli* and *Staphylococcus saprophyticus*.[14] That familiar culprit *E. coli* is responsible at least 80 percent of the time.[15] *E. coli* comes from the intestinal tract. It lingers at the vaginal opening and around the urethral area, and from these locations it can easily get up into the bladder to cause infection. Women who are susceptible to UTIs have more bacteria colonizing these sites and more sites for bacterial attachment on the bladder surface compared with women without UTIs. Genetic, hormonal, and other factors probably influence the ability of bacteria to stick. Natural defenses against bacterial adherence—local antibodies produced by the urinary tract, competing bacteria, and normal patterns of urination—may be genetically determined.[16]

RECURRENT UTI

A great many women with UTI have symptoms come back at some point or another. This is known as *recurrence*. Recurrences are most often infections with a new bug (reinfection), not infection with the same bug that never got wiped out. These reinfections rarely represent a serious problem. Recurrences often develop with several clusters over six to twelve months.[17] Recurrences are especially common in the groups at highest risk for UTI (sexually active women, postmenopausal women, and women who use a diaphragm with spermicide).

IT'S BACK!	Which Kind of UTI Is It?
Is your UTI old or new? Here are the main differences between the same old bug (a relapse) and a new kid on the block (recurrence). Either kind can be dealt with successfully.	
Same Old Bug (Relapse)	**New Kid on the Block (Recurrence)**
Original infecting bacteria, usually within two weeks after completing therapy	Different species or strain of bacteria, usually more than two weeks after completing therapy
If long-term (2–6 weeks) antibiotics are not helpful, urological referral is important	Referral to urologist is not routinely indicated; clinician may suggest a change if the woman uses a diaphragm and spermicide
No relation to intercourse	Related to intercourse
Antibiotics 2–3 times per week for prevention	Antibiotics after intercourse for prevention; patient-initiated therapy for symptoms

Less frequently, symptoms come back from persistence of the same bacteria that has never gone away. This is called *relapse*. If there is a short interval of time between infections, such as ten to fourteen days, there is a possibility that the kidneys or ureter (upper urinary tract) may have an infected place that is sending bacteria down to the bladder. When the same bacteria cause an infection over and over again, an abnormality of the urinary tract, such as a narrowing of the tract or a stone, needs to be looked for. Stones (which occur when mineral salts clump together) can occur anywhere in the urinary tract—the kidney, the ureter, or the bladder. Stones are famous for causing terrible pain. But a stone can also develop silently, acting as a sort of magnet for bacteria, which nest around it and then cause infection. Stones can usually be found by ultrasound or by an X-ray study using dye to outline the urinary tract.

The difference between recurrence from reinfection and relapse from persistent bacteria is important in management because women with recurrence usually *do not have* an underlying abnormality of the urinary tract and usually require long-term medical management. They do not

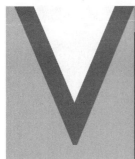

Good catch!

The best way to provide a clean-catch urine sample is to first clean around the urinary opening (usually the clinician will provide a disposable sterile pad for this), then start to urinate. Don't collect your sample right away. Wait until the midportion of the urination.

need a trip to a urologist and all kinds of special studies. They just need a course of long-term antibiotics. On the other hand, women with relapse from persistent bacteria are usually cured by identifying and surgically removing an anatomical problem such as a narrowed place or a stone.[18]

Untreated bladder infection can progress to kidney infection *(pyelonephritis),* but the majority of women with bladder infections don't go on to develop this problem. Whether or not kidney infection develops depends on how powerful the bacteria are in causing disease and how good they are at sticking to surface cells. Abnormalities of the urinary tract, a weakened defense system, and having had procedures such as catheterization are other contributing factors.

DIAGNOSING UTI

As I said, you can wait twenty-four hours (in the absence of fever or pain) to see if the problem clears up on its own. If not, though, you should have an exam. Your clinician can make sure there is no other cause for the symptoms, such as vaginitis. Diagnosing UTI also requires a clean-voided urine sample, sometimes called a clean catch, for testing.

Normal urine is sterile and should not contain any bacteria, red blood cells, or white blood cells. There are two ways to test the urine, with a dipstick in the office or with a more formal urinalysis in the lab. Urine dipsticks provide a quick and inexpensive method for detecting red blood cells and white blood cells. Dipsticks also test for leukocyte esterase, a chemical indication of the presence of white blood cells, and nitrite that is released by bacteria in the urine. Formal urinalysis uses urine that has been spun in a centrifuge to separate any solid materials from the water. This spun sediment is then viewed under the microscope. Red and white cells as well as bacteria can actually be counted. Pus in the urine (pyuria) is defined by ten or more white blood cells per microscope field. The majority of women with UTIs will have pus cells in the urine.

A urine culture is a test to see if bacteria grow from a small amount of urine put on special material to promote growth in the lab. Infection is present when a urine culture shows a hundred or more clumps or colonies

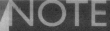

You came to Aruba to see the beach, not the gyn

UTI or yeast infection can spoil a honeymoon or vacation. I send all my brides off with medicine to cover a bladder or yeast infection. If you've had these problems before, if you have never had sex, or if you have a new partner, ask for prescriptions before you leave.

of bacteria per milliliter (about ten drops) of urine.[19] When infection is suspected, culture is not always necessary. The leukocyte esterase dipstick is accurate enough that some clinicians feel that it is not necessary to send a culture to a lab; if the woman has symptoms and a negative leukocyte esterase test, a culture can be done.

For many years it was believed that to diagnose bladder infection, a significant number of bacteria (100,000 or more organisms per milliliter of urine) had to be present in the urine. Clinicians have since learned that although half of women with bladder infections do have this particular level of bacteria, a third of women with the same symptoms have fewer bacteria. These women too have a bladder infection.[20] If the culture is negative even though the woman has acute symptoms and pus in the urine, she may have urethritis caused by chlamydia. She needs to be evaluated for chlamydia in the cervix and treated with the medication that works best against chlamydia, tetracycline.

If you have a history of repeated infection, a sensitivity test to see what kind of antibiotic works best against the bacteria that grow in the culture can be done. The drug that works best against the bugs growing in your sample can then be used.

Proceed with caution if you have frequent bladder infections and are sent to a urologist for a detailed evaluation. This may include a special X-ray study of the kidneys (intravenous pyelogram, or IVP), a look into the bladder through a cystoscope, and enlarging the urethra (dilatation). A great deal of money is spent on unnecessary and uncomfortable tests for women who have nothing more than reinfection brought on by sexual intercourse. In healthy women with reinfections (as opposed to women with relapse of the same infection), it's very rare that something would be wrong with the kidneys and ureters, so these tests are not needed.[21] Before these tests are done on a woman with no other health problems or complaints beyond UTI, a trial of preventative antibiotics (described in the following section) should be undertaken first.

Studies *should* be done for women who keep getting reinfected by the same bacteria (relapse), to look for problems such as a stone. Studies also need to be done for women who have pain, who need to urinate frequently, who need to get to the bathroom quickly, or who are up at night more than once or twice, if these symptoms occur when a woman does not have a UTI.[22]

Also consider a second opinion if a urethral dilatation is recommended. In the past, narrowing of the urethra (stricture) was widely believed to be the cause of recurrent UTI, so opening up of the urethra (dilatation) was frequently done. But clinicians are no longer sure that repeated infection is related to a narrow urethra, and the helpfulness of stretching the urethra has come into question.[23] Recently trained urologists are using it less frequently.[24]

TREATMENT COURSES FOR BLADDER INFECTION

Circumstances	Route	Drug	Dosage (mg)	Frequency per dose	Duration (days)
Uncomplicated infection in healthy women	Oral	TMP-SMX	160–800	Every 12 hours	3
		TMP	100	Every 12 hours	
		nitrofurantoin	100	Every 6 hours	
Complicated: Symptoms more than 7 days, recent UTI, age over 65, diabetes, diaphragm use	Oral	TMP-SMX	160–800	Every 12 hours	7
		fluoroquinolone	250–400	Every 12 hours	
Pregnancy, breast-feeding	Oral	amoxicillin	250	Every 8 hours	7
		cephalexin	500	Every 6 hours	
		nitrofurantoin	100	Every 6 hours	
		TMP-SMX	160–800	Every 12 hours	

TREATING UTI

Many studies have been done in recent years to find the best treatment for uncomplicated bladder infection—that is, an isolated, nonrecurring bladder infection in a healthy, nonpregnant woman with no known urinary tract problems.[25] Most UTIs respond rapidly to a variety of antibiotics. The oral antibiotics that are most effective in fighting the infection while preserving the balance of good bacteria in the vagina and intestine include trimethoprim-sulfamethoxazole (TMP-SMX), trimethoprim alone, nitrofurantoin, cephalexin, and the fluoroquinolones. Amoxicillin is seldom used because *E. coli,* the most common cause of infection, is usually

WHAT ABOUT CRANBERRY JUICE?

Many women routinely drink cranberry juice in the belief that it can prevent bladder infections. This belief is grounded in some truth. We know that cranberry juice cuts down on the ability of bacteria to stick to the cells of the urinary tract. (It does not work by acidifying the urine, as is commonly thought.) If you're going to rely on cranberry juice, though, you should know that in the study that proved it worked, it took four to eight weeks before it started reducing the bacteria found in the urine. And it's a preventative measure—not a cure once you already have a bladder infection. You should also know that the women in the study drank a tall 10 ounces per day. Watch out for the calories, or choose an artificially sweetened drink.

Source: A. E. Sobota, Inhibition of bacterial adherence by cranberry juice: potential use for the treatment of urinary tract infections, *J Urol* 1984:131:1013.

resistant to it [26] For single-dose therapy, the best results have been achieved with TMP-SMX.[27] With most antibiotics, three-day regimens appear best, with success rates similar to seven-day regimens but with fewer side effects (such as rash and yeast infection) and lower cost.[28] Single-dose therapy can also be used, but it generally results in lower rates of cure and more frequent recurrences, especially with drugs such as amoxicillin and other drugs that are rapidly eliminated from the body.[29] Because the fluoroquinolones (e.g., ciprofloxacin) are expensive and cannot be used in pregnancy, their use is favored only when there is bacterial resistance to other drugs or the woman cannot tolerate the other available choices. Studies show that the concentration of trimethoprim and the fluoroquinolones in vaginal secretions is high, wiping out *E. coli* but minimally altering normal vaginal bacterial residents.[30]

One of the main ways to try to help women who have recurrent UTI is preventative use of antibiotics (prophylactic therapy). This approach decreases recurrences by almost half.[31] A woman takes a small dose of an antibiotic daily, generally at bedtime, for six to twelve months. The big problem is

NOTE

Quick reminder for repeated bladder infections

Recurrence means the later infections are unrelated to the first one. *Relapse* means the same bug you had in the first place comes back; it never really went away.

that while there may be some improvement for a while after the end of the treatment, there is no long-lasting effect, probably because the reason the woman gets infected in the first place hasn't been eliminated (e.g., a short urethra, a genetic background that makes your bladder cells "stickier" so bacteria can latch on better).[32] Some women need to stay on long-term *low-dose* antibiotics; there are also alternatives.

Another way to deal with the problem is to pop a pill after sex. Antibiotics such as nitrofurantoin, cephalexin, or TMP-SMX taken as a single dose after intercourse help reduce the possibility of a related UTI.[33] Unfortunately, many clinicians do not offer this to women, or women are afraid to take the antibiotics. This single dose is unlikely to cause yeast.

A third possibility, if a woman doesn't want to take the six-month antibiotic prophylaxis or the postsex prophylaxis, is to manage UTI symptoms as soon as they start.[34] In this method, women identify episodes of infection based on their symptoms and treat themselves at the beginning of their symptoms with a single dose of TMP-SMX.

All of these methods for the woman with reinfection (not relapse with the same bug) involve antibiotics.

PREVENTING UTI

The following advice can help reduce your odds of bladder infection.

- ▼ Drink plenty of fluids each day; a glass of water every two to three hours is a good rule of thumb. Not only does it help to flush bacteria from your bladder, it's a generally healthy way to live.
- ▼ Eat well, obtain adequate rest, and exercise to keep up your resistance.
- ▼ Be sure to drink at least 10 ounces of cranberry juice cocktail daily if you are using it as a preventive measure against UTI.
- ▼ Practice clean sex. Reduce the odds of introducing bacteria by being sure you and your partner have clean hands and clean bodies prior to sex. Take care that fingers or the penis do not travel from the anus

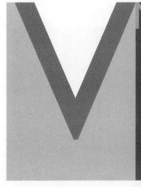

Preventing future bladder infections

Strategies on the horizon may include chemicals that prevent bacteria from sticking to the bladder, and the right kind of lactobacilli (human) to promote the normal state in the vagina. A vaccine against UTI is in development.

Source: S. Langerman, S. Palaszyunski, M. Barnhart et al., Prevention of mucosal *Escherichia coli* infection by FirmH-adhesin-based systemic vaccination, *Science* 1997:276:607.

to the vagina without being washed first. Make sure you have adequate lubrication, because little cracks around the urethra can be a place for bacteria to enter. Urinating after sex may help flush bacteria out of the urethra.

▼ If you have frequent UTIs, consider single-dose preventative antibiotics, especially if you have a new partner. Bring along these antibiotics on your honeymoon or on vacation when you anticipate increased sexual activity.

▼ If you use a diaphragm and have frequent UTIs, consider a smaller diaphragm or another form of birth control.

▼ If you are postmenopausal and experience frequent UTIs, consider estrogen. Used in the form of a vaginal ring, it will stay in the vagina and not be carried anywhere else in the body. Estrogen cream can also be used in a safe manner so that it does not enter the bloodstream in large amounts.

▼ Use herbs cautiously. People have long been drinking teas made of goldenseal, bayberry, uva ursi, horsetail, corn silk, cleavers, echinacea, or lemon balm to prevent or treat UTIs. Unfortunately, there are no medical studies on these.

▼ See a doctor if you develop a fever or back pain along with your urinary symptoms; these might indicate a kidney infection, and that's more serious than a bladder infection.

Interstitial cystitis (IC)

Interstitial cystitis (say "IN-ter-STI-she-al sis-TIE-tis") deserves an in-depth look here because it's a confusing and underdiagnosed problem in women. IC is a chronic inflammatory bladder disorder resulting in a feeling of needing to go often and immediately, as well as bladder pain. While cystitis involves infection in the bladder itself, the inflammation of interstitial cystitis extends through the lining and into the wall of the bladder. The name comes from this location: The bladder wall is known as *interstitium*.

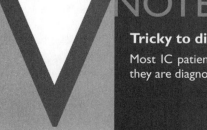

Tricky to diagnose

Most IC patients report having seen several physicians before they are diagnosed correctly, usually in midlife.

Of the 450,000 Americans estimated to have IC, the majority are Caucasian.[35]

We're not sure what causes IC. It's definitely not infection. It is probably not an autoimmune disease. A popular theory suggests that the protein building blocks forming the bladder lining are defective and leaky, allowing irritating urinary substances to pass out of the urine into the bladder wall.[36] Another leading theory suggests that some kind of insult to the bladder (no one knows what) stirs up nerve fibers in the bladder wall, triggering an inflammatory process. Release of inflammatory chemicals turns on mast cells (part of the body's normal defense system), which release more inflammatory substances, resulting in greater inflammation, cell and tissue damage, and scarring in some places on the bladder wall.[37] The scarring can make the bladder capacity smaller.

THREE URINARY PROBLEMS THAT AREN'T INFECTIONS

When a woman has irritative urinary symptoms and a urine culture is negative, she is said to have urethral syndrome. This problem is not well understood, but generally it can be divided into three subgroups:

1. Urethral irritation caused by chlamydia, gonorrhea, mycoplasma, or herpes. The underlying problem is diagnosed by culturing for these organisms and treating them if they are found.

2. Interstitial cystitis (IC), a painful bladder disease of unknown cause that involves inflammation in the bladder. It occurs in women of all ages. This inflammatory condition causes symptoms similar to UTI, but cultures are negative and antibiotics do not help. Clinicians believe that IC may be related to vulvar vestibulitis, since many symptoms overlap and the two conditions often occur together. IC is best diagnosed by cystoscopy under anesthesia so that the bladder can be filled up with enough fluid to see the areas that are abnormal.

3. "Pure" urethral syndrome, which is probably part of vulvodynia. Women experience burning or stinging with urination, or spasm or pain around the urethra or "up inside." (See Chapter 17.)

The inflammation of the bladder and its wall causes symptoms that feel like a UTI at first, but urine cultures are negative. As the inflammation continues, so do the symptoms. It's not unusual for a woman with IC to void sixteen times a day, even up to forty times daily.[38] Other signs of IC include getting up to go to the bathroom three or more times a night, although not everyone has this. Pain with urination and in the abdomen, bladder, and/or vagina are common. Pelvic pain and pain with intercourse are part of IC for many women. The pain is worse when the bladder is full and is relieved by emptying the bladder.[39] Loss of control of the urine (incontinence) and blood in the urine (hematuria) are not usually seen in IC.

IC usually starts slowly, then accelerates to a peak of severe symptoms, and finally cools down. Flare-ups alternate with times of well-being. Flares are associated with diet, illness, stress, and the menstrual cycle.[40] Low levels of estrogen in the second part of the cycle and in the perimenopausal and postmenopausal periods may contribute to the problem.

IC can be confused with recurrent UTI, overactive bladder, and endometriosis.[41] Bladder cancer may also mimic IC.[42]

DIAGNOSING IC

Because it can develop subtly, be mild as well as severe, and mimic other diseases, IC often eludes diagnosis. In fact, women with IC frequently are not diagnosed for many years in spite of many clinician visits. On top of its variable nature, IC isn't well understood by clinicians, and its symptoms, which can be hard to pinpoint, overlap with other problems. There is no single diagnostic test.

At least diagnosis may be getting easier. In the past, IC was not diagnosed unless a physician saw certain classic bladder changes, including a reduced bladder volume, by looking into the bladder with cystoscopy. To do this, the bladder often has to be filled with fluid and stretched (distended) past its usual capacity. Such stretching is painful and not well tolerated; usually it has to be done under general anesthesia in an operating room.

Other studies of bladder size and function, or cystometrics (say "sis-toe-MEH-tricks"), used to be the last word in diagnosis. If a woman didn't have a small bladder capacity, she was thought not to have IC.[43] But now some clinicians think that bladder volume testing is not that helpful—someone in the early stages of IC may not show a small bladder capacity at all or may never have had inflammation bad enough to develop it.[44] Unfortunately, a lot of cystometric studies and many office cystoscopies are still carried out; without full distension, the abnormalities may not be

A PROMISING NEW TEST

A new diagnostic test for IC, the potassium sensitivity test, was introduced in 1998. This is an office test that may identify patients with a leaky bladder lining, a possible cause of IC. Two solutions, salt water and a potassium solution, are put into the bladder, one after the other. After each instillation, patients rate their sense of needing to go (urgency) and pain on a scale of 0 to 5, with 5 representing the greatest urgency and pain. A score of 2 or more in response to the potassium solution is considered a positive finding, meaning that the potassium has leaked through the bladder wall to cause pain. The physicians who developed this test found that it was positive in three-quarters of IC sufferers but only 4 percent of those who did not have IC. This test may become the new way to diagnose IC if further work with it confirms these findings.

Source: C. L. Parsons, M. Greenberger, L. Gabal, et al., The role of urinary potassium in the pathenogenesis of interstitial cystitis, J Urol 1998:159:1862.

seen, and women who may have IC, with the history and the symptoms, are told they do not.

Cystoscopy under anesthesia is valuable and important to make sure there is nothing else wrong with the bladder, such as urethral abnormalities, bladder stones, and tumors. But increasingly, clinicians make the diagnosis of IC by taking a woman's history and doing some simple office tests. The history includes asking about urinary complaints, voiding patterns, pain description, and the time frame for the problem. Some physicians ask women to keep a voiding diary. The history includes questions about gynecology or other conditions that might cause bladder symptoms. A physical examination is less helpful, although tenderness over the bladder and under the urethra and bladder base may be found on pelvic exam. The exam is important, however, to rule out other causes of the symptoms such as endometriosis, pelvic mass, vaginitis, or urethral disease. Vulvar vestibulitis and vulvodynia are common in IC patients.[45]

With the combination of the history, the voiding log, the elimination of other possible diagnoses that are confused with IC, and the finding of bladder neck tenderness on exam, a clinician may suspect IC. To confirm this, a urinalysis, urine culture, and evaluation of the urine for precancerous cells (cytology) are done. Urethral and cervical cultures are sent to labs as well to ensure that chlamydia, mycoplasma, and gonorrhea aren't present. A wet prep is done to rule out vaginitis.

TREATING IC

Since the cause of IC remains uncertain, the treatment is based on trial and error and usually involves more than one approach. The main prongs of treatment are described below.

Self-Help, Education, and Behavioral Modification

Any treatment works better when patients understand the whole picture of their problem and know what they can do to help themselves. Patient education and self-help are well recognized as vital for the chronic pain of IC. (See Resources for information and support groups.)

Behavioral therapy involves timed voiding, which is particularly useful when frequency of urination is the main problem.[46] Women also benefit from stress-reduction techniques, relaxation skills, massage, and acupuncture, especially when combined with other therapies.

Dietary Changes

Although good scientific proof is lacking, changing one's diet can help a lot. Since caffeine, alcohol, acidic foods, and carbonated beverages top the list of foods associated with worsening of IC symptoms, avoiding these and other problematic foods may decrease symptoms.[47] (See box on page 362.)

Drug Treatment

Drugs instilled into the bladder have been used to treat IC for many years. Dimethyl sulfoxide (DMSO), heparin, hydrocortisone, and silver nitrate have been used in this fashion with varying results. DMSO has been well studied; it provides relief in half to almost all of patients.[48] One-third to one-half of those who respond will develop symptoms again after a month or two, but about 50 percent of these relapsers respond when the treatment is repeated.[49] Mixtures of different drugs have been used with some success; a common combination includes

AVOID THESE FOODS IF YOU HAVE IC

Chocolate	Alcoholic beverages
Soy sauce or tamari	Spicy foods
Fruits, esp. citrus	Coffee, tea, all caffeine
Citric acid	Avocado
Artificial sweeteners	Cheese, esp. aged
Brewer's yeast	Corned beef
Fava beans	Mayonnaise
Lima beans	Onions in large amounts
Pickled herring	Vitamins with aspartate
Rye bread or rye products	Vitamins with yeast
Yogurt	Vitamins with ergosterol or ergocalciferol (synthetic vitamin D)
Sour cream	
Meals high in animal protein	Fermented foods
Vinegar and vinegar products	Tap water
Sprouts of any kind	Foods with molds
Foods with chemical additives	Foods containing sugar or honey
Yeast foods (bread, food with nutritional yeast added)	Smoked or barbecued foods
	Fried foods
Hydrogenated fats, including margarine and shortening	

Source: K. E. Whitmore, Self-care regimens for patients with interstitial cystitis, Urol Clin N Am 1994:21(1):121.

DMSO, heparin, hydrocortisone, a local anesthetic, and sodium bicarbonate weekly for six weeks.[50]

A recent study reported significant success with bladder training and instillation of oxybutynin, an antispasmodic with local anesthetic properties.[51] Oxybutynin has been used orally for years in the treament of overactive bladder.

Antihistamines were among the first drugs used in the treatment of IC, and they work pretty well when you have a strong history of allergy. One study reports a 40 percent improvement in IC symptoms with the use of hydroxyzine (Atarax), which lessens activity from the mast cells.[52] Women often don't like Atarax because it makes them tired, but frequently this fatigue diminishes if you hang in there for a few weeks.

Amitriptyline, an antidepressant belonging to the tricyclic family, keeps the bladder's nerve supply from getting overstimulated and blocks the histamine churned out by the mast cells.[53] Both it and its cousins (nortriptyline and desipramine) are good first-line treatments.

The most recent addition to the armament of treatments for IC is pentosan (Elmiron). This is a molecule similar to the building blocks found on the surface of the bladder lining. Clinicians initially thought Elmiron corrected a defect in the bladder lining, building up its barrier ability and thus preventing irritating substances in the urine from reaching the bladder wall.[54] A recent report, however, suggests that Elmiron works as a powerful antihistamine, blocking release of histamine, a chemical that causes pain and inflammation.[55] So far, it's reported to help anywhere from about 20 to 50 percent of the women who try it.[56] Side effects are infrequent.[57] Because it takes a long time to repair the leaky bladder lining, Elmiron is not a quick fix; three to six months of continuous therapy are needed to build up the bladder wall.

Other Treatments

Stretching the bladder with fluid (hydrodistension) under anesthesia is used for treatment as well as diagnosis of IC. The distension must be held for ten minutes in order to be effective. Stretching the bladder probably causes mechanical damage to the stretch receptors with a lessening of pain and urinary frequency. Stretching improves symptoms for six months or less.[58]

When IC is not responsive to other treatment, clinicians use long-acting painkillers and pain relief through transcutaneous electrical nerve stimulation (TENS). Surgical approaches (removal of the bladder or diversion of urinary drainage to another site at the skin or bowel) are reserved for the most severe cases (fortunately fewer than 5 percent).

IC BOTTOM LINE

Let me emphasize again that the rules for diagnosing IC may be changing. Your history alone (or in concert with some simple tests) may be used to make the diagnosis. If you think you might have IC, search out the most knowledgeable physician you can find. Use the Interstitial Cystitis Association to find names (see Resources), or call a teaching hospital in a large city. A urologist who has recently completed training is likely to be familiar with the new thinking, though many experienced clinicians work hard to keep current. Try the diet and use all the self-help guides available. Contact others who have the problem through the Interstitial Cystitis Association. Work with your physician on all the available medications and treatments. Remember that it is often a combination of things you do (meds, bladder distension and instillation, physical therapy, acupuncture, massage therapy) that can make the difference.

▼

CHAPTER 20

The Lifetime Virus
Living with Genital Herpes

O f all the unhappiness that vulvar conditions can bring, perhaps the most dismay comes from genital herpes caused by the herpes simplex virus (HSV). You're smart to find out everything you can about genital herpes if you've been diagnosed with it, because the virus takes up permanent residence in the nerve endings near your vulva. That's right; it's not going to go away. From time to time, it can cause painful sores and then recede, although outbreaks vary tremendously from one woman to the next. The good news, though (yes, there is some), is that treatment has come a long way. The outbreaks can be controlled effectively, even during pregnancy.

Unpleasant as these prospects may be, your worries and hurt feelings when you learn you have herpes are likely to be far worse than any physical problems you experience. *How could this happen to me? How will I ever deal with its impact on my life? What does this mean as far as having children is concerned?* I hear these questions all the time.

Herpes first arrived on the sexual scene in the 1960s and 1970s. Because of its lifelong nature, it created more paranoia than any of the other sexually transmitted diseases then becoming household words. (This was before AIDS, which now makes herpes look relatively benign and manageable in comparison.) Far from being a problem of the past, though, genital herpes cases are rising. In 1991 about forty-five million Americans were infected with genital herpes; ten years later the number had grown to fifty million, many of whom simply don't know enough

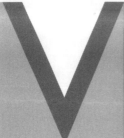

Keeping them straight

HSV-1 is short for herpes simplex virus type 1, which mostly causes cold sores on the mouth; HSV-2 is short for herpes simplex virus type 2, which causes genital herpes. Both can show up in either area of the body, though.

about it.[1] Record numbers of babies have also been born with herpes in the past two decades.[2]

We're talking about a very common problem. Think you're not playing fast and loose enough to be affected? Unlike some other fellow sexually transmitted viruses, herpes isn't necessarily a disease of sexual promiscuity. Herpes is highly contagious. It takes only one contact with someone who may not even know that he is infected.

How herpes works

Herpes simplex viruses are present all over the world. Unlike other viruses, such as the one responsible for the common cold, they do not vary with the season or by country. Humans are the only hosts attacked by herpes.[3] There are two types of the virus, HSV-1 and HSV-2. Most genital herpes (about 80 percent) is caused by HSV-2. HSV-1 accounts primarily for fever blisters or cold sores on the mouth and lips, though it can also cause genital herpes if the virus is passed from the mouth to the genitals during oral sex. The reverse is also true: Cold sores and blisters can be caused by HSV-2 as the virus is passed from the genitals to the mouth. And it's possible for a person with HSV-1 in the mouth to spread the virus to her own genitals with her hands. Cultures can show which virus you have.

The virus is introduced directly into cells in the top layer of the skin; for genital herpes this occurs either during intercourse or with contact of mouth to genitals. Infection occurs, the virus takes over the cells and kills them after using their cell machinery to assemble new particles of virus.[4] With progressive destruction of the cells in the skin, fluid leaks into the tissue, and watery blisters (called *vesicles*) form within the skin layer. These are the telltale blisters of herpes.

About twenty-four hours after the blisters appear, the virus begins to spread from the infected cells along sensory nerve fibers to nerve centers (ganglia) outside the spinal cord. They infect the ganglia, then enter an inactive period. This latency persists indefinitely. Reactivation—the process of the virus getting out of the nerve centers and back in the skin as the hallmark blisters of repeated herpes—can occur at any time in the subse-

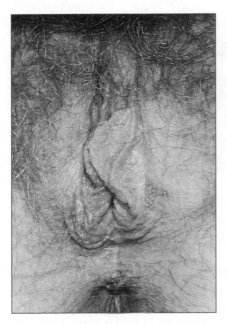

FIG. 48 Herpes. The watery blisters, or vesicles, have ruptured, causing tiny ulcers.

quent days, months, or years. Recurrences are often unpredictable but can be related to intercourse, stress, or menstruation. HSV-2 infections are more likely to come back (60 to 80 percent of cases recur) than HSV 1 (14 to 25 percent of cases recur).[5]

The big question

Among the first things that patients with herpes inevitably ask me is "Where did I get this?" or "Who gave it to me?" Sometimes the answer is clear. You knew that your partner had herpes and now you have come down with it too. Or you ask your partner and he admits that he has herpes and never told you. Or perhaps he admits that he didn't tell the truth when you asked about his history. Lots of the time, however, it is not at all clear where the infection came from. How about if you've been in the same relationship for years and suddenly you come down with herpes? Or if your partner swears up and down that he has never, ever had anything resembling herpes? Is he lying? Or what if you're a widow and you haven't been sexually active since your partner died? Just had a baby and had no new partner in years? Herpes is possible for all these. How can this be?

Medicine doesn't yet have any test that can answer your questions for sure, but let's explore the possible answers. You'll need to understand some more about herpes first, beginning with some information about how our immune systems work (immunology).

Our immune systems fight off disease in two ways. With the first way, we make antibodies. Some antibodies do the active fighting that can sometimes destroy the invading foreigners; other antibodies do not fight and serve only as markers that an invader (such as the herpes virus) has entered the body. Antibodies to the herpes virus can be detected by several methods. Their presence does not appear to have any influence on the development of recurrent infection, but it's thought that as they circulate through the bloodstream, they have some protective effect. HSV-1 antibodies lessen the severity of the first episodes of HSV-2 infection, for example, and can prevent infection with HSV-2 entirely.[6] The problem with looking at antibodies in blood tests is that the antibodies are present forever once infection has occurred, and most tests have not been able to tell

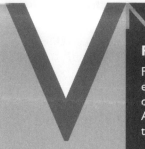

Risk factors for genital herpes

Factors that increase your risk of contracting herpes include early age at first sexual intercourse, multiple sexual partners, increasing years of sexual activity, a history of other STDs, being African American or Hispanic, lower levels of income or education, and being single or divorced.

the difference between antibodies to HSV-1 and HSV-2. Therefore a woman who has an HSV-1 infection with cold sores will test positive for herpes even if she is not infected with HSV-2. New tests are coming out that are more specific, but these will not be generally available until we know that they are completely reliable.

The second way that antibodies combat disease is by making special white blood cells that can fight off the invader (a process called *cell-mediated immunity*). The fighter and killer cells of the immune system seem essential in preventing or lessening genital herpes, but the role of cell-mediated immunity is not understood.[7] No one knows why some people exposed to herpes never develop it, or why some have so many more outbreaks than others.

So how does this give us any clues about who gave what to whom? Accurate blood testing is on the horizon. Many Americans have had cold sores caused by HSV-1 and therefore have antibodies to HSV-1. As mentioned, these antibodies can do enough active fighting to lessen the severity of the first episode of herpes caused by HSV-2, to the point that the person doesn't know an outbreak of herpes has occurred. So now that person has herpes and sheds the virus and can infect others without realizing that he himself (or herself) has herpes. This person is one type of what's known as a silent shedder (or *asymptomatic shedder*), a person who has herpes, sheds the virus, but does not know that he or she has the disease and is infecting others.

There are other types of asymptomatic shedders. Most individuals who transmit HSV to their sexual partners, even in retrospect, do not have a typical attack of genital herpes around the time of transmission.[8] In this case, the person knows that he or she has had herpes at some point in the past but doesn't have any blisters or symptoms during the current episode of sexual activity. For example, in a study checking on the individuals who had been in contact with sixty-six people with newly acquired genital herpes, only one-third of the contacts had a history compatible with a recent genital herpes infection. Of the remaining contacts, one-third had a history of genital symptoms that were not typical of genital herpes, and another third were found to be HSV-2 antibody positive but never had any prior symptoms.[9]

This stealthiness explains why the most common sources of genital herpes are people who have no idea that they have herpes and people who have had herpes in the past but have no symptoms at the time of sexual encounter.

Genital herpes infections are more likely to occur without symptoms than with symptoms.[10] About 1 percent of individuals previously infected with HSV-2 reactivate their infection, without symptoms, on any given day, and up to 80 percent of these people will never have experienced a clinically evident infection.[11] So, as you can see, there is a very large number of asymptomatic shedders contributing to the transmission of HSV.[12] This explains why herpes infections are on the rise and are not easy to figure out. You can appreciate the danger of a virus that can work so silently.

It's possible that you yourself could have had a silent first outbreak of herpes at some point and are only now having a symptomatic episode (probably because of some change in your immune function). Or your partner could be an asymptomatic shedder and now you have come down with the infection. This can happen many years after the initial attack, so people can have long-established relationships or be into old age when the herpes shows up.

Another common way for someone to get herpes is to receive HSV-1 through oral-genital sex with someone who has cold sores. Many people do not realize that oral sex can cause illness. Cold sore blisters contain active virus. So if your partner does not have genital herpes but does have cold sores, you can still come down with genital herpes yourself.

What symptoms are like

What are herpes infections like when they produce symptoms? They vary a great deal depending on whether they are first or recurrent attacks. Stay with me here, and don't let the long names throw you.

FIRST EPISODE PRIMARY HERPES VULVOVAGINITIS

The classic severe first episode occurs in about one-third of women who have no preexisting antibodies against HSV-1 or HSV-2. The incubation pe-

NOTE

Equal-opportunity infection
Herpes is as common in men as women, although women tend to have more obvious and severe symptoms.

V

VOICES

"I'm one of what I suspect are the many clueless veterans of the '60s and '70s who thought she just had a very bad yeast infection the first couple of times. About a year later it flared up again when I happened to have a gyn appointment, and the doc took one look, palpated the lymph node in my groin, watched me hit the ceiling, and gave me the news.

"That he was matter-of-fact about it, and that this happened when the specter of AIDS had just become clear, helped me keep it in a better perspective than I might have otherwise. But it wasn't easy, and I'm mortified to say that to this day I don't know who gave it to me or exactly when I got it, though I subsequently did what I could to be responsible with any partners I thought might be affected.

"It's sometimes not as bad as the descriptions make it out to be, which is part of the problem. Acyclovir works, it will be okay, get on with your life. And if you visit the online bulletin boards in this area, have a stiff drink handy."

—Frances, 54, who has herpes

riod for a first attack of genital herpes is between two and ten days. Burning or itching may come two or three days before the appearance of the lesions. These lesions are at first red, then turn into little fluid-filled blisters, which eventually break open to form tiny, shallow ulcers that are painful. In women, herpes are most often seen on the labia majora and minora, clitoris, perineum, and perianal areas. Swelling of the labia is common, and the pain can make an examination almost impossible. In 80 percent of first cases, the cervix is involved.[13] There will also be vaginal discharge as ulcers on its surface drain. Painful urination is also common, either because the urine stings as it hits the blistered vulva or because of herpetic ulcers around the urinary opening. Urination may be so painful that women have to sit in a bathtub full of water in order to urinate. Tender, enlarged lymph nodes in the groin appear during the second week of the primary herpes outbreak and are generally the last sign to go away.[14] Women often have flulike symptoms too: headache, fever, and a general sense of not feeling well.

The symptoms of primary genital herpes reach their worst after seven to ten days and then gradually diminish. The ulcers begin to crust, and after fourteen to twenty-one days, healing may be virtually complete. But in some women the blisters appear in crops, so recovery takes longer. Yeast can also invade as a secondary development and cause more trouble. Although less common, bacterial infection can complicate herpes as well.[15]

A first attack is not always so dramatic, though. Some women don't even know they are being affected. And at the other extreme, it can be much worse. Herpes isn't always limited to the genital tract. The virus enters the bloodstream. You may get off easy—just a generalized infection (it could pass as the flu) with fever, vomiting, muscle aches, and sore throat (the same blisters as seen on the genitals can be found in the throat), or a generalized infection plus involvement all through the lower genital tract. But some women have to be hospitalized for these symptoms. And one-third of women with a first infection will get viral meningitis, requiring treatment with intravenous antiviral drugs.[16]

FIRST EPISODE NONPRIMARY HERPES VULVOVAGINITIS

Almost half of patients who are seen with their first outbreak of genital herpes have existing antibodies to the virus.[17] Remember, in some people the illness can be so mild that it is not recognized the first time. Then, when the next infection occurs and is recognized, it's referred to as first episode nonprimary, typically caused by HSV-2 in the presence of antibodies to HSV-1. These patients have fewer systemic symptoms, a shorter duration of pain, fewer blisters, and a shorter healing time compared with patients with true primary infections.

RECURRENT HERPES VULVOVAGINITIS

A quarter of patients or fewer will have a recurrence after the first genital infection caused by HSV-1, while 70 to 80 percent of cases will recur after genital HSV-2 infection.[18] Here, unlike our bladder infection discussion in Chapter 19, recurrent means the same virus—either HSV-1 or HSV-2 is at work. The average interval between a first episode of infection and an initial recurrence is about 120 days. Subsequent recurrences occur more quickly, however, with an average interval between them of only 42 days.[19] Factors involved in bringing on a recurrent attack include emotional stress, menses, and sexual intercourse.[20] More than half of recurrences occur without a clear preceding cause, though.

One of the few silver linings in this condition is that symptoms of recurrent genital herpes are much milder than first-episode infections. Almost

Viral relatives

Genital herpes is in the same family of viruses as chickenpox, shingles, cold sores, and mononucleosis.

half of patients experience some preliminary warning symptoms lasting several hours to three days.[21] These vary from mild tingling to severe shooting pain. A small number of patients have constitutional symptoms such as headache and muscle aches, and these are mild. Blisters are not widespread and are on one side in most cases. The cervix is involved only 12 percent of the time. Blisters usually increase in size for the first three days, reach a steady state between four to eight days, then rapidly go away. Tender lymph nodes, painful urination, and vaginal discharge are all much less than was seen with the first outbreak. Complications are rare.

Getting a diagnosis

If a woman is seen when she has painful blisters on the vulva, the diagnosis of herpes can be made by inspection alone. A special herpes culture is taken for confirmation. But many women are seen *after* the blisters have progressed to ulcerations or are crusted over. No one can look at them and say exactly what they are. These lesions must be differentiated from other sexually transmitted diseases and diseases that cause ulcers on the vulva. In that case, a culture also must be taken, along with other cultures and blood tests to identify other sexually transmitted diseases that cause genital sores.

Herpes cultures are the gold standard for diagnosing genital herpes infection.[22] Without a positive culture it is hard to say with confidence that a person has herpes. But the culture if it is negative is not foolproof. Whether or not the virus grows in culture depends on the stage of the lesion when it is sampled. Virus can be isolated from about 94 percent of blisters, 87 percent of pustules, 70 percent of ulcers, and 27 percent of crusted areas.[23] This means that if a culture is done after a lesion has been around for several days, the virus might not grow.

When herpes is suspected and a culture is negative, a woman may have to come back for another office visit at the beginning of the next outbreak in order to receive confirmation.

As HSV cannot be reliably recovered even from new blisters, a blood test to diagnose persons with HSV-2 would be helpful. Unfortunately, many currently available commercial blood tests do not accurately distinguish between HSV-1 and HSV-2 infection.[24] Blood tests in the past have been the source of great distress; a negative test has been fine, as it means no exposure to herpes. But a positive test can range from someone who has a cold sore from time to time to one who has antibodies to genital herpes and is left wondering who, how, where. Accurate type-specific blood tests that would allow identification of subclinical HSV infection, confirmation of previous clinical diagnosis, or diagnosis of symptoms that are atypical of HSV have not existed in the past but are soon to be available.[25] If you have reasons for wanting to be tested for herpes, talk with your clinician about available blood tests and how specific they are. *Make sure you know exactly what the test will tell before you have it.*

Treating first infections

The antiviral drug acyclovir works. Usually it's given by mouth. For severe first infections, it can be given intravenously. Its effect on first-episode infections is impressive: Fever and general body symptoms are reduced within forty-eight hours of beginning treatment, and symptoms from the blisters also lessen. It shortens the course of herpes when taken. Treatment with acyclovir is recommended for all patients with clinical first-episode genital HSV infection who are seen with blisters. Treatment should be started in patients suspected of having primary genital herpes even before laboratory results are available, as the greatest benefit will be realized if treatment is started early.[26] The medication can be stopped if genital herpes is not the diagnosis.

But acyclovir does not change the pattern of any following recurrent disease. People treated with acyclovir for a first outbreak of genital herpes will still experience recurrent infections.

It has been standard to use 200 mg of acyclovir five times a day for ten days to treat herpes. Taking that many pills is a nuisance. A different schedule, 400 mg three times a day, appears to work just as well.[27] Higher doses of 800 mg five times a day do not offer any greater benefit, though.[28] New oral forms, valacyclovir (Valtrex) and famciclovir (Famvir), were introduced recently. These need to be given only twice a day, making them more con-

A HERPES SUCCESS STORY

Hilda has genital herpes and she's known it a long time. She got it from the only sexual encounter she had had, about three years before I met her. She told me that when she got the diagnosis, she was floored, to the point that she avoided going out with men for some time. But a really great guy came along, and when Hilda came for her annual exam she had been living with him for about a year—without telling him about the herpes. She considered it her deepest, darkest, most miserable secret. She couldn't bring herself to mention it, even though she had recently agreed to marry him. She took acyclovir to keep the virus as suppressed as possible and insisted on condoms.

We talked. We talked about the unbelievable burden she was carrying with her secret. We spoke of the risk that Freddy might find her acyclovir pills, or what might happen if Freddy developed herpes. We wondered how she'd continue to keep her secret from him during a pregnancy. And we discussed the risk of losing Freddy if she told him, and the capacity of people who care for each other to deal with dark and embarrassing information. It was her call. I was just the pros-and-cons person.

When a little flowering plant arrived for me about a week later, I figured things had gone well. The card said she'd blurted it all out the night after our talk. Freddy said he wished she'd told him sooner because he didn't like to think about all the suffering she had gone through.

I received an invitation to the wedding a few months later.

Mind healing

Dealing with the psychological aspects of this disease is as important as taking care of the physical symptoms. Many people with herpes find that talking to other people with the problem, especially in the setting of a support group, helps them feel less alone and makes it easier to cope with the disease. There are several good online groups, which offer support anonymously and in the privacy of your own home. See Resources.

venient to take. While these drugs are probably as safe and effective as acyclovir, further studies need to be done to establish their role.

Acyclovir in an ointment has been available and widely used, but the current makeup of the topical drug is just not as effective as any of the oral medications.[29] Using the topical version with the oral acyclovir provides no additional value, so it's not recommended for either a first episode or recurrent infection.[30]

Millions of Americans take the oral drugs without problems. Stomach upset and headache are the most frequent side effects. Less frequent are diarrhea, dizziness, lack of appetite, fatigue, swelling, skin rash, leg pain, swollen glands in the groin, and a mediciney taste in the mouth.

Special attention is needed for the treatment of the considerable discomforts of a first episode of herpes. Headache, body aches, and fever respond to Tylenol. Cool compresses or soaks in temperate water soothe the blisters. Exposing the sores to the air as much as possible is also valuable. Topical numbing agents, such as Xylocaine gel, may help as well. If urinating is painful, try pouring warm water over the vulva while urinating, or urinating while sitting in a tub of warm water.

Antibiotics are of no help since they cannot work against viruses. Your clinician will check for other STDs (since they often travel in packs), however, and may simultaneously treat them with antibiotics.

Treating recurrent infections

Oral acyclovir helps to reduce the length of recurrent attacks; healing time is improved by about two days and viral shedding is lessened by one day. The effect on pain and itching is less than the effect on shedding and healing, though.[31] Physicians often don't want to treat mild recurrent attacks because there is less effect on the blisters, but patients who have frequent recurrences, six or more a year, benefit from acyclovir if it is started at the earliest stage of a recurrent attack. The dose of acyclovir for recurrence is 400 mg two or three times a day or 200 mg three to five times a day.

If a woman is having outbreaks every month or more, long-term suppression with acyclovir (400 mg twice a day) eliminates the misery of skin blisters and fissures and cuts down on viral shedding that could pass the virus to a sexual partner. Unfortunately, suppression with acyclovir does not guarantee that a woman cannot pass the virus to a partner, but it does lessen the amount of shedding. Viral suppression makes a big difference in comfort. After a year of therapy, patients are encouraged to go off the drug for three to six months because the frequency and severity of recurrent genital herpes can vary over time. If the attacks are still frequent, suppressive therapy may be resumed. Individual plans of therapy often need to be worked out. Topical acyclovir is of no value in treating recurrent herpes.[32]

Recent studies show that the clinical benefit of treatment of recurrences may be greater than previously appreciated and should receive more attention.[33] Important note: Asymptomatic viral shedding (infecting others though you have no obvious symptoms) is not eliminated with suppressive acyclovir; the infection can still be passed on from persons receiving acyclovir suppressive treatment.[34]

Acyclovir's long-term safety has been demonstrated.[35] Famciclovir and valacyclovir have been proven safe to take for as long as one year and will probably be shown to have the safety record of acyclovir. So far only acyclovir has been shown to reduce viral shedding, although information about shedding with the newer agents should be available soon. Work to develop a vaccine against genital herpes has brought disappointing results to date, but other vaccines are currently undergoing clinical testing.[36]

One of my patients, Nancy, got herpes from her husband and started having frequent outbreaks. He was opposed to her taking acyclovir, saying that if she used it, there would be nothing available to treat her if she ever developed widespread life-threatening herpes. (His concerns were completely baseless; genital herpes does not progress in this fashion.) By the time she got to me she had vulvodynia, probably as a result of multiple outbreaks of herpes. (The two problems can go hand in hand, a scenario called postherpetic neuralgia.) Acyclovir and Elavil got her disease under control.

In contrast, Olivia hasn't told her partner that she has herpes, convinced he'd leave her if he knew. Nothing I say sways her. Finally, afraid he'd find her pills, she went off acyclovir. I worry about the relationship issues she has not dealt with.

A special case: herpes and pregnancy

One aspect of genital herpes merits special attention, especially by women of childbearing age: its impact on childbirth. HSV in newborns is, fortunately, quite rare. Various studies suggest a rate of transmission from mother to newborn that ranges from 1 in 3,000 live births to 1 in 20,000

V NOTE

Small but potent

Viruses are smaller than bacteria, too small to be seen with a regular microscope.

live births.[37] Nevertheless, it's of concern because the increasing numbers of herpes infection in adults during recent years appears to be mirrored in growing rates of newborn herpes infections.[38] Herpes in the newborn (neonatal herpes) can be a very severe disease. Typically, infection is confined to the skin, eyes, and/or mouth and can be successfully treated with acyclovir. But herpes can also cause inflammation of the brain (encephalitis) in a baby or can cause generalized infection in multiple organs. Of the babies having widespread infection, half will not survive even if treatment is given; survival following brain infection is almost always associated with brain damage.

To try to avoid transmission to the newborn, it's recommended that pregnant women with visible genital blisters or warning symptoms of herpes outbreaks at labor be delivered by cesarean section within four hours of rupture of the bag of waters. This practice has meant that numerous unnecessary c-sections are done simply because there is a history of herpes in a pregnant woman who has no symptoms. Yet c-section does not always prevent newborn herpes.[39] Why not? Because there are women with herpes who don't know they have it, so they don't get c-sections. And even in women with herpes who had c-sections, there are unfortunately a few cases of babies who got herpes anyway. Somehow the virus got across to the baby either by the bloodstream or up through the cervix. We don't know exactly how.

It's important to keep in perspective that the risk of giving the virus to the baby is really low (less than 2 percent) among women who are known to have herpes. Nor does a mother who gets a new case of herpes in the first or second trimester of pregnancy increase the chance of problems for her baby.[40] The highest rate of transmission of the virus from the mother to the baby appears to occur when the mother develops HSV-2 for the first time during *late* pregnancy. If this happens to you, ask for consultation with an expert in high-risk pregnancy or infectious diseases. Clinicians are starting to use acyclovir during pregnancy with some success.[41] As indicated, while cesarean delivery is thought to decrease the risk of herpes in the newborn, it does not eliminate it completely.

Recurrent episodes of genital herpes are very common in pregnant women who have an established herpes infection. Among women with a history of symptomatic recurrent genital herpes prior to pregnancy, 84 percent experienced a recurrence during pregnancy.[42] Recurrences with symptoms occur more frequently during pregnancy, tend to last longer, and produce more symptoms as pregnancy advances.[43] First-ever symptomatic recurrences in the latter half of pregnancy among HSV-2 antibody-positive women, on the other hand, may be hard to figure out—is this the first-ever infection (primary) or is this the first time there are symptoms of herpes that has been around a while (nonprimary)? In these unique situations, special testing may be needed to find out whether this is primary or recurrent disease, since, as we've said, primary infection has a much higher risk of transmission to the baby.

So if both primary and recurrent herpes are problems in pregnancy, what can be done? In a word, acyclovir.

Acyclovir has an effect only on cells infected with HSV. It works by acting as an incomplete building block in the assembly line of viral production, terminating the process. It is this unique activity of acyclovir that makes it effective against the virus and safe for all other cells. Traditionally, clinicians have been reluctant to give acyclovir in pregnancy because no one knew whether or not it is safe for the baby and because they worried that it would mask obvious herpes outbreaks

---

THE BOTTOM LINE IF YOU HAVE HERPES

Although it's your burden to learn to live comfortably and peaceably with the virus, this is entirely within your reach. Millions of people lead normal lives despite the virus. It's also your responsibility to avoid infecting others.

Some advice:

▼ Keep the information about your disease to yourself, if you like, with one big exception: *You must let your sexual partners know, since herpes is contagious.*

▼ Practice safe sex. Use condoms and/or abstain during outbreaks.

▼ For comfort's sake during outbreaks, try warm baths. But don't use the same towel on other parts of your body that you use on your genitals, to avoid the spread of infection. Wash the towel promptly so that no one else uses it. Talk to your clinician about other care measures.

▼ Wash your hands after using the toilet. Avoid rubbing your eyes.

▼ Maintain your overall health—it's especially important if you have herpes, to help fight infections.

▼ Be good to yourself. Shame, embarrassment, and remorse aren't productive. You're still the same person; you simply have an infection that you've got to learn how best to live with.

▼ Above all, don't let denial or fear of a partner's finding out lead you to quitting the treatment you need.

▼ Do talk to your clinician about your symptoms and suppressive antiviral therapy. It's of help in cutting down on shedding by up to 75 percent, although its ability to decrease transmission of the virus is unproven.

THE BOTTOM LINE IF YOU DON'T HAVE HERPES

Avoiding herpes first requires acknowledging that it exists; you simply can't stick your head in the sand like an ostrich. Ideally:

▼ Have only one partner and practice safe sex.

▼ Learn your partner's sexual history.

▼ Avoid sexual contact with persons who have active herpes sores. Of course, people with herpes can be shedding virus at any time, regardless of the presence of ulcers. *It's a myth that people cannot spread the virus if they're symptom-free.*

▼ Always use a condom; although condoms do not provide complete coverage, they are better than nothing. Female condoms may do a slightly better job against transmission. This is still being studied. Sexual partners who are in a monogamous relationship and who are both already infected with herpes do not need to take precautions.

▼ Share your knowledge about herpes with your friends and family, especially the fact that it can be acquired from someone who does not appear to have symptoms. The world needs to know about this challenging problem!

but not stop the asymptomatic shedding of virus, which could be passed on to the baby at delivery. Recent work, however, suggests that in the newborn, including premature babies, acyclovir is a safe and effective treatment, even at high doses.[44]

A recent study demonstrated that pregnant women whose first clinical episode of genital herpes occurred during pregnancy were helped by doses of acyclovir that prevented herpes outbreaks. These doses were given during the last month of pregnancy until delivery. The study patients had fewer recurrences of genital herpes at delivery as well as fewer cesareans for herpes than did those who got a placebo (i.e., just sugar pills).[45] These findings supported an earlier study from 1990.[46] In both studies, the treatment with acyclovir significantly decreased the number of herpes outbreaks without increasing the frequency of asymptomatic shedding. The study numbers were small but results were encouraging; more studies are needed.

In addition, on follow-up, there were no apparent ill effects in any of the newborns who had exposure to acyclovir before birth. In fact, information from an agency set up to collect information about the use of acyclovir in pregnancy (the Acyclovir in Pregnancy Registry) suggests no bad outcomes from acyclovir in more than six hundred babies who were exposed to the drug before birth, no matter how far along the pregnancy was.[47] In addition, we know that both full-term and preterm babies treated daily with intravenous acyclovir tolerate the drug well.[48]

If you have herpes and are pregnant or planning to be pregnant, you will want to talk with your physician about confirming the diagnosis of herpes, plans for delivery, and the possible use of acyclovir.

▼

CHAPTER 21

The Crafty Virus

HPV Causes Warts, Abnormal Paps, Cervical Cancer—and Nothing

Talk about the man with many faces! You might first hear about human papillomavirus (HPV) in connection with an abnormal Pap smear. It causes all cervical cancer and precancerous conditions detected by the Pap. Or you might be told you have HPV when you go into the clinician's office to find out about the bumps on your vulva, which turn out to be genital warts. Then again, you might have HPV and not even know it. The virus affects as many as six in ten sexually active women, though the majority have no symptoms at all; the virus simply hangs out in your otherwise healthy body doing nothing.[1]

Quite a range of effects, isn't it? Fortunately, more women are becoming aware of HPV as it gains a higher profile. The number of cases *with* symptoms has increased more than 500 percent in the last fifteen years, growing most rapidly among adolescents and young adults.[2] It's reaching epidemic proportions because this crafty virus is highly contagious. Frustratingly, there's no effective way to determine when a person with HPV is contagious. But HPV is not necessarily a disease of sexual promiscuity. It takes only one sexual contact with someone who may not even know that he or she is infected. On the positive side, if you become HPV-savvy ahead of time, you can head it off at the pass.

Should you turn out to be among the one million women diagnosed with HPV this year, you absolutely must realize that genital warts or an abnormal Pap indicating cervical precancer do not inevitably condemn you to cervical cancer. In fact, in the majority of women, HPV infection

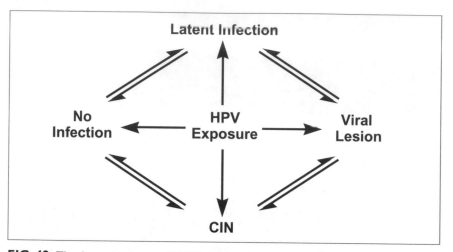

FIG. 49 The dynamic nature of HPV infection. There are more than one hundred types of HPV; nearly thirty different types affect the genital and anal areas.

Source: T. V. Sedlacek, Advances in the diagnosis and treatment of human papillomavirus infection, *Clin Obstet Gynecol* 1999; 42(2):206.

means that the virus is present silently in the skin and goes away on its own within three to six months.[3]

We haven't got an ideal cure yet, but treatment has come a long way. Also on the up side, clinicians now have a huge amount of experience detecting and treating all HPV-related problems when women come for regular care. (Reason 9,789 to make and keep a checkup appointment!)

The kinds of effects you experience depend on which of the more than one hundred HPV types you have.[4] The types are numbered in order from the first identified; thus, HPV type 1 was the first, type 16 was the sixteenth, and so on. Nearly thirty different HPV types infect the genital and anal areas. Some are very aggressive in causing quick and extensive warts. Only about a dozen are clearly associated with cancer. The majority are low-level, nonthreatening nuisances.

Warts from HPV

The wart *(condyloma acuminatum)* is the most common bump on the vulva. All warts in the body are caused by one strain or another of HPV. Like most viruses, this one infects only skin and mucous membranes such as the mouth and vagina.[5] Some strains cause warts on the hands or feet; others prefer the moist areas of the vulva, vagina, and cervix.

You can be perfectly healthy and get genital warts, though conditions that favor their development include diabetes and having a suppressed immune system from cancer, HIV, lupus, or pregnancy.[6] Age, chronic illness, sexual partners, smoking, alcohol, antibiotic use, steroids, and other STDs all can play a role.

Most women with HPV don't develop warts. Instead they have what's called latent infection—the virus is in the tissue but causes no symptoms. The way an HPV infection shows itself and the way a woman responds to treatment depend on how her immune system is working. Thus the virus can lie inactive in the skin for long periods, later causing symptoms as a result of an illness or other stress on the immune system. Sexual contact with a new partner who is carrying a different HPV type may lead to an outbreak of warts.[7] Latent disease can also disappear entirely with time. The HPV virus may be more readily passed on when warts are present, but it also can be transmitted by someone who not only shows no sign of HPV but may be entirely unaware that he or she carries the virus.[8]

While most HPV is passed on by sexual contact, it's also possible to contract warts in other *rare* ways.[9] They include transmission from mother to child (a baby passing through a vagina filled with warts may develop warts on the vocal cords, which show up months or years after birth) and transmission of nongenital warts to the genital area. Most of the time, as with herpes, you can't be sure how you got it. The amount of time it takes a wart to develop (its incubation period) varies, making the source of infection impossible to trace. Warts on the male can go unnoticed because they are so small, or a man can have a wart, pass the virus on to the woman, then have his wart clear up just as she discovers hers. Or, as mentioned, a person can have the virus silently in the skin and pass it on.

Unfortunately, condoms are of limited use in preventing HPV spread since the condom covers only the penis, while the exposed skin of the scrotum can harbor the virus. With new partners, condom use is associated with only a 35 percent reduction in transmission rates.[10] But 35 percent is better than nothing.

RISK FACTORS FOR HPV

Factors That Increase Risk of Getting HPV	By How Much
More than 5 sex partners in last 1–4 years	12 times
Age 20–29 years	5 times
Warts on partner	3 times
More than 5 sexual partners in lifetime	2.5 times
Intercourse more than 4 times weekly	2 times
Smoking	2 times

Source: T. V. Sedlacek, Advances in the diagnosis and treatment of human papillomavirus infection, *Clin Obstet Gynecol* 1999; 42(2):206.

And since clinicians can seldom say with any assurance when someone got the virus, or from whom, it's important to look at the risks for developing any HPV infection. (See box on page 381.)

Diagnosing warts

Warts appear a few days to weeks after exposure. They start as an irritation or itching, then progress to a red bump that becomes irregular and pebbly in appearance with pointed ends. Ancient Romans used the term *acuminate* (sharply pointed) to describe the fingerlike projections seen with new warts that are just starting to grow. Warts come in a variety of shapes, sizes, and appearances. Young warts are pale and have the classic "pointy" surface. Their coating of the uppermost skin surface (keratin) gives them a gray to white look. As they grow older, those that arise from skin that has pigment coloring to it tend to become darker, while those that come from mucosal surfaces appear purple because of the partially visible blood vessel supply. The shape also changes with age: The pointed surface of the young wart changes to a stalk (pedicle) or plump (polypoid) growth. Very old growths may flatten out and spread over wide areas.

Warts may be present on the vulva, in the vagina, or on the cervix. The most common site in the woman is the vulvar region (in 66 percent of cases), including the vaginal opening (introitus), labia majora, and labia minora. The next most common location is the vagina

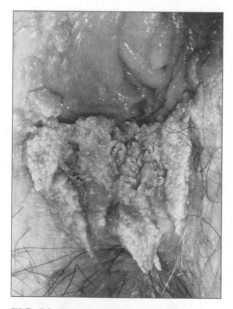

FIG. 50 The multiple young warts on this patient's perineum are characterized by their "pointy" appearance and irregular surface.

Courtesy of Raymond H. Kaufman, M.D.

(in 37 percent of cases). Warts may also commonly occur on the perineum (29 percent) and in the anal area (23 percent). Warts in more than one place are common; the vulva and the cervix are often involved together.

Sometimes the appearance of a wart is classic, making identification easy. But sometimes warts can be confused with other kinds of genital lesions. These may include such normal things as papillae (pillarlike structures) of the vestibule and sebaceous glands that sometimes appear after yeast infections, and other conditions that cause a similar appearance, such as molluscum, seborrheic keratosis, lichen planus, skin tags, and moles. (See Chapters 15 and 16 for more on nonwart skin conditions.) Your clinician may need to take a small sample of the tissue. Biopsy is also important to be sure that lesions are warts before starting chemical or surgical therapy to the vulva or the vagina. Papillae were once frequently mistaken for warts, leading to extensive but unnecessary treatment. Some of these treatments can cause ongoing vulvar pain or irritation.

> **NOTE**
>
> ### Harmful but not hurting
> Remember that no matter how extensive, warts or the wart virus in the skin do not cause vulvar pain (vulvodynia). Itching, yes. Slight irritation, yes. But most of the time, you feel next to nothing—and certainly nothing approaching real pain.

Women with vulvar warts have a 50-50 chance of having the virus in the cervix. When vulvar warts are found, the cervix needs to be checked too. Therefore, a Pap smear and examination of the vulva, vagina, and cervix with a bright light and magnification (colposcopy) are standard practice.

Compounding a woman's misery, vaginitis often accompanies warts. Since warts are usually sexually transmitted, other sexually transmitted diseases need to be checked for. The cause of the vaginitis must be diagnosed and treated. Until the warts are eliminated all sexual partners should wear condoms to prevent reinfection or transmission.

Treating warts

No 100 percent effective cure exists, for warts are difficult to treat and often return.[11] The virus, once in the skin, may be inactive for a time, then reappear. To help cope with the frustrating phenomenon of recurrence, consider the dandelion analogy. Everyone is familiar with the little yellow weeds that spring up in even the most closely tended lawns. When they bloom, we attack them with chemical poisons, root cutters, and flame throwers. Yet

TREATMENTS THAT DESTROY OR REMOVE WARTS

Name	Mechanism of Action	Application Frequency	Clearance Rate	Major Advantages	Drawbacks	Other Comments
Podophyllin resin	Toxic to viral cell by inhibiting mechanism of division (mitosis)	1–2 times per week for 4 weeks	32–79%	Inexpensive, minimally painful.	Skin reactions have been seen; failure common. Not for pregnancy. Small potential for systemic toxicity.	Clinician applied. Contains ingredients that with sustained use have been linked with cancer. Cannot be used in pregnancy.
Podofilox	Same	2 times per day, 3 days per week, for 2–4 weeks	44–88% with liquid; 37–68% with gel	Low toxicity, minimal irritation.	Patient has to be able to see warts to apply it. Not for use in pregnancy.	Patient applied. Active element of podophyllin but not linked with cancer. Not for use in pregnancy. Expensive.
Trichloroacetic acid/ bichloroacetic acid	Chemical destruction	1–2 times per week for 4–8 weeks	70–81%	Inexpensive, low toxicity. Can be used in pregnancy.	Depth of penetration difficult to control, can ulcerate. Can be painful.	Clinician applied.
Tissue-destructive therapies	Physical removal or destruction	Usually one treatment, but possibly more	Removal in one session, but recurrence rates are as high as 50%	Except for cryotherapy treatment, complete in one session. Safe in pregnancy.	Expensive; requires long office visit or trip to the OR. Requires special training for provider. Prolonged healing time (weeks).	Includes local surgical excision, cryotherapy (freezing), laser, electrosurgery, infrared coagulator (IRC). Laser or surgery is generally used for extensive warts.

TREATMENTS THAT DESTROY OR REMOVE WARTS

Name	Mechanism of Action	Application Frequency	Clearance Rate	Major Advantages	Drawbacks	Other Comments
Interferon	Works through the immune system (antiviral effects, exact mechanism not understood)	5 IU (international units) three times per week for 3 weeks, injected into warts or intramuscularly	19–62%		Flulike symptoms. Possible depression. Expense. Possible liver or white blood cell changes. Injections. Impractical for extensive warts.	Very expensive.
Imiquimod (Aldara)	Works through the immune system (stimulates production of tissue chemicals [cytokines] with antiviral effects)	3 times per week for 16 weeks	33–72%	Patient applied.	Mild to severe skin reactions.	Expensive.

Sources: Condylomata International Collaborative Study Group, A comparison of interferon alfa-2a and podophyllin in the treatment of primary condylomata acuminata, Genitourin Med 1991:67:394; K. M. Stone et al., Human papillomavirus infection and genital warts: update on epidemiology and treatment, Clin Infect Dis 1995:20(1)suppl.:S91; A. Ferenczy, Epidemiology and clinical pathophysiology of condylomata accumirata, Am J Obstet Gynecol 1995:172:1331; Mortality and Morbidity Weekly Report 1993:42(RR-14):83.

we're not surprised to find new weeds springing up again within a few weeks of such treatments. The seeds are presumed to be underground where they can't be seen until they sprout. Only then does direct treatment become possible. It's just the same with warts.[12]

Warts can be destroyed or removed. Clearance rates range from 30 percent to 90 percent with the best results from therapies that physically destroy the warts such as laser, cryotherapy (freezing), and excision. But these too have recurrence rates. (See box on pages 384–85.)

If the wart doesn't go away after treatment, it may not be a wart. If you didn't have a biopsy before treatment, doing so would be a wise precaution.

All of these treatments need to be tailored to your individual needs. For a few warts, topical chemicals administered in the office or at home can be tried. Combining topical treatment with freezing is often successful. Extensive warts need surgery or laser. The combination of laser or surgery plus interferon looks promising for treatment of warts that have not responded to other methods.

A once-popular cream called Efudex (5-FU) to destroy warts has fallen into limited disuse for good reasons. This highly caustic cream can be terribly painful on application and even cause bad scarring in the vagina with repeated use. Vulvovaginal experts believe that with extensive use, it may produce vulvodynia. Some clinicians do use it for vaginal warts if they feel they can clear the lesions with a limited number of applications.

HPV and Pap smears

Now that you know all about HPV and warts, you need to know about HPV and cervical cancer. There's certainly good news: Cancer of the cervix

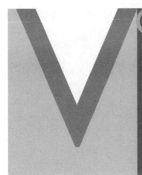

OICES

"I haven't had a Pap test in years. When I was having my children, of course, I saw my ob-gyn a lot. But after my kids were born, who has the time? Besides, I have felt healthy. But when I learned that the kind of cancer that the Pap test screens for is so slow-growing, I got to thinking that maybe I shouldn't be so cavalier. Better safe than sorry, as they say."

—Maria, 62

is on the decline in the United States. But there's also bad news: Precancerous conditions of the cervix, which can be distant early-warning signs of these cancers, are being found in increasing numbers of women.

Luckily, these early phases can be detected through testing, even though they give no symptoms. That's why we gyns are always harping about the importance of regular Pap smears—the best test we have to screen for cervical cancer—and regular pelvic exams.

Important recap: You can find a full discussion about Pap smears in Chapter 9. There I talk about how Paps are declared to be either normal or abnormal, and how the situation is further evaluated when the finding is abnormal. Some abnormal Paps indicate a low-grade or a high-grade type of cervical precancer (called cervical intraepithelial neoplasia, or CIN), caused by HPV. This chapter will describe how those conditions are treated.

Before you panic at the very word *cancer,* it's very important to understand the difference between cancer and precancer. Actually, the correct term for any new growth or mass of cells in the body is *neoplasm.* A

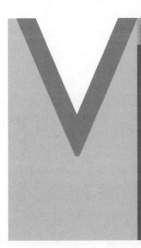

NOTE

Woman to woman

Women who have sex with women are not necessarily "low risk" for acquisition of HPV and should receive Pap smear screening according to current guidelines. Genital HPV has been detected on the fingertips of subjects, so the virus could be introduced with digital-vaginal contact between partners. Most women who have sex with women have had sex with men, and many continue to have sex with men.

Source: J. M. Marrazzo, K. Stine, L. A. Koutsky, Genital human papillomavirus infection in women who have sex with women: a review, *Am J Obstet Gynecol* 2000:183(3):770.

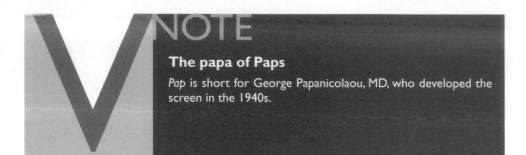

malignant neoplasm means a new mass of tissue that grows beyond and out of coordination with the normal tissues around it. The neoplasm continues to grow excessively even after the end of whatever stimulus started it growing in the first place. (We usually don't know what that stimulus is.) We're talking about renegade cells that do not behave in the orderly fashion of the organ in which they originated; they don't have the same controls, they don't follow the rules. Eventually these wild cells take over enough of the organ to choke out the normally functioning cells, with disastrous results.

Cancer is the common term for all malignant neoplasms, that is, the wild growths whose uncontrolled expansion without regard to normal functions gives them the potential to kill.

Cervical cancer almost never strikes out of the blue in women who have regular checkups. Half of cervical cancer occurs in women who don't have regular Pap smears. There is a lengthy warning period. Treatable precancerous stages produce a variety of changes in the tissues usually extending over many years before the actual cancer develops. Cancers have precursor cells, confined to the top layer of tissue. These precursor cells—*intraepithelial neoplasia* (say "IN-tra-epi-THEEL-ial nee-o-PLAY-see-ah)—are abnormal, but they have not yet broken away from the top layer in disorderly growth. When in the cervix, these cells are called *cervical intraepithelial neoplasia* (CIN). Another general term you might hear is *dysplasia*.

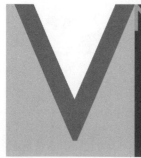

NEW HPV TESTING

Remember, the Pap test only screens for cells that don't look right, inviting further testing to verify cervical cancer or precancer (CIN). A promising new test screens specifically for HPV, the virus that causes cervical cancer and CIN. Doctors are still debating how HPV testing should best be used. Some clinicians advocate routine HPV testing along with the Pap test. Others—including me, at least until the test's accuracy improves—feel that HPV testing is best used to help evaluate abnormal Pap smears. The idea is that if your Pap is suspicious but your HPV test is negative for high-risk HPV, then you can be reassured that you have a low-risk virus that will probably go away on its own. If your HPV test is positive, then you can be monitored every four months for signs of problems.

The test works by looking for the DNA of the HPV virus in cervical cells obtained through a ThinPrep Pap test. (Chapter 9 discusses ThinPrep, which is basically a different way of collecting the sample.) Two different HPV tests are available. One is the FDA-approved Virapap. The other test is called polymer chain reaction (PCR).

As with the Pap, there are accuracy problems. The Virapap has a significant false-negative rate, meaning that the test can be negative when HPV is really in the sample. There are similar problems with the PCR test. One of the high-risk HPV types, type 16, can be present in women who have no evident disease. But women with a normal Pap smear and a test positive for high-risk HPV type could be tested more often to determine whether they eliminate the virus or go on to develop an abnormal Pap smear.

In 1999, a huge study of more than 46,000 women, 973 of whom had suspicious Paps, led the researchers to conclude that HPV-based testing would provide equally sensitive detection of high-grade dysplasia (HSIL), fewer colposcopy exams, and fewer follow-up visits than current practices. Furthermore, the savings from decreased visits and procedures offset the added costs of the ThinPrep method for all routine screening. Other experts emphasize the value of a negative HPV test in relieving patient anxiety and physician apprehension in the presence of an abnormal Pap. On the other hand, it's also been argued that most women who test positive for HPV don't have serious disease, and their positive HPV test can lead to more anxiety than a positive Pap test.

Meanwhile, HPV testing continues to improve in accuracy. A recent report shows that HPV testing is as sensitive as the Pap test for detecting HSIL. The tests are currently available for women who wish to pay for it. If you fall into a high-risk group, talk with your physician about the pros and cons of HPV testing for your particular situation.

Sources: C. J. L. M. Meijer, L. Rozendaal, J. C. van der Linden, et al., Human papillomavirus testing for primary cervical cancer screening, in *New Developments in Cervical Cancer Screening and Prevention,* E. Franco, J. Monsenego, eds. (Oxford: Blackwell Science, 1997), 338; J. T. Cox, A. T. Lorincz, M. H. Schiffman, et al., Human papillomavirus testing by hybrid capture appears to be useful in triaging women with cytologic diagnosis of atypical squamous cells of undetermined significance, *Am J Obstet Gynecol* 1995:172:946; C. P. Crum, P. T. Taylor, Intraepithelial squamous lesions of the cervix, in *Gynecologic Oncology,* R. C. Knapp, R. S. Berkowitz, eds. (New York: McGraw-Hill, 1993), 179; C. Bergeron, D. Jeannel, J. D. Poveda, et al., Human papillomavirus testing in women with mild cytologic atypia, *Obstet Gynecol* 2000:95:821; M. M. Manos, W. K. Kinney, L. B. Hurley, Identifying women with cervical neoplasia: using human papillomavirus DNA testing for equivocal Papanicolaou results, *JAMA* 1999:281(17):1605; B. A. Krumholz, Value of human papillomavirus testing [letter], *Am J Obstet Gynecol* 2000:182(2):479; R. H. Kaufman, E. Adam, Value of human papillomavirus testing [reply to letter], *Am J Obstet Gynecol* 2000:182(2):479; T. C. Wright, L. Denny, A. Pollack, A. Lorincz, HPV DNA testing of self-collected vaginal samples compared with cytologic screening to detect cervical cancer, *JAMA* 2000:283:81; L. Denny, L. Kuhn, A. Pollack, et al., Evaluation of alternative methods of cervical cancer screening for resource-poor settings, *Cancer* 2000:89:826.

HPV and cervical precancer (CIN)

Remember that the cervix—the mouth of the womb, located at the top of the vagina—is entirely different from the more familiar rest of the uterus—so different, in fact, that clinicians consider the cervix a separate organ. In order to understand how CIN exists and is evaluated, you need to understand how the cervix is constructed. The top layer, where CIN develops, is the epithelium. The cells here come in two forms, rugged *squamous epithelium,* which covers the outside surface of the cervix, and more delicate mucus-producing cells that line the cervical canal, *columnar epithelium.* The point at which the two meet is called the *squamocolumnar junction* (SCJ).

The SCJ is a very important meeting point. The canal cells in this area are constantly changing into surface cells in response to estrogen levels. Because of their constantly changing state, the cells are susceptible to the invasion of HPV. It is at the SCJ that precancer and cancer most frequently develop.

Unlike a fixed landmark where a couple might arrange to rendezvous for date after date, however, the SCJ keeps moving around. Its location varies according to a woman's age and estrogen status. In young adults, there is a moderate amount of estrogen around, and the canal cells meet the surface cells right on the surface of the cervix just outside the opening. During pregnancy and right after childbirth, large amounts of estrogen stimulate many of the canal cells to grow out of the canal onto the surface and get changed into surface cells. The SCJ enlarges and is found located farther away from the canal opening, out on the cervix. After menopause, and without estrogen, the cells of the canal retreat up through the opening, making the junction high up in the canal (in a woman who is not taking estrogen).

When HPV attacks these highly vulnerable cells in the SCJ, it deactivates some proteins that control cell division. Cells reproduce rapidly without regulation. This is the beginning of CIN.

To help you visualize all this, take a pear and look at the end with the stem coming out. You can imagine the pear as the

---

YOU'RE MORE LIKELY TO DEVELOP CIN IF . . .

▼ You have multiple sex partners

▼ You became sexually active at a young age

▼ You've been exposed to a "high-risk man"; that is, a man with a history of promiscuous sexual activity and/or sexual exposure to a partner who develops genital neoplasia

▼ You smoke (nicotine from tobacco probably promotes the growth of the virus)

Source: M. J. Arends, C. H. Buckley, M. Wells, Aetiology, pathogenesis, and pathology of cervical neoplasia. *J Clin Pathol* 1998:51:96–103.

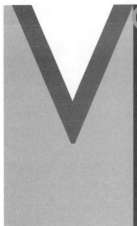

uterus. The neck of the pear with the stem is like the cervix. Now look at the surface of the pear just around the stem. The pear skin there is like the rugged surface covering of the cervix. Pull the stem off (your cervix doesn't have a stem!). The hole left represents the cervical canal that you can imagine goes on up into the body of the pear (a pear has no open cavity inside, like a balloon would, but your uterus does). The place where the pear skin meets the stem hole is like the SCJ. You can easily see it.

Now take the cardboard cylinder from a toilet paper roll. Put the stem end of the pear at one end. The cardboard cylinder represents the vagina. If you look at the stem end of the pear through the other end of the cardboard cylinder "vagina," you've got the view of the cervix that a clinician sees through the speculum or colposcope. You can see all of the surface and the canal opening. While you're at it, notice that there's no place for anything to get lost up there.

HPV is not like the herpes virus, which stays in the body for life. To date it appears that HPV infections do not persist over a lifetime.[13] Most women have no apparent clinical evidence of disease and show no symptoms, and the infection eventually goes away without treatment.[14] In other situations, the women do have signs of disease; low-grade CIN is diagnosed and eventually goes away on its own. Only a minority of women exposed to HPV develop CIN that persists.[15]

This bears repeating: *Most early CIN will go away on its own without treatment.*[16] The term *CIN* means only that it *may* progress to cervical cancer. CIN and dysplasia both mean the same thing: that there are cells with abnormal maturation in the cervix with potential to progress to cancer *or* potential to go away spontaneously. The Pap smear is designed to find these abnormal cells.

There are three different grades of CIN. If the abnormal cells are present only in the outer one-third of the epithelium, the lesion is called CIN 1

Wendy was a junior at a small college when a routine exam at the student health service turned up an abnormal Pap. With colposcopy, the doctor found an area on her cervix that he said might be precancerous. He told her it was the result of a sexually transmitted virus. Wendy just heard the word *cancerous* and was petrified. She'd had intercourse with only one partner in her life, and now she had cancer!

She had a meltdown on the phone with her parents, who flew into town to see her. They got her Pap smear and biopsy slides and arranged for me to see her. It looked like moderate dysplasia, which is something to treat, but certainly not a reason to put your affairs in order. I sat down and explained the facts of HPV and precancer to Wendy. She had a LEEP (an excision procedure described under "Treating CIN"), done with a local anesthetic in my office. The tissue taken indeed showed moderate dysplasia, and the problem spot was completely removed. Wendy went back to college and finished with a 4.0 average and a normal Pap.

(mild). If the cells reach to the middle third, the lesion is CIN 2 (moderate), and if the cells involve the entire thickness of the cervical epithelial layer, the lesion is CIN 3 (severe), also referred to as carcinoma in situ. Once the cells grow through the membrane that separates the top layer from the underlying layers, invasive cancer has occurred.

If you have CIN of any grade, what is the chance that it will progress to cancer? Of course there's no one answer, but overall, the progression to invasive cancer is quite slow. It can take many months or years to occur, and odds are good that it might not happen at all.[17] We know this from recent studies of mild and moderate cervical dysplasia, where researchers used Pap smears and biopsies to follow women over a twenty-year period.[18] A return to normal from *mild* dysplasia occurred in 62 percent of the cases. That's almost two-thirds, which is good news. Progression to more severe dysplasia occurred in 16 percent, and the remaining 22 percent had mild dysplasia that just held steady. In the cases of *moderate* dysplasia in the study, regression occurred in over half the cases over six years. Just under a third progressed to severe dysplasia, and 16 percent had persistent disease. The risk of high-grade CIN progressing to cancer seems to be higher, though it too can go away on its own.[19]

Treating CIN

Treatment is designed to destroy the abnormal cells in a given area, allowing healthy new cells to grow in. There are several ways of doing this, including surgically cutting the area out, freezing (cryosurgery), laser treatment, and cutting it out with an electrically wired loop. This last method has another one of those names that sound complicated, but all those syllables are just defining what it is: loop electrosurgical excision procedure (LEEP).

Freezing, laser, and LEEP are all about the same in terms of success rate (about 90 percent) and few complications.[20] Just remember what I said about HPV being a "crafty virus" that can come back. There's a 10 percent chance the precancerous conditions will return with any of these treatments, severe dysplasia being more likely to come back than mild or moderate dysplasia.[21] Whatever you have, you need to keep having a Pap every few months until you have at least four normal ones in a row.

Remember that the treatment of CIN doesn't end with a single procedure. Since CIN has a 10 percent recurrence, follow-up is essential for years to come.

There are some ground rules that clinicians are expected to follow before destroying any cervical abnormality:

▼ The Pap, colposcopy, and biopsy must all agree that there is no evidence of cancer.

▼ The abnormal area is on the outer cervix, and all of it can be seen.

▼ There is no disease in the cervical canal, as confirmed by colposcopy and scrapings taken from the canal.

CRYOTHERAPY

Freezing by cryotherapy destroys the top layer of the cervix with the dysplasia in it by turning water inside the cells into ice crystals, destroying the cell. Nitrous oxide or carbon dioxide is used to cool a two-inch metal circle to 20 to 30 degrees below freezing. This cold metal probe is placed against the cervix until the clinician can see ice crystals form a short distance around the probe circle.

Freezing has been used a long time, so it's safe and has few problems associated with it. It's readily available in most doctors' offices. The patient is first given some ibuprofen to relieve the moderate cramping that occurs. The thing women dislike the most is that freezing causes lots of watery discharge that goes on for two to four weeks after the procedure. Cryotherapy can change the appearance of the cervix, so future evaluations may be a little harder for your clinician.

Cryotherapy is effective, but its cure rate depends on the abnormality (it provides a better chance of a cure with CIN 1 than with CIN 3), as well as the size of the abnormal area.[22]

LASER

The laser machine makes a beam of light that can be aimed at abnormal tissue to zap it—transform it into air and make it disappear. The clinician can control how deep and how wide the zap goes by looking through the colposcope. Neighboring healthy tissue is therefore not injured. The tissue repairs itself within ten days.[23]

Laser is particularly helpful for large patches of dysplasia that a freezing probe cannot cover. These include an irregular cervix that a flat freezing probe doesn't fit well, dysplasia that has extended off the cervix to the vagina, and disease shown on biopsy to go deep into the cervical glands.[24]

Besides destroying abnormal tissue, the laser can be used for fine-tuned excision, so that a specimen of tissue can be cut out for examination in the laboratory. Laser excision may be used for a cone excision (see below) when the lesion extends up the canal out of view. Laser cone excision can be combined with ablation for an abnormality that is on the surface of the cervix and also extends up the canal.

Laser has few complications. When performed under local anesthesia, there is little pain. Bleeding is usually minimal.[25] Unfortunately, laser is not available everywhere.

LOOP ELECTROSURGICAL EXCISION PROCEDURE (LEEP)

LEEP can be used for both diagnosis and treatment during one visit.[26] A loop of wire is used with electrical current to remove from the cervix a circle of tissue containing the abnormality. The shallow crater left after the

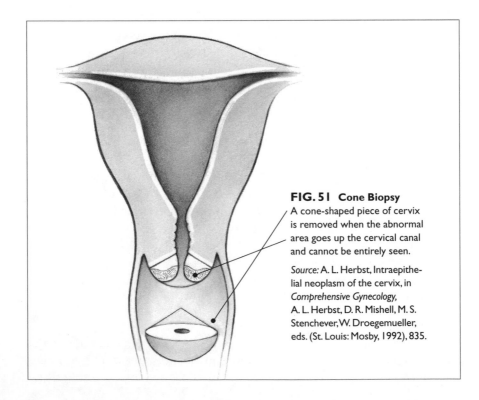

FIG. 51 Cone Biopsy
A cone-shaped piece of cervix is removed when the abnormal area goes up the cervical canal and cannot be entirely seen.

Source: A. L. Herbst, Intraepithelial neoplasm of the cervix, in *Comprehensive Gynecology,* A. L. Herbst, D. R. Mishell, M. S. Stenchever, W. Droegemueller, eds. (St. Louis: Mosby, 1992), 835.

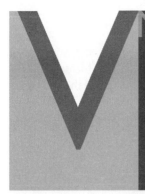

Fine-tuning

Right now few women are tested to see which of the hundred-plus HPV types they have. Most, remember, aren't harmful. But doctors have learned that cervical cancers caused by type 18 have double the mortality rate of cancers caused by other strains. This kind of pinpointing could lead to vaccines or other treatments based on the specific strain that seems to be involved in a particular woman's case.

excision is then cauterized to prevent bleeding. The procedure is performed in the office under local anesthesia and has a low rate of complications.[27] Recurrence following LEEP is low, ranging from 2 to 4 percent, making it a safe and effective procedure.[28] Clinicians also like the procedure because it gives a specimen for examination in the lab. (We always like to know we got it all.)

CONIZATION

Conization of the cervix involves taking a cone-shaped piece of tissue from the cervix for both diagnosis and treatment. Conization used to be the standard method of evaluating an abnormal Pap smear, but now its use is reserved for diagnosis in women who have HSIL with a lesion that cannot be entirely seen with colposcopy, or in whom the SCJ cannot be seen on colposcopy. Usually these areas cannot be viewed because they are high up in the cervical canal. Conization is also done if scrapings from the canal show CIN 2 or CIN 3, or if a high-grade lesion on the Pap cannot be confirmed with biopsy. The figure on preceding page shows what a cone biopsy looks like.

Conization was originally done in the operating room using a

THE LAST WORD: BE HPV-SAVVY

As we've seen, HPV can cause a lot of grief. It can cause you to break out in warts. It can make your Pap abnormal, requiring years of monitoring, Pap smears, colposcopies, biopsies, and LEEPs. It could even lead to cervical cancer. Most of the time it will go away completely, but you can't know in advance how it will turn out for you. Best advice? Keep it away!

▼ Practice sexual smarts. Save sex. Wait for Mr. or Ms. Right. Find out a sexual history. Use a condom (it's all we have).

▼ Strengthen your immune system to do battle with the virus. Stop smoking. Eat a well-balanced diet. Get some exercise. Learn how to practice stress management.

▼ Monitor for the presence of the virus with a vulvar self-exam for bumps, and have a regular Pap smear.

▼ If your Pap has ever been abnormal, listen to your physician's advice and have regular follow-up.

surgical scalpel to cut out a cone-shaped piece of cervix. Risks included bleeding during or after the procedure, or secondary hemorrhage occurring five to fourteen days after the procedure. There was also the risk that the cervix would be altered enough to become "incompetent" to hold a pregnancy, leading to miscarriage or premature delivery. This risk is related to the size of the cone specimen.[29]

Then cone excisions started to be done with the laser, and now by LEEP, making it possible to do the procedure in most cases on an outpatient basis.

HYSTERECTOMY

For many years the most severe form of CIN was treated very aggressively with hysterectomy, though this is no longer the case. Some women with HSIL may be candidates for hysterectomy, however, especially if childbearing is completed, the problem is recurrent, or they have lesions that cannot be treated adequately with local therapy.

▼

CHAPTER 22

V Cancer and Precancer

Reassuring Facts About Uncommon Conditions

Before you panic about the words *vulvar* and *cancer* appearing together, please let me assure you that this kind of cancer is rare. In twelve years of V specialization, I have seen only two cases. Vaginal cancer is even rarer. Meriting more concern are precancerous conditions of the vulva. These are on the rise thanks to the HPV virus, described in Chapter 21. (Actual vulvar cancer, though, is not increasing.) Not that V precancers are cause for excessive alarm either. As is true of changes in the cervix found during a Pap smear, precancerous changes in the Vs are distant early-warning signs; they do not signal that cancer is inevitable. With the right care, vulvar precancer can be dealt with safely, effectively, and almost always completely. What's more, these treatments are simpler than ever before.

Chalk up the possibility of V precancer as yet another reason for annual exams. Often a clinician notices something suspect on a routine exam, or on the follow-up of another gyn problem, before you experience a single symptom. Of course, you should also report itching or other problems as they arise; in the unlikely event that it's cancer-related, early intervention is key. If you notice a bump, point it out. It's probably not a V precancer, but you'll have peace of mind (and proper treatment for whatever it is).

Vulvar precancer (VIN)

Usually long before cells in the vulvar skin go on the warpath toward cancer, they send up smoke signals. The cells grow in number and make a little raised or slightly discolored place on the skin; under the microscope, these cells look different from normal cells. Doctors call them atypical cells. We've already talked about a similar situation in the cervix. The condition in the vulva is known as *vulvar intraepithelial neoplasia* (VIN) or dysplasia. (Say "IN-tra-EP-ee-THEEL-EE-al NEE-oh-PLAY-zee-ah"). Its long name, just as we discussed with the cervix, describes the situation exactly: *Vulvar* tells you where it is (not in the vagina, not on the cervix), *intra* means within (not on top or under), *epithelial* refers to the top layer of skin, *neo* means new, and *plasia* is growth. So we have a tiny little patch of vulva with new growth of cells that shouldn't be there in the top layer of skin. Another word for this precancerous change in the tissue is dysplasia.

VIN is divided into categories based on the extent of the problem.

▼ *VIN 1 (mild dysplasia):* abnormal cells are in about one-third of the top layer of the skin (epithelium) of the affected area

▼ *VIN 2 (moderate dysplasia):* the atypical cells involve about two-thirds of the top layer

▼ *VIN 3 (severe dysplasia/carcinoma in situ):* the abnormal cells have replaced more than two-thirds of the top layer of skin in the affected area

If the abnormal cells grow out of the top layer and enter neighboring tissue underneath, the precancer becomes cancer (carcinoma).

Younger VIN, older VIN

Curiously, VIN is seen in two completely different groups of women: one mostly young and one almost always older. The younger group (average age 35) have VIN caused by the HPV virus. They have little wartlike areas containing the virus; half have it in more than one place on the vulva.[1] These women often have had genital warts caused by the virus too. Smokers are most vulnerable.[2]

The previous chapter explained how there are different types of HPV. VIN caused by a low-risk type of HPV may just go away, especially if it's mild (VIN 1).[3] VIN 2 can also go away.[4] But, just as you might expect, VIN 3, especially when caused by a high-risk type of HPV, is less likely to disappear on its own and has an increased risk of moving on to cancer.[5] To add to the challenge, both low-risk and high-risk forms of the crafty virus can be found in the same area on the vulva.[6] And VIN 1, 2, and 3 can be found together on the vulva. The virus can be in any place where sexual activity occurs. About a third of patients (30 percent) with VIN also have a problem in the cervix (CIN). One-fifth (20 percent) are affected in the anal area (because a substantial number of sexually active women have anal intercourse). A few (4 percent) also have vaginal precancer (VAIN; see page 407), and a very few will have the condition everywhere.[7]

An entirely separate group of VIN sufferers are women mainly over 50, who have a single little patch of precancerous cells that does not contain the HPV virus.[8] Clinicians don't know what causes this kind of VIN but suspect that it's related to chronic irritation. Fortunately, it progresses from the VIN 3 level to cancer in just 2 to 4 percent of cases.[9] That certainly doesn't mean that this VIN can be ignored, but it's good to know that it's not a wildly aggressive condition. *The fact that vulvar precancer can be found in women over 50 makes it essential for you to realize that regular gyn exams are as important as ever after menopause!*

Diagnosing VIN

How does your doctor know if you have VIN, which kind it is, and what level it's at? There's no one symptom, not even necessarily a telltale lump, such as often alerts one to breast cancer. Women sometimes complain of vulvar itching, maybe some discomfort with sexual intercourse, possibly some bleeding or pain. Others have no symptoms until they find a small bump that may be anywhere on the vulva.[10] As mentioned above, younger women tend to have several areas of abnormal tissue, whereas women over 50 tend to have just one spot. Sometimes the VIN is discovered on a routine examination or during a follow-up exam for an abnormal Pap.

When a clinician looks at the vulva, he or she can see flat or raised areas with color changes ranging from white to red to dark shades of brown. Taking a small sample of tissue (a biopsy) is necessary to find out what these bumps are. Sometimes it's necessary to take several if there are a number of different places with skin changes.

If the biopsy samples are normal, it isn't VIN. As I describe in Chapter 16, dozens of different conditions appear as bumps on the vulva, since it's made of skin. VIN is most frequently confused with warts. If a woman has warts that are not clearing in a reasonable amount of time with usual treatment, I take a biopsy before I keep going with another wart treatment.

If a biopsy shows VIN, though, a second step is needed to learn the extent of the problem. HPV loves the skin and mucous membranes of the entire genital area. Your clinician needs to look at all the places HPV can hang out to see if there is anything else going on. Follow-up tests therefore include a Pap smear and a colposcopy (if it hasn't already been done) of the cervix, vulvar, and anal areas. The tissue is washed with vinegar (acetic acid) and the colposcope, with its bright light and magnifying glass, is used to check all these areas for different-looking tissue that suggests an HPV hangout. Again, several tiny skin samples may be necessary in order to obtain a complete picture of what is going on.

A good lab and an experienced, board-certified pathologist are important for an accurate diagnosis. You can ask your clinician about the quality of the lab he or she uses. You can arrange to have your biopsy slides sent to a major teaching hospital's lab for a second opinion. This would be important if you have VIN in several places over the vulvar skin and you've been told you need extensive treatment of all these areas.

You can see how important it is to have itching evaluated. Here's another example of the fact that everything that itches is not a yeast infection. Nor, of course, is everything that itches vulvar precancer or cancer. If you have vulvar itching, go to the clinician, have an exam, and do as he or she suggests for a short period of time (up to twelve weeks). If what has been prescribed isn't working week after week, see if your doctor thinks a vulvar colposcopy—more accurately, a vulvoscopy—is something you should have.

NOTE

Why no VSE?

While regular breast self-exam (BSE) has become a standard component of women's health, vulvar self-exam needs to catch on. You probably won't find cancer, but you might find something else that needs attention. Become familiar with what your healthy vulva looks like and be alert to any possible changes, such as bumps or raised areas, color changes, or rashes (whether or not you feel other symptoms). Then you can point out any change to your doctor. So next time you do BSE, make a quick detour farther south as well. Tell your mother and grandmother that they need to do it too!

TREATING VIN

Whenever you have a problem such as VIN, which has the potential to be anything from no big deal to a very big deal, you need to make sure that you have the right diagnosis and know exactly what the extent of the problem is. And then you pursue the most minimal, yet most effective, treatment appropriate.

The first question you want to ask is "Is treatment necessary?" It's now widely accepted that VIN 1 represents a mild HPV-induced change in the skin and will often go away on its own. Watching carefully may be all that's needed. That means vulvoscopy and possibly biopsy in another three to six months to make sure the mild VIN is not progressing to a more advanced stage. If the decision is made to watch, it's absolutely essential that these tests be done.

Most other precancerous changes, VIN 2 or VIN 3, are usually removed surgically. In the past, removing large portions of the vulva (vulvectomy) was used to treat VIN 3. Today this extensive surgery has been replaced by two highly precise techniques designed to clear up the VIN without removing neighboring normal vulvar tissue: laser surgery and wide local excision (the removal of the patch of VIN along with a little extra tissue around it as a safety zone). Both methods seem equally effective, though laser is probably the most popular method today.[11] The laser beam can be used like a knife with great precision. Laser therapy is not successful for treatment of VIN in areas of the vulva where hair grows, however, since the precancerous cells can go down the hair shaft and hide.

Successful laser surgery depends on a clinician who has advanced laser skills and access to a high-powered, pulsed carbon dioxide laser. (For use of the laser machine, there is basic and advanced training. Basic equips the clinician to deal with superficial problems such as warts. Advanced training is required for VIN; it gives the physician a detailed knowledge of landmarks and tissue layers of the vulvar skin so that he or she lasers to sufficient depth to get rid of the VIN, which is more deeply seated than a wart.) Laser treatment that goes too deep can destroy oil, sweat, and mucus glands. Such destruction leads to dryness and painful intercourse. Do not accept laser treatment of VIN from anyone without advanced laser training and experience with VIN treatment.

For VIN that goes down deep into tissue (as determined by the pathology report on the biopsies) or that extensively involves the hair-bearing areas of the vulva, excision may be preferred. There are also many towns where a laser is not available and excision of the VIN is regularly done.

Newer techniques include the loop electrosurgical excision procedure (LEEP), another way of surgically removing a single area of abnormal tissue (described in Chapter 21). The Cavitron ultrasonic aspirator (CUSA) uses ultrasound to treat VIN. Two medications used to treat warts, imiquimod (say "im-ICK-qwee-mod") (Aldara) and interferon, an antiviral and immune-system-boosting substance, are also being used to treat VIN. No data are available yet about the successes of these newer methods, but ask, if you are exploring your options.

In the past, VIN was treated with 5-FU (5-fluorouracil) cream. This caused a great deal of pain because it peeled off the vulvar skin, and sometimes led to chronic vulvar discomfort. It is no longer recommended for VIN; ask for another opinion if it is recommended for you.[12]

Your therapy must be individualized for you, depending on what degree of VIN is present, how deep it goes, what area of the anatomy it involves, and any other history you have. Your clinician must be confident that he/she has evaluated all the problem spots completely enough with biopsies to say that no cancer is present, only VIN. You will need to have careful discussions with your clinician about why he or she is recommending your treatment method, what the advantages are, what problems might be encountered, and what success rates can be expected. Ask about the track record of anything that's offered.

Here's a cautionary tale about why it's important to be thorough. Sylvia came to see me for a second opinion on laser treatment for VIN 1. Her story had begun with some warts on her perineum. Her primary-care provider gave her some topical wart medicine to use at home. Upset that this had happened to her, Sylvia went all out to get rid of the warts, applying the medicine more frequently than prescribed. She burned her skin. It eventually healed, leaving a suspicious thickened spot. This had been biopsied: VIN 1. Sylvia and I went over things. She didn't smoke and had never had any other HPV-related problems. Her Pap was normal and colposcopy/vulvoscopy showed only this one area on the perineum, which looked like tissue that was healing after a big insult. Sylvia agreed to come back for another look in three months. I gave her some cortisone cream to use in the meantime to quiet the inflammation. After three months a repeat biopsy showed just a little inflammation, and at six months I couldn't find anything that needed to be biopsied when I looked with the scope. Success: Sylvia was spared an unnecessary laser treatment.

Regardless of what treatment is used, VIN can come back in as many as one-third of women because that's the way intraepithelial neoplasia behaves.[13] There are a lot of unruly cells, and they don't give up easily. For example, Cindy had had only one partner, but one night she learned that he had been sleeping with someone else. When she went to be tested for STDs, some brownish bumps were noted around the introitus and over the perineum. I followed up on these with a Pap smear and a vulvar and cervical colposcopy, with biopsy of the bumps. Her Pap was atypical and she had VIN 3. I treated her with laser, but two weeks later at her postop check the bumps were back. It took two other laser procedures combined with interferon injections to strengthen her immune system, but to date she is clear of VIN. Her Pap is still atypical; we will follow with Pap and colposcopy until this crafty HPV is cleared.

Once again, just because it *can* come back doesn't mean

PREGNANCY AND VIN

Pregnancy's a time when your immune system is turned down so that it won't go after the cells of the developing baby. (As much as you want the baby, your immune system regards the fetus as a "foreigner" and could try to attack if Mother Nature didn't arrange for your immune system to chill out to some degree for nine months.) So without the watchdog efforts of the immune system to keep something like VIN at bay, it can grow more rapidly during pregnancy. At the same time, lots of perfectly normal changes in the skin pop up in pregnancy because all of your body systems are revved up. Moles come out and little loose flaps of skin (skin tags) can develop. So new little spots could be ignored or chalked up to skin changes of pregnancy. It's perfectly safe to do both colposcopy/vulvoscopy and biopsy in pregnancy, and these need to be done if you or your clinician has a question about a bump or color change.

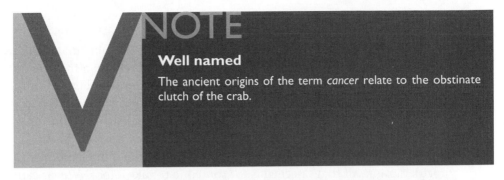

Well named

The ancient origins of the term *cancer* relate to the obstinate clutch of the crab.

that it always does. Recurrence is more common in women with advanced VIN in several places on the vulva. If the problem comes back or shows up in a new place, repeat evaluation needs to be done, and then a treatment plan made based on what's found and what the woman's particular story is. After any VIN treatment, a woman will need to have regular exams and colposcopy/vulvoscopy on a schedule that her clinician recommends.

Vulvar cancer

Precancerous bumps may not be unusual, but actual vulvar cancer is downright rare. It occurs in 1.9 women in 100,000—accounting for about 5 percent of all kinds of gynecological cancers.[14] Of the two cases I've seen in the past twelve years, both were women in their sixties who hadn't seen a clinician in years (they didn't think they needed regular gyn checkups after menopause) and came in with lumps.

As I mentioned in the previous section on VIN, it's possible (albeit unlikely) for HPV-caused precancer to evolve into cancer, especially in younger women. But what about women with the other kind of precancer, the type that strikes women over 50? For a long time doctors had no idea why they got it. Now there's been a breakthrough. Careful questioning of these women often reveals a long history of V symptoms, especially itching. It seems that chronic V irritation and inflammation from various V skin problems, unrecognized and untreated, may after many years—but not always—lead toward cancer.

That means vulvar cancer is probably preventable. If you accurately diagnose and treat all the V irritants, inflammations, and infections at age 25 or 30, you can make a difference in what shows up at age 50 or 60 or 70. Vulvar cancer tends to be diagnosed late because of the combination of delay on the part of the women who have itching and/or bumps for ages and don't speak up, and on the part of clinicians who for one reason or another do not make the diagnosis promptly.

Let me be clear: It's not that all itching can lead to cancer (no way!) but that *abnormal* skin that itches is *linked to* cancer. Vulvar cancer arises from abnormal skin. But just because you have an itchy skin disease does not mean you're going to have cancer. Treat the skin and you significantly reduce the *already small* risk of cancer development.[15]

Most vulvar cancers develop in the skin itself—on the labia majora, the labia minora, the clitoris, and in the vestibule. Cancers seen in the skin elsewhere on the body, such as melanoma and basal cell carcinoma, may also develop on the vulva.

Of all female cancers, vulvar cancer may be the easiest to screen for; it occurs as a lump, a thickened raised area, or an ulcer (where the skin is worn away) that can be seen by the woman or by her clinician during a regular exam. All that's needed is for someone to take a look. Vulvar cancer typically grows slowly.

If you have a bump that is biopsied and shows cancer, your doctor will refer you to a gyn cancer expert. In the past, extensive surgery with removal of the vulva (vulvectomy) and lymph nodes in the groin was routine. Fortunately, in recent years, we've had a revolution in vulvar cancer management with a much more conservative approach (same as with the breast—breast removal is now done much less often). Treatment has become individualized, and in most cases just the lump can be removed with enough tissue around it to make sure all the cancer has been taken out. Radiation is used if there is any cancer in the lymph nodes. The results have been excellent. But if the cancer is large enough to require vulvectomy, we now have reconstruction with plastic surgery, similar to what can be done if a breast is removed.

Paget's disease

This problem is not cancer but has a small association with other cancers. Like VIN, Paget's disease is another kind of intraepithelial neoplasia, which simply means that cells multiply, develop a weird appearance, and have the ability to go places they shouldn't be. It's rare, but I want to mention it because it produces awful itching and women with Paget's have suffered a lot. Paget's has to be considered in any workup of itchy skin patches.

No one knows what causes Paget's disease, and no one is exactly sure what cell in the skin starts this off. A skin biopsy, however, will show distinctive cells called Paget's cells; the pathologist recognizes their size, shape, and other characteristics.

Paget's disease is almost always seen in white women between 50 and 70. It's been found in younger women and in the African American population, but not very much.

Itching and soreness are the main complaints. The itching is intense and responds poorly to cortisone or other anti-itch medications. Embarrassed, women often delay seeing a clinician, so that the disease is present for months prior to diagnosis. On the vulva, Paget's makes a fiery red area

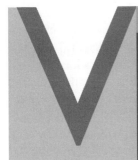

with little islands of thickened skin giving a white speckled appearance. There may be just a small patch, or Paget's can be pretty widespread over the labia and/or in the skin around the anus. Paget's disease is frequently confused with yeast on the skin, but antifungal cream does absolutely nothing for it. Paget's disease is also confused with a number of other conditions such as VIN and with vulvar skin problems such as eczema and lichen sclerosus. Biopsy is necessary to make the diagnosis and will reveal those classic Paget's cells.

If you have a biopsy that shows Paget's, you'll need some studies of other areas of the body before any treatment is done. In the past, the presence of Paget's cells in the vulva was believed to signal the presence of cancer elsewhere—in the vulvar glands under the skin with Paget's in it, in other skin, or in the breast, lung, or colon—in about one-fifth of patients.[16] Now it seems that these other cancers with Paget's are rare.[17] Nevertheless, a thorough check is in order so that nothing else is missed.

Paget's disease is difficult to treat because the abnormal cells can spread horizontally under skin that looks perfectly normal on the surface, and they can spread vertically deep into the tissue below. You need a surgeon with experience treating Paget's, often a cancer surgeon. Ask for a referral to a large teaching center and find a physician with experience treating this tricky disease.

In the past, vulvectomy was routinely done for this problem, but once again this drastic surgery has been abandoned in favor of tailoring individual treatments using the most limited surgery possible to remove the diseased tissue. If there is no evidence of an underlying cancer, removing the affected patch of skin with a wide margin around it is the usual approach. The edges of the removed tissue can be checked under the microscope in the operating room to try to make sure all of the Paget's has been removed. If there is a cancer deep in the tissue under the Paget's area, removal of the patch with even wider margins is necessary, and lymph nodes in the groin are taken out with a separate incision. Laser therapy is also being tried out for some cases of Paget's.

IF YOU'VE BEEN EXPOSED TO DES

Diethylstilbestrol (DES), a manufactured (not natural) estrogen, was given to several million pregnant women in the United States and Europe from 1938 to 1971 to prevent miscarriage and premature birth. In 1971, use of the drug stopped when doctors started to see a rare type of vaginal cancer in the daughters of women who took DES. Clear cell carcinoma, one of the rarest of the rare, is a kind of cancer that arises in glandularlike tissue in the vagina. If you remember, the vagina has no glands. But DES is able to stimulate the formation of glandularlike tissue in the vagina, from which this rare cancer develops.

A recent study has shown that women exposed to DES in the womb show no increased risk of other cancers. However, DES has proved responsible for other abnormalities in the cervix and uterus (a cervix with a ridge of tissue looking like a cockscomb, and a small T-shaped uterine cavity). Difficulty becoming pregnant and ectopic pregnancy are more frequent in DES-exposed women. The youngest DES-exposed patient to develop clear cell cancer was 7 years old at the time of diagnosis, and in 1992 the oldest patient was 42 years.

The DES scare is not over, since the last women to receive the drug in 1971 only turned 30 in 2001. Just because your mom took DES does not mean that you are guaranteed to have any of these problems, though. It simply means that you should be especially vigilant about your gynecological health. Any woman who has been DES-exposed should be followed yearly with a special Pap smear that includes sampling of both the cervix and vaginal walls, a colposcopy of the cervix, and careful feeling of the vaginal walls for any lumps.

Sources: E. E. Hatch, J. R. Palmer, L. Titus-Ernstoff, K. L. Noller, Cancer risk in women exposed to diethylstilbestrol in utero, JAMA 1998:280(7):630; A. L. Herbst, Diethylstilbestrol and adenocarcinoma of the vagina, Am J Obstet Gynecol 1999:181(6):1576.

The challenge of Paget's is that even with careful effort to remove all disease, it frequently comes back because of the ability of the cells to tunnel and burrow under normal-appearing skin.[18] So all women with Paget's need to be followed closely with regular evaluations to make sure the disease is not coming back.

If Paget's returns, a woman has the choice of more surgery or laser therapy. Promising work is now being done with the medicine that I mentioned earlier that treats warts, imiquimod (Aldara). Paget's has no connection with warts, but Aldara can stimulate your own fighter cells to attack Paget's cells and eliminate them. If you have recurrent Paget's, find a dermatologist in a large teaching hospital who works with this and ask about it.

I take care of two women who have had Paget's disease with surgery some years ago. Iris has recurrent disease. The itching is miserable, not helped by any of our standard cortisone or anti-itching medications. She is unwilling to have any more surgery because she has lost faith in its ability to help her. She feels that if the disease came back once, it will come back again. She has started to use Aldara with remarkable improvement so far.

Meanwhile, Mara has not had any recurrence of her disease. But she has vulvodynia that probably developed after the trauma of the surgery she had to remove the Paget's. And the burning from this makes her worry constantly that Paget's has returned. Estrogen cream helps her considerably, but she does not wish to take the tricyclic antidepressant that would probably help her pain.

Vaginal precancer (VAIN)

A counterpart to CIN in the cervix and VIN in the vulva is a condition called *vaginal intraepithelial neoplasia* (VAIN). Much less common and therefore not as well studied as CIN, it's seen in patients who have been previously treated for CIN 3 with hysterectomy. It appears that VAIN, like VIN and CIN, is caused by HPV.[19] For this reason, a Pap smear of the vagina, taking a smear from the wall of the vagina, is recommended for women who have had a hysterectomy for malignant or premalignant disease. Almost all VAIN shows no symptoms, but it may be found when colposcopy is done for other reasons. It is treated by cutting out or removing with a laser the small area that is involved.

Vaginal cancer

Vaginal cancer develops in the top layers of the vagina *(squamous epithelium)*. It is one of the rarest cancers in the human body. Most vaginal cancers spread to the vagina from the cervix. The epithelium of the vagina itself seems almost immune to developing malignant change on its own. The commonest symptom is vaginal bleeding. Treatment depends on the extent of the disease; radiation has been the main treatment. If you are diagnosed with vaginal cancer, you need to be in the hands of a gyn cancer specialist.

▼

CHAPTER 23

V Is for Voice

Some Parting Thoughts

S o now you know things about your body that you may never have known before. Even though this information is basic to me—after all, it's what I deal in day after day—I still manage to be pretty amazed by the intricate forces at work in the Vs. I hope you've been impressed too, or at least have found useful nuggets to improve your health and quality of life. Perhaps all of this information has been a bit frightening because it is new. Certainly if you have a specific problem—or an undiagnosed or unresolved one—it can seem overwhelming before it seems familiar. Rest assured, though, that there is no V condition without help or hope.

What I want you to do

Now what? Imparting good information is my main goal, but it's not my only one. Now I want you to act on what you've learned.

▼ *Consider yourself lucky.* Less than a generation ago, this information was barely talked about in doctors' offices, let alone anywhere else. This is the best time ever for women to be in charge of their bodies and their health. And if you do have a V problem, your odds of being helped are greater than ever before as well. Not since primitive peoples found the yoni something to celebrate has there been this much good news for the "lowly" vulva and vagina!

▼ *Look at yourself.* Basic but important. Whether for the very first time, or as part of regular self-exams, I hope that, at a minimum, you'll familiarize yourself with what your own visible body parts look like. Being comfortable with your own body is where it all starts. And—I can't emphasize this enough—by knowing what's what when things are normal, you'll be ahead of the game in explaining symptoms in case something should go awry. Know yourself.

▼ *Be good to yourself.* Follow the V-friendly guidelines found throughout this book. They can help prevent problems, or minimize further discomfort if you already have some kind of trouble.

▼ *Be an active participant in your health care.* This notion has, thankfully, been drilled into women's heads in recent years. But when it comes to V care, that message is particularly true. Your clinician—even a trusted person you've been seeing for a long time—may do a great job delivering your babies and dealing with your irregular periods but may not be up on the very latest V tests and treatments. Not a day goes by that I don't hear about a misdiagnosis, an ineffective or inappropriate treatment, or a problem that was mishandled for too long. I'm not suggesting that you routinely second-guess your care provider, but rather that you take nothing for granted. Ask questions. Understand why certain procedures are being done, and follow up on the results. Bring this book to your appointment. If an invasive treatment is recommended, or if the problem persists despite attempts at treatment, get a second opinion from a clinician with vulvovaginal experience. Be proactive.

▼ *Think twice before you grab that yeast cream.* I know, it's easy. But you now know that yeast is not the only cause of V problems, and more harm than good can come from overreliance on self-diagnosis. Better to be sure first.

▼ *Ask your mom or grandmother when she last had a gynecological checkup.* Sadly, it's all too common for women to tune out on V care after menopause. But as you now know, gynecology is about more than periods and babies! There are plenty of reasons to continue monitoring vulvovaginal health all through life. Sometimes a nudge from a younger and wiser relative can bring comfort or maybe even save a life.

▼ *Talk about this stuff with your friends.* Girlfriends exchange tips and tidbits all the time about diets, doctors, and such. Many younger women, especially, dish to one another about sex. Isn't it weird to exclude V health problems from this roster of topics? The more we talk about things such as yeast infection myths, abnormal Paps, assorted vaginitis, and V pain, the more information can be learned and put to use.

▼ *If my words have helped you, help advance V care in general.* What can the average woman do? Plenty, as a matter of fact. Some suggestions follow.

Advancing V care

Despite the massive strides of medicine as a whole, vulvar disease toddles forward with baby steps. Here are the problems it faces and here's what you can do to help.

Problem: Women don't know that vulvar disease is not well understood or taught in the medical community. Traditionally, it simply wasn't considered important. Yet we're not talking about some obscure corner of the body here, or some narrow range of problems that affect only a few hundred people a year. Every woman has a vulva. Every woman has a vagina. And every woman has something mess up there at some point in her life. The $600 million spent annually on yeast cream tells us something about the need out there. Yet the typical medical student spends just a few days learning about female genitalia—hardly enough time to really learn everything found between the covers of this book. Most ob-gyn residents receive catch-as-catch-can instruction, without formal focus on this essential area. Twelve years ago when I started my specialization, I had to scratch for every scrap of information. Today women with serious problems still need to scratch to find a clinician who is truly experienced in vulvovaginal problems. At a time when almost every other area of women's health is zooming forward, this is not right.

Approach: Vulvovaginal disease needs equal time—or at least proportional time—starting with its inclusion in medical school curricula and residency programs. If you feel strongly about this matter, you can make phone calls or write letters to medical school deans and nursing school deans, to directors of ob-gyn programs and nurse-practitioner programs, and to the American College of Obstetricians and Gynecologists to encourage more and better V education for their pupils. Tell the directors of all the ob gyn departments and programs that boast about their prowess in women's health in the twenty-first century that without V care, their initiative is woefully deficient. Ask them to sponsor graduate continuing medical education programs on vulvovaginal disease.

Ask your HMO or medical associates group to train a V specialist, an interested gyn who would spend a few weeks precepting with a known expert and pick up the ball. (Your trump card with your insurance providers is that accurate diagnostic work up front saves money in the long run. If you receive a prompt and accurate diagnosis, you won't have to have repeated visits and unnecessary prescriptions.) Endow a lecture series on vulvovaginal care at your hospital's ob-gyn grand rounds. Endow a V professorship or chair at a medical school.

Problem: Funding to study vulvovaginal problems has been minimal, compared with the generous grants other aspects of women's health have received over the last decade. Without solid research, we're left without many of the answers women sorely need, as I've pointed out again and again in these pages.

Approach: Let your legislative representatives know that we need money to go toward V study. Give to the International Society for the Study of Vulvovaginal Disease. Send money to the National Vulvodynia Association, the women largely responsible for the current NIH funding for the study of vulvar pain.

Problem: Clinicians often lack a financial incentive to specialize in this arena. V problems require diagnostic work—time spent figuring out what's wrong—as opposed to specialized procedures or surgeries to repair a problem. Because insurance does not reimburse well for diagnostic work, as opposed to procedures, a clinician cannot make a living doing V work. Some exist by not accepting insurance. While diagnostic reimbursement has started to improve, this problem is far from fixed.

Approach: Understand that a clinician who does not accept insurance is not a bad guy. It's the only way he or she can make ends meet.

▼ ▼ ▼

The future of V care lies with us. We all know the power of the consumer. And we all know the power of a woman. We are no longer knocked

V NOTE

V is for . . .

Vulva, vagina, vestibule,
valuable, valid, very, vital,
variety, velvety, vellum, violet, vermillion, variegated, vanity,
vivid, vivacious, vigorous, voluptuous, verdant, Venus,
virgin, valentine, vamp, vixen, virile, vibrator, volcano, voltage,
    vroom,
venereal, virus, vaginitis, vulvodynia,
veiled, vague, Victorian, vanish, vacuum, vamoose,
violate, victim,
vigilante, vigilant, veracity,
voyage, viable, visible, valiant, validation,
visionary, vanguard, vogue,
verge, victory,
V-day, V-8, VIP,
viva,
Voice.

out and tied down to have our babies. We have amazing assistance when we have trouble conceiving. Technology is fast eliminating the heavy bleeding that once kept woman homebound. Menopause clinics have sprung up everywhere. Let it be the same with the vulva—the same expertise, the same ingenuity. I hope you'll join me in my quest.

When I opened my discreetly named Stewart-Forbes Specialty Service, I never would have dreamed that a play called *The Vagina Monologues* would become a smash hit off-Broadway, winning an Obie award and having A-list actresses clamoring to appear in its cast. Or that a memoir about a woman's bout with vaginal pain (*The Camera My Mother Gave Me,* by Susanna Kaysen) would be published. Or that the word *vulvodynia* would be said on the popular TV series *Sex and the City.*

Such developments make some people cringe and others merely blush. Still others remain oblivious. But I consider growing interest in the Vs to be reason to cheer. Letting them see a bit of daylight (metaphorically, of course!) makes it easier to get the current, rock-solid, comprehensive information that women need—this book—into your hands.

▼

resources

Alternative Medicine

Alternative Medicine Homepage

www.pitt.edu/~cbw/altm.html

Herbs, faith healing, meditation, AIDS links

Doc Weil Database

http://www.hotwired.com/drweil

Harvard-educated Andrew Weil, M.D., specializes in complementary medicine and the mind-body connection. The site includes several search engines, menus, alternative medicine information, and "Ask Dr. Weil." Combines information from traditional and alternative modalities.

National Center for Complementary and Alternative Medicine (NCCAM), National Institutes of Health

http://nccam.nih.gov

NCCAM conducts and supports basic and applied research and training and puts out information on complementary and alternative medicine. Phone inquiries: 888-644-6226.

Birth Control/Contraception

Chalker, Rebecca. *The Complete Cervical Cap Guide.* New York: Harper & Row, 1987.

Hatcher, Robert, et al. *Contraceptive Technology,* 17th. New York: Irvington, 1998.

Mauck, Christine K., et al., eds. *Barrier Contraceptives: Current Status and Future Prospects.* New York: Wiley-Liss, 1994.

Treiman, K., L. Liskin, A. Kols, and W. Rinehart. "IUDs—An Update." Population Reports, Series B, no. 6 (December 1995). Available from Population Information Program, Johns Hopkins University, 327 St. Paul Street, Baltimore, MD 21208.

Weschler, Toni. *Taking Charge of Your Fertility: The Definitive Guide to Natural Birth Control and Pregnancy Achievement.* New York: HarperCollins, 1995.

Cancer

Information on diagnosis, treatment, and support for gynecologic cancers

www.eyesontheprize.org

Drysol Antiperspirant

May be purchased through www.canadadrugs.com

Female Circumcision

For information from the American College of Obstetricians and Gynecologists, contact:

Shirine Mohagheghpour
Manager, Health Care for Underserved Women
American College of Obstetricians and Gynecologists
410 12th Street, SW
Washington, DC 20024-2188
Phone: 800-673-8444, ext 2469

For legal information and questions:

Center for Reproductive Law and Policy (CRLP)
120 Wall Street
New York, NY 10005
Phone: 212-514-5534
Fax: 212-514-5538
www.crlp.org

For information on local community groups and community education material:

Research, Action and Information Network for the Bodily Integrity of Women (RAINBO)
915 Broadway, Suite 1109
New York, NY 10010
Phone: 212-477-3318
Fax: 212-477-4154
www.rainbo.org

For listing of published and unpublished literature on FC/FGM:

The FGM Resource Group
The Population Information Program of the Johns Hopkins Center for Communications Programs
POPLINE
111 Market Place, Suite 310
Baltimore, MD 21202-4012
Phone: 410-659-6300
Fax: 410-659-6266
www.jhuccp.org

Genital Herpes

American Social Health Association (ASHA)

resources

P.O. Box 13827
Research Triangle Park, NC 27709
Phone: 800-230-6039
www.ashastd.org

ASHA is a nonprofit organization dedicated to STD prevention. Its Web site has a wealth of information; you can call for educational materials on herpes. Ask for *Managing Herpes: How to Live and Love with a Chronic STD* by Charles Ebel. ASHA's special site for teens is www.iwannaknow.org.

Centers for Disease Control and Prevention (CDC)

http://www.cdc.gov

General information sponsored by Novartis

www.cafeherpe.com

Herpes support

www.herpeszone.com

National Institute of Allergy and Infectious Diseases
Send postcard to: Genital Herpes
NIAID, Office of Communications
31 Center Drive, MSC 2520
Building 31, Room 7A50
Bethesda, MD 20892-2520

National Herpes Hot Line: 919-361-8488
(Monday–Friday, 9 A.M. to 7 P.M., EST)

Herpes Resource Center
American Social Health Association
P.O. Box 13827
Research Triangle Park, NC 27709-9940
800-230-6039
http://jama.ama-assn.org/issues/v280n10/fpdf/jpg0909.pdf

Hair Removal

Facts on laser hair removal

http://www.fda.gov/cdrh/consumer/laserfacts.html#hair

Information on hair removal techniques

http://www.cfsan.fda.gov/~dms/cos-hrem.html

Laser Devices

http://www.fda.gov/cdrh/databases.html

Access this site to learn if a specific laser manufacturer has received FDA clearance for hair removal. You will need to know the manufacturer or device name of the laser. You can also call FDA's Center for Devices and Radiological Health, Consumer Staff at 1-888-INFO-FDA or 301-827-3990, fax your request to 301-443-9535, or send an e-mail to *DSMA@cdrh.fda.gov.*

List of licensed and certified electrologists

International Guild of Professional Electrologists
202 Boulevard Street, Suite B
High Point, NC 27262
Phone: 800-830-3247

Herbs

Medicinal Herb FAQ

http://www.ibiblio.org/herbmed/faqs/medi-cont.html

This privately maintained Web site and chat room has anecdotal information on medicinal herbs and their uses.

Hormones and Hormone Replacement Therapy

Online Resources

Hormone Foundation

http://www.hormone.org

Consumers may download a free 32-page pamphlet about hormones and health.

National Cancer Institute, National Institutes of Health

http://www.nci.nih.gov

Contains a full listing of information on the effects of hormones on breast cancer and the use of antiestrogens such as selective estrogen receptor modulators (SERMs). Has decision tree software for determining relative risk for breast cancer within the next year and by age 90.

To Read

Rako, S. *The Hormone of Desire.* New York: Three Rivers Press, 1996.

Vliet, E. L. *Screaming to Be Heard: Hormone Connections Women Suspect and Doctors Still Ignore.* New York: M. Evans and Company, 2001.

resources

Human Papillomavirus (Genital warts)

American Social Health Association (ASHA)
Phone: 800-230-6039
www.ashastd.org

ASHA is a nonprofit organization dedicated to STD prevention. Its Web site has a wealth of information; you can call for educational materials on human papillomavirus. Its special site for teens is www.iwannaknow.org.

Interstitial Cystitis

Online Resources

Interstitial Cystitis Association
51 Monroe Street, Suite 1402
Rockville, MD 20850
Phone: 301-610-5300; 800-HELP-ICA
www.ichelp.org

Interstitial Cystitis Network Web site

www.ic-network.com

To Read

Chalker, Rebecca, and Kristene E. Whitmore, M.D. *Overcoming Bladder Disorders: Compassionate, Authoritative Medical and Self-Help Solutions for Incontinence, Cystitis, Interstitial Cystitis, Prostate Problems and Bladder Cancer.* New York: Harper and Row, 1990.

Brody, Jane. "Interstitial Cystitis: Help for a Puzzling and Extraordinarily Painful Illness of the Bladder." *The New York Times* (January 25, 1995):B7.

Laboratory Standards

For lab qualifications and practice guidelines go to the Web site of the College of American Pathologists

http://www.cap.org

Massage Therapy

American Massage Therapy Association (AMTA)
820 Davis Street, Suite 100
Evanston, IL 60201
Phone: 847-864-0123
www.amtamassage.org

Web site explains requirements for licensing and certification (now required in twenty-nine states and the District of Columbia) and tells where you can find a certified massage therapist.

Medical Information and Literature

MEDLINEplus

http://medlineplus.nlm.nih.gov

This site from the National Library of Medicine helps consumers find answers to health questions, mostly by government or professional organizations. It offers access to MEDLINE, which finds articles in the medical literature about specific topics. Spanish resources available.

Menopause

Patient information brochures available from the American College of Obstetricians and Gynecologists (ACOG)
The Menopause Years
Midlife Transitions: A Guide to Approaching Menopause
Preventing Osteoporosis
Hormone Replacement Therapy
Phone: 800-410-ACOG
www.acog.org

Available from the North American Menopause Society (NAMS)
Menopause Guidebook
"MenoPak"
Reading List: Suggested Reading for Informed Decision-Making, a list of booklets, books, newsletters, and magazines on menopause recommended by NAMS. NAMS Web site lists questions and answers frequently asked about menopause.
Phone: 800-774-5342
www.menopause.org

Available from the American Academy of Family Physicians
Menopause: What to Expect When Your Body Is Changing
Osteoporosis in Women: Keeping Your Bones Healthy and Strong

resources

Phone: 800-944-0000

Available from the National
Osteoporosis Foundation (NOF)
*Boning Up on Osteoporosis: A Guide to
Prevention and Treatment*
*Be BoneWise Exercise: NOF's Official
Exercise Video*
How Strong Are Your Bones?
*Style Wise: A Fashion Guide for Women
with Osteoporosis*
Fax: 202-223-2237
www.nof.org

Menstrual Products

Museum of Menstruation

www.mum.org

Food and Drug Administration

http://www.fda.gov

Huge government site contains vast
information on food, drugs, cosmetics,
and related resources. Also has many
links and facts. Phone inquiries: 888-
INFO-FDA (888-463-6332).

The Padette
Athena Medical Corporation
10170 SW Nimbus Avenue, Suite H-1
Portland, OR 97223
Phone: 503-968-8800

The Keeper
The Keeper Inc., Box 20023
Cincinnati, OH 45220
Phone: 513-631-0077

Instead
Ultrafem Inc.
500 Fifth Avenue, Suite 3620
New York, NY 10110
Phone: 212-575-5740; 800-INSTEAD

InSync Miniform
A-Fem Medical Corporation
10180 SW Nimbus Avenue
Portland, OR 97223
Phone: 503-968-8800

Terra Femme

www.web.net/terrafemme

Natracare

www.natracare.com

To Read

"Tampons and Pads: Should You Use What
Mom Used?" *Consumer Reports.* January
1995, 51–55.

Mental Health: Depression, Conflict

American Association for Marriage and
Family Therapy
1133 15th Street NW, Suite 300
Washington, DC 20005
Phone: 202-452-0109; 888-AAMFT-99
http://www.aamft.org

American Mental Health Counselors
Association
801 N. Fairfax Street, Suite 304
Alexandria, VA 22314
Phone: 703-548-6002; 800-326-2642
E-mail: amhcahq@pie.org

**American Psychological Association
(APA)**

http://www.apa.org

Includes search engines, professional
associations, testimonials on emotional
problems.

Mental Health Server

http://www.mentalhealth.com

Offers help and testimonials on mental
health issues. Includes referrals and a
question-and-answer forum.

Nutrition

American Dietetic Association (ADA)

http://www.eatright.org

Professional and classified listings on
nutrition

**International Food Information
Council (IFIC)**

http://ificinfo.health.org

IFIC tries to bridge the gap between
science and consumers by collecting and
distributing scientific information on
food safety, nutrition, and health. Works
with scientific experts to translate
research into understandable and useful
information.

**National Agricultural Library (NAL),
US Department of Agriculture**

http://www.nal.usda.gov

The Food and Nutrition Information
Center (FNIC) is one of several
information centers at the NAL. It has
access to all FNIC resource lists and many

resources

other food and nutrition-related links. Includes Dietary Guidelines for Americans.

Pain and Painful Intercourse (*see* Vulvodynia)

Physical Therapy for the Pelvic Floor

To find a physical therapist knowledgeable about the pelvic floor, call the American Physical Therapy Association, 800-999-APTA. From the menu choices, select Women's Health. Ask for a regional representative to help you locate a therapist in your area. The APTA has a network of reps who know every therapist in a given geographical zone.

Sexual Abuse

National Child Abuse Hotline
P.O. Box 630
Los Angeles, CA 90028
Phone: 800-422-4453

A 24-hour hotline for adult survivors as well as children.

National Coalition Against Domestic Violence
119 Constitution Avenue, NE
Washington, DC 20002
Phone: 202-544-7893

National Domestic Violence Hotline
Phone: 800-799-SAFE

To Read

Bass, Ellen, and Laura Davis. *The Courage to Heal: A Guide for Women Survivors of Child Sexual Abuse*. New York: HarperPerennial, 1994.

Dolan, Yvonne. *Resolving Sexual Abuse: Solution-Focused Therapy and Ericksonian Hypnosis for Survivors*. New York: Norton, 1991.

Herman, Judith. *Trauma and Recovery*. New York: Basic Books, 1992.

Jack, Dana Crowley. *Silencing the Self: Women and Depression*. Cambridge, MA: Harvard University Press, 1991.

Louden, Jennifer. *The Woman's Comfort Book: A Self-Nurturing Guide for Restoring Balance in Your Life*. San Francisco: Harper, 1992.

Maltz, Wendy. *Sexual Healing Journey: A Guide for Survivors of Sexual Abuse*. New York: HarperCollins, 1992.

Renzetti, Claire M. *Violent Betrayal: Partner Abuse in Lesbian Relationships*. Newbury Park, CA: Sage Publications, 1992.

Sexual Health and Education

American Association of Sex Educators, Counselors, and Therapists (AASECT)
P.O. Box 238
Mt. Vernon, IA 52314
Phone: 319-895-8407

The organization assists in locating resources for sex therapy in your area.

Kinsey Institute for Research in Sex, Gender and Reproduction Information Service
Indiana University
313 Morrison Hall
Bloomington, IN 47405
Phone: 812-855-7686

Offers a free list of bibliographies on many aspects of sexuality. List available for a fee at www.indiana.edu/~kinsey.

The Sexual Health Network
One Tamarac Ridge Circle
Huntington, CT 06484
Phone: 203-924-4623
www.sexualhealth.com

Provides information, educational materials, referrals to sexual health professionals knowledgeable about disabilities and chronic diseases.

Sexuality Information and Education Council of the United States (SIECUS)
130 West 42nd Street, Suite 2500
New York, NY 10036-7802
Phone: 212-819-9770
Fax: 212-819-9776
www.siecus.org/pubs

Publishes a journal, bibliographies, brochures, and pamphlets related to sexuality research, education, and legislation.

resources

To Read

Barbach, Lonnie G. *For Each Other: Sharing Sexual Intimacy.* New York: Signet, 1984.

Barbach, Lonnie G. *For Yourself: The Fulfillment of Female Sexuality.* New York: Doubleday/Anchor Books, 1976.

Berman, Jennifer, and Laura Berman. *For Women Only: A Revolutionary Guide to Overcoming Sexual Dysfunction and Reclaiming Your Life.* New York: Henry Holt and Company, 2001.

Davis, Elizabeth. *Women, Sex, and Desire: Exploring Your Sexuality at Every Stage of Life.* Alameda, CA: Hunter House, 1995.

Dodson, Betty. *Sex for One: The Joy of Selfloving.* New York: Crown Publishing Group, 1992.

Due, Linnea. *Joining the Tribe: Growing Up Gay and Lesbian in the '90s.* New York: Anchor Books, 1995.

Heiman, Julia, and Joseph LoPiccolo. *Becoming Orgasmic.* New York: Fireside, 1992.

Kitzinger, Sheila. *Woman's Experience of Sex.* New York: Penguin Books, 1985.

Villarosa, Linda, ed. *Body and Soul: The Black Women's Guide to Physical Health and Emotional Well-Being.* New York: HarperCollins, 1994.

Online Resources

Dr. (Ruth) Westheimer's Web site

http://www.drruth.com

Extensive site covers sex education and sex issues.

Go Ask Alice!

http://www.goaskalice.columbia.edu

Site includes a wealth of information on sexual health, relationships, physical health, and sex-related questions from viewers. Sponsored by Columbia University's Health Education Department.

Sexually Transmitted Diseases (STDs)

American Association of Retired Persons (AARP)
Phone: 800-424-3410
www.aarp.org

The AARP sells an AIDS-prevention video, *It Can Happen to Me.*

American Social Health Association (ASHA)
Phone: 800-230-6039
www.ashastd.org

ASHA is a non-profit organization dedicated to STD prevention. Its Web site has a wealth of information; you can call for educational materials on herpes and human papillomavirus. Its special site for teens is www.iwannaknow.org.

Centers for Disease Control and Prevention (CDC)

http://www.cdc.gov

Large government site focused on studies of disease causes and cures. Links to related sites. Phone inquiries: 800-322-3435 and 404-639-3534.

CDC National STD Hotline
Phone: 800-227-8922

Planned Parenthood Federation of America
Phone: 800-230-PLAN
www.plannedparenthood.org

Numerous informational materials on STDs and contraception

Urinary Tract Infection

American College of Obstetricians and Gynecologists
409 12th St, SW
Washington, DC 20024
Phone: 800-762-2264
www.acog.org

Publishes *Urinary Tract Infections,* ACOG Patient Education Pamphlet AP050.

American Academy of Family Physicians
8880 Ward Parkway
Kansas City, MO 64114-2797
Phone: 800-944-0000
www.aafp.org

Publishes *Urinary Tract Infection: A Common Problem for Some Women.*

National Institute of Diabetes and Digestive and Kidney Diseases
National Kidney and Urologic Diseases Information Clearinghouse
3 Information Way
Bethesda, MD 20892-3580

resources

Phone: 301-654-4415
www.niddk.nih.gov/health/endo/
endo.htm
Publishes *Urinary Tract Infection in Adults*.

Vaginitis
There are many sources that conflict with what I've given you in *The V Book*. I've worked hard to make *The V Book* the most complete and accurate source available.

Violence Against Women
Online Resources

The Family Violence Prevention Fund
www.fvpf.org/

SafetyNet Domestic Violence Resources
www.cybergrrl.com/planet/dv

To Read

Davis, Angela. *Violence Against Women and the Ongoing Challenge to Racism*. Latham, NY: Kitchen Table Women of Color Press, 1987.

Fairstein, Linda. *Sexual Violence: Our War Against Rape*. New York: Berkley Publishing, 1995.

Fortune, Marie M. *Sexual Violence: The Unmentionable Sin: An Ethical and Pastoral Perspective*. New York: Pilgrim Press, 1983.

Levy, Barrie, ed. *Dating Violence: Young Women in Danger*. Seattle: Seal Press, 1991.

Martin, Del. *Battered Wives*. New York: Simon & Schuster/Pocket Books, 1990.

Rush, Florence. *The Best Kept Secret: Sexual Abuse of Children*. New York: McGraw-Hill, 1992.

Vulvodynia and Related Pain Problems

Endometriosis Association
8585 N. 76th Place
Milwaukee, WI 53223
Phone: 800-992-3636
www.EndometriosisAssn.org

Fibromyalgia Association of Greater Washington
P.O. Box 2373

Centerville, VA 22020
Phone: 703-790-2324

International Society for the Study of Vulvovaginal Disease
20 W. Washington Street, Suite 1
Hagerstown, MD 21740
Phone: 301-733-5418
Fax: 301-733-5775
www.issvd.org

Interstitial Cystitis Association
51 Monroe Street, Suite 1402
Rockville, MD 20850
Phone: 301-610-5300; 800-HELP-ICA
www.ichelp.org

National Vulvodynia Association
P.O. Box 4491
Silver Spring, MD 20914-4491
Phone: 301-299-0775
Fax: 301-299-3999
www.nva.org

Vulvar Pain Foundation
Post Office Drawer 177
Graham, NC 27253
Phone: 910-226-0704

Information for women suffering from vulvodynia, frequently asked questions, chat room, mailing list from Dr. Howard Glazer, originator of biofeedback for treatment of vulvodynia.

www.vulvodynia.com

Vulvovaginal Specialists

International Society for the Study of Vulvovaginal Disease
20 West Washington Street, Suite 1
Hagerstown, MD 21740
Phone: 301-733-5418; 800-787-7227
Fax: 301-733-5775
E-mail: khall@asccp.org
www.issvd.org

Women's Health
Online Resources

American College of Obstetricians and Gynecologists (ACOG)
http://www.acog.org

Excellent resource for everything from vaginitis to sexual abuse. Includes book lists and many e-mail addresses for different resources.

resources

American Medical Association, Women's Health Information Center

http://www.ama-assn.org/women

Part of the AMA's large Web site.

Female Health Links

http://www.femalehealthlinks.com

Has links to magazines, journals, and conferences on women's health.

Harvard Women's Health Watch (newsletter)

http://www.med.harvard.edu/ publications/pubs/html (click on "Harvard Health Publications," then "Harvard Women's Health Watch")

Online newsletter sponsored by Harvard University Medical School features questions and topics of interest to women, researched by doctors specializing in the field. Includes many Harvard links.

Healthfinder

http://www.healthfinder.gov

Site has wide range of topics on women's health, with links to many sites on consumer health and human services.

Health Web

http://www.healthweb.org

Supported by the National Library of Medicine, the site provides links to Internet resources selected by librarians and information professionals at leading midwestern academic medical centers.

Mayo Health Oasis

http://www.mayohealth.org

From the renowned Mayo Clinic, this interactive site features a search engine, question forum and library, and health-related resources.

National Women's Health Information Center

http://www.4woman.org

Includes many resources on women's health. Frequently Asked Questions (FAQ) section includes interstitial cystitis, STDs, vaginal infections, information for women of color and lesbian women. Extensive links to disease-specific sites.

MediSpecialty.com

www.obgyn.net

Ob-gyn topics include information and discussion forums, though no vulvovaginal information.

Women's Health

http://www.feminist.com/resources/ links/links_health.html

Includes reproductive health section (Gynecology 101 and Sexuality), emotional-support articles, information for women of color.

To Read

Boston Women's Health Book Collective. *Our Bodies, Ourselves for the New Century: A Book by and for Women.* New York: Touchstone, 1998.

Doress-Worters, Paula B. and Diana Laskin Siegal, in cooperation with the Boston Women's Health Book Collective. *The New Ourselves, Growing Older.* New York: Touchstone, 1994.

Yeast

There are many sources that conflict with the information in *The V Book.* I have made every effort in Chapter 10 to give you the most up-to-date and medically documented information available.

Journal Abbreviations

If you're interested in doing further research, the following is a list of medical journals I have cited in this text along with their abbreviations for easy reference. Some of these journals can be accessed for free online at the websites I've provided below (others require a paid subscription).

Abbreviation	Journal Name
Acta Anat	Acta Anatomica Journal
Acta Cytologica	Acta Cytologica
Acta Derm Venereol (Stockholm)	Acta Dermatolgica Venereologica (Stockholm)
Acta Obstet Gynecol Scand	Acta Obstetrica et Gynecologica Scandanavica Journal
Advance for Nurse Practitioners	Advance for Nurse Practitioners Journal
Age and Aging	Age and Aging
Allergy Proc	Allergy Proceedings
Am J Epidemiol	American Journal of Epidemiology
Am J Health Syst Pharm	American Journal of Health Systems & Pharmacology
Am J Obstet Gynecol	American Journal of Obstetrics and Gynecology
Am J Public Health, AJPH	American Journal of Public Health
Am J Psych	American Journal of Psychiatry
Am Fam Phys	American Family Physician
Anal Chem	Analytical Chemistry
Ann Allergy	Annals of Allergy
Ann Rev Sex Research	Annual Review of Sex Research
Ann Int Med	Annals of Internal Medicine
Antimicrob Agents Chemother	Antimicrobial Agents & Chemotherapy
Applied and Env Microbiol	Applied and Environmental Microbiology
Arch Dermatol	Archives of Dermatology
Arch Sex Behav	Archives of Sexual Behavior
Arthritis Rheumatol	Arthritis & Rheumatology
Australas J Dermatol	Australasian Journal of Dermatology
Aust NZ J Obstet Gynaecol	Australia New Zealand Journal of Obstetrics and Gynaecology
Br J Cancer	British Journal of Cancer
Br J Clin Pract	British Journal of Clinical Practice
Br J Obstet Gynaecol	British Journal of Obstetrics and Gynaecology
Br J Surg	British Journal of Surgery
BMJ	British Medical Journal
Can Med Assoc J	Canadian Medical Association Journal
Clin Dermatol	Clinical Dermatology
Clin Exp Dermatol	Clinical & Experimental Dermatology
Clin Obstet & Gynecol	Clinical Obstetrics & Gynecology
Colposcopy & Gynecol	Colposcopy and Gynecology
Comprehensive Ther	Comprehensive Therapy
Contact Derm	Contact Dermatology
Contemp Ob/Gyn	Contemporary Ob/Gyn
Contraception	Contraception
Dermatology	Dermatology
Dermatol Surg	Dermatologic Surgery
Dis Colon Rectum	Diseases of the Colon and the Rectum
Endocrinology	Endocrinology
Epidemiology	Epidemiology
Eur J Dermatol	European Journal of Dermatology
Eur J Obstet Gynecol Reprod Biol	European Journal of Obstetrics, Gynecology and Reproductive Biology
Fam Plann Perspect	Family Planning Perspectives
The Female Patient	The Female Patient
Fertil Steril	Fertility and Sterility
Genitourin Med	Genitourinary Medicine
Gynecol Obstet Invest	Gynecological & Obstetrical Investigation Journal
Health Psychol	Health Psychology
Immunology	Immunology

Infect Immun	Infection & Immunity	J Periodical Res	Journal of Periodical
Infect in Med	Infections in Medicine		Research
Int J Cancer	International Journal	J Psychosom Obstet	Journal of
	of Cancer	Gynaecol	Psychosomatic
Int J Dermatol	International Journal		Obstetrics &
	of Dermatology		Gynaecology
Int J Fertil	International Journal	J Reprod Med	Journal of
	of Fertility		Reproductive
Int J Gynecol Obstet	International Journal		Medicine
	of Gynecology and	J R Soc Med	Journal of the Royal
	Obstetrics		Society of Medicine
Int J Gyn Path	International Journal	J Sex & Marital Ther	Journal of Sex &
	of Gynecologic		Marital Therapy
	Pathology	J Urol	Journal of Urology
Int J Impotence	International Journal	Lancet	Lancet
Research	of Impotence	Maturitas	Maturitas
	Research	Mayo Clinic	Mayo Clinic
Int J Sexol	International Journal	Proceedings	Proceedings
	of Sexology	Med Clin North Am	Medical Clinics of
Isr J Obstet Gynecol	Israeli Journal of		North America
	Obstetrics and	Med J Austr	Medical Journal of
	Gynecology		Australia
Isr Chem	Israeli Chemistry	Menopausal Medicine	Menopausal Medicine
J Adv Med	Journal of	MMWR	Morbidity and
	Advancement in		Mortality Weekly
	Medicine		Review
J Allergy Clin	Journal of Allergy and	Mycoses	Mycoses
Immunol	Clinical	N Engl J Med	New England Journal
	Immunology		of Medicine
J Am Acad Dermatol	Journal of the	Neurourol Urodyn	Neurological
	American Academy		Urodynamics
	of Dermatology	Nurs Stand	Nursing Standards
J Am Ger Soc	Journal of the	Obstet Gynecol	Obstetrics and
	American Geriatric		Gynecology
	Society	Obstet Gynecol Clin	Obstetrics and
JAMA	Journal of the	North Am	Gynecology Clinics
	American Medical		of North America
	Association	ObG Management	ObG Management
J Eur Acad Dermatol	Journal of the	Obstet Gynecol Surv	Obstetrics &
Vener	European Academy		Gynecology Survey
	of Dermatology and	Persp Allergy	Perspectives in Allergy
	Venereology	Postgrad Med J	Postgraduate Medical
J Clin Microbiol	Journal of Clinical		Journal
	Microbiology	Practitioner	Practitioner
J Clin Pathol	Journal of Clinical	Proc Roy Soc Med	Proceedings of the
	Pathology		Royal Society of
J Clin Res Drug Dev	Journal of Clinical		Medicine
	Research in Drug	Psych Clin North Am	Psychiatric Clinics of
	Development		North America
J Cutan Path	Journal of Cutaneous	Psychom Med	Psychosomatic
	Pathology		Medicine
J Clin Endocrinol	Journal of Clinical	Rev of Infec Dis	Review of Infectious
Metab	Endocrinology and		Diseases
	Metabolism	Scand J Infect Dis	Scandinavian Journal
J Fam Pract	Journal of Family		of Infectious Diseases
	Practice	Sem Dermatol	Seminars in
J Gen Microbiol	Journal of General		Dermatology
	Microbiology	Sex Trans Dis	Sexually Transmitted
J Infect Dis	Journal of Infectious		Diseases
	Diseases	Sex Trans Infec	Sexually Transmitted
J Natl Cancer Inst	Journal of the		Infections
	National Cancer	Southern Med J	Southern Medical
	Institute		Journal
J Lower Genital Tract	Journal of Lower	Transactions St John's	Transactions of St
Dis	Genital Tract Disease	Dermatol Soc	John's
J Neurosurg	Journal of		Dermatological
	Neurosurgery		Society
J Pediatr	Journal of Pediatrics	Urol	Urology

Web sites:

http://www.harcourthealth.com
http://www.lib.uiowa.edu/hardin/md/ej.html
http://www.achoo.com/features/refsources/journals.asp

Introduction

1. H. C. Wisenfelf, and I. Macio, Evaluation of vulvovaginal symptoms by women's health care providers. Presented at the Annual Meeting of the Infectious Diseases Society for Obstetrics and Gynecology, Jackson Hole, Wyoming, August 5–8, 1998.

Chapter 1: The Mind

1. G. Steinem, Introduction, in Eve Ensler, *The Vagina Monologues* (New York: Villard, 1999), ix.
2. R. Eisler, *The Chalice and the Blade* (San Francisco: Harper & Company, 1988).
3. J. C. Webster, Progress in obstetrics and gynecology, in *Harrington Lectures* (Buffalo: Medical Faculty of the University of Buffalo, 1910).
4. J. V. Ricci, *The Genealogy of Gynaecology* (Philadelphia: Blakiston, 1943),147.
5. Webster, Progress in obstetrics and gynecology.
6. Ricci, *The Genealogy of Gynaecology.*
7. N. Angier, *Woman* (Boston: Houghton Mifflin, 1999), 84.
8. Ricci, *The Genealogy of Gynaecology.*
9. Ibid.
10. Webster, Progress in obstetrics and gynecology.
11. Roy Porter, *The Greatest Benefit to Mankind: A Medical History of Humanity* (New York: W. W. Norton, 1997), 676.
12. Webster, Progress in obstetrics and gynecology.

Chapter 2: The Vulva

1. F. H. Sillman, M. G. Muto, The vulva, in *Kistner's Gynecology,* K. J. Ryan, R. S. Berkowitz, R. L. Barbieri, eds. (St. Louis: Mosby, 1995), 50.
2. C. K. Hong, H. G. Choi, Hair restoration surgery in patients with hypotrichosis of the pubis: the reason and ideas for design, *Dermatol Surg* 1999:25(6):475.
3. W. S. Lee, I. W. Lee, S. K. Ahn, Diffuse heterochromia of scalp hair, *J Am Acad Dermatol* 1996 Nov:35(5 Pt 2):823.
4. E. J. Wilkinson, I. K. Stone, *Atlas of Vulvar Disease* (Baltimore: Williams & Wilkins, 1995).
5. A. Toesca et al., Immunohistochemical study of the corpora cavernosa of the human clitoris, *J Anat* 1996:188:513.
6. B. R. Komisaruk, B. Whipple, The suppression of pain by genital stimulation in females, *Ann Rev Sex Research* 1995:6:151.
7. A. B. Berenson, A longitudinal study of hymenal morphology in the first 3 years of life, *Pediatrics* 1995:95:490.
8. J. E. Emmans, E. R. Woods, E. N. Allred, and E. Grace, Hymenal findings in adolescent women: impact of tampon use and consensual sexual activity, *J Pediatr* 1994:125:153.
9. N. Jeffcoate, Hypertrophy of the labia minora "Spaniel ear nymphae," in *Principles of Gynaecology,* 4th ed. (London: Butterworths, 1975), 151.

Chapter 3: The Vagina

1. M. Hilliges, C. Falconer, G. Ekman-Ordeberg, O. Johansson, Innervation of the human vaginal mucosa as revealed by PGP 9.5 immunohistochemistry, *Acta Anat* 1995:153:119.
2. C. J. Dewhurst, *Integrated Obstetrics and Gynaecology for Postgraduates,* 2nd ed. (Oxford: Blackwell Scientific Publications, 1973); R. L. Dickinson, *Control of Conception* (Baltimore: Williams & Wilkins, 1938).
3. M. J. Godley, Quantitation of vaginal discharge in healthy volunteers, *Br J Obstet Gynaecol* 1985:92:739.
4. N. Dusitsin, A. T. Gregoire, W. D. Johnson, et al., Histidine in human vaginal fluid, *Obstet Gynecol* 1967:29:125.
5. I. Sjoberg, S. Cajander, E. Rylander, Morphometric characteristics of the vaginal epithelium during the menstrual cycle, *Gynecol Obstet Invest* 1988:26:136.

6. D. P. Wolf, L. Blasco, M. Khan, et al., Human cervical mucus: V. Oral contraceptives and mucus rheologic properties, *Fertil Steril* 1979:32:166.

7. A. B. Onderdonk, B. F. Polk, N. S. Moon, et al., Methods for quantitative vaginal flora studies, *Am J Obstet Gynecol* 1977:128:777.

8. S. Faro, Bacterial vaginitis, *Clin Obstet & Gynecol* 1990:34:582.

9. B. Watt, M. J. Goldacre, N. Loudon, et al., Prevalence of bacteria in the vagina of normal young women, *Br J Obstet Gynaecol* 1981:88:588.

Chapter 4: At Different Ages

1. C. P. Goplerud, M. J. Ohn, R. P. Galask, Aerobic and anaerobic flora of the cervix during pregnancy and the puerperium, *Am J Obstet Gynecol* 1976:126:858.

2. J. Paavonen, Physiology and ecology of the vagina, *Scand J Infect Dis* 1983:S40:31.

3. C. C. Tsai, J. P. Semmens, E. C. Semmens, et al., Vaginal physiology in post-menopausal women: pH value, transvaginal electropotential difference, and estimated blood flow, *Southern Med J* 1987:80(8):987.

4. S. Leilblum, G. Bachman, E. Kemmann, et al., Vaginal atrophy in the post-menopausal woman: the importance of sexual activity and hormones, *JAMA* 1983:249:2195.

5. R. B. Greenblatt et al., Evaluation of an estrogen, androgen, and estrogen-androgen combination, and a placebo in the treatment of the menopause, *J Clin Endocrinol Metab* 1950:10:1547; C. H. Birnberg, R. Kurzrok, Low-dosage androgen-estrogen therapy in the older age group, *J Am Ger Soc* 1955:III:656; H. S. Kupperman et al., Contemporary therapy of the menopausal syndrome, *JAMA* 1959:171:103.

6. B. B. Sherwin, M. M. Gelfand, W. Brener, Androgen enhances sexual motivation in females: a prospective, crossover study of sex steroid administration in the surgical menopause, *Psychom Med* 1985:47:339.

7. L. Cardozo et al., The effects of subcutaneous hormone implants during climacteric, *Maturitas* 1984:6:177; H. G. Burger et al., The management of persistent menopausal symptoms with oestradiol-testosterone implants: clinical, lipid and hormonal results, *Maturitas* 1984:6:351; B. B. Sherwin, Changes in sexual behavior as a function of plasma sex steroid levels in post-menopausal women, *Maturitas* 1985:7:225.

8. J. Berman, L. Berman, *For Women Only: A Revolutionary Guide to Overcoming Sexual Dysfunction and Reclaiming Your Sex Life* (New York: Henry Holt, 2001).

9. E. L. Vliet, *Screaming to Be Heard: Hormone Connections Women Suspect and Doctors Still Ignore* (New York: M. Evans, 2001).

10. Ibid.

11. Ibid.

Chapter 5: V Smarts

1. M. J. Thornton, Use of vaginal tampons for absorption of menstrual discharges, *Am J Obstet Gynecol* 1943:46:259.

2. Thornton, 1943.

3. M. T. Osterholm, J. P. Davis, R. W. Gibson, et al., Toxic shock syndrome: relation of catamenial products, personal health and hygiene and sexual practices, *Ann Int Med* 1982:96(6):954.

4. A. W. Chow, R. H. See, Microbiology of toxic shock syndrome: overview, *Rev of Infec Diseases* 1989:11(1S):S55.

5. S. M. Garland, M. M. Peel, Tampons and toxic shock syndrome, *Med J Austr* 1995:163(1):8.

6. M. Meadows, Tampon safety, *FDA Consumer,* March–April 2000.

7. E. G. Friedrich, Tampon effects on vaginal health, *Clin Obstet Gynecol* 1981:24(2):395.

8. T. J. Williams, The role of surgery in the management of endometriosis, *Mayo Clinic Proceedings* 1975:50:198; J. C. Weed, J. B. Holland, Endometriosis and infertility: an enigma, *Fertil Steril* 1977:28:135; V. C. Buttram, Conservative surgery for endometriosis in the infertile female: a study of 206 patients with implications for both medical and surgical therapy, *Fertil Steril* 1979:31:177.

9. W. P. Dmowski, E. Radwanska, Current concepts of pathology, histogenesis, and etiology of endometriosis, *Acta Obstet Gynecol Scand Suppl* 1984:123:29.

10. J. A. Sampson, Peritoneal endometriosis due to the menstrual dissemination of endometrial tissue into the peritoneal cavity, *Am J Obstet Gynecol* 1927:14:422.

11. S. L. Darrow, J. E. Vena, R. E. Batt, et al., Menstrual cycle characteristics and the risk of endometriosis, *Epidemiology* 1993:4:135.

12. D. W. Cramer, Epidemiology of endometriosis, in *Endometriosis*, E. A. Wilson, ed. (New York: Alan R. Liss, 1987).

13. R. Dickinson, Tampons as menstrual guards, *JAMA* 1945:128:490.

14. S. J. Emans, E. R. Woods, E. N. Allred, E. Grace, Hymenal findings in adolescent women: impact of tampon use and consensual sexual activity, *J Pediatr* 1994:125:153.

15. M. A. Farage-Elawar, N. A. Enane, S. Baldwin, et al., A clinical method for testing the safety of catamenial pads, *Gynecol Obstet Invest* 1997:44:260.

16. A. M. Geiger, B. Foxman, Risk factors for vulvovaginal candidiasis: a case control study among university students, *Epidemiology* 1996:7:182.

17. S. M. Dawkins, J. M. B. Edwards, R. W. Riddell, Yeasts in the vaginal flora: their incidence and importance, *Lancet* 1953:1230; C. A. Morris, D. F. Morris, Normal vaginal microbiology of women of childbearing age in relation to the use of oral contraceptives and vaginal tampons, *J Clin Pathol* 1967:20:636.

18. B. Watt, M. J. Goldacre, M. Loudon, et al., Prevalence of bacteria in the vagina of normal young women, *Br J Obstet Gynaecol* 1981:88:588.

19. Tampons and pads: should you use what Mom used? *Consumer Reports,* January 1995: 51–55.

20. S. Wysocki, New options in menstrual protection, *Advance for Nurse Practitioners* 1997 Nov:51.

21. R. M. Soderstrom, Latest developments in menstrual protection, *Contemp Ob/Gyn* 1996 Apr:91.

22. Wysocki, New options in menstrual protection.

23. I. A. Elegbe, M. Botu, A preliminary study on dressing patterns and incidence of candidiasis, *Am J Public Health* 1982:72:176.

24. I. A. Elegbe, I. Elegbe, Quantitative relationships of *Candida albicans* infections and dressing patterns in Nigerian women, *Am J Public Health* 1983:73:450.

25. Geiger and Foxman, Risk factors for vulvovaginal candidiasis.

26. A. E. Washington, P. Katz, Cost of and payment source for pelvic inflammatory disease: trends and projections, 1983 through 2000, *JAMA* 1990:263:1936.

27. B. A. Mueller, M. Luz-Jiminez, J. R. Daling, Risk factors for tubal infertility: influence of history of prior pelvic inflammatory disease, *Sex Transm Dis* 1992:19:28.

28. M. J. Rosenberg, R. S. Phillips, Does douching promote ascending infection? *J Reprod Med,* 1992:37(11):930.

29. W. H. Perloff, E. Steinberger, In vivo survival of spermatozoa in cervical mucus, *Am J Obstet Gynecol* 1964:88:439.

30. W. H. Chow, J. R. Daling, N. S. Weiss, et al., Vaginal douching as a potential risk factor for tubal ectopic pregnancy, *Am J Obstet Gynecol* 1985:153:727; J. R. Daling, N. S. Weiss, S. M. Schwartz, et al., Vaginal douching and the risk of tubal pregnancy, *Epidemiology* 1991:2:40; J. M. Chow, M. L. Yonekura, G. A. Richwald, et al., The association between *Chlamydia trachomatis* and ectopic pregnancy, *JAMA* 1990:263:3164.

31. J. S. Kendrick, H. K. Atrash, P. M. Strauss, P. M. Gargiullo, Vaginal douching and risk of ectopic pregnancy among Black women, *Am J Epidemiol* 1995:141:S25 (abstract).

32. R. S Phillips, R. E. Tuomala, P. J. Feldbaum, et al. The effect of cigarette smoking, *Chlamydia trachomatis* infection, and vaginal douching on ectopic pregnancy, *Obstet Gynecol* 1992:79:85.

33. J. Zhang, A. G. Thomas, E. Leybovich, Vaginal douching and adverse health effects: a meta-analysis, *Am J Public Health* 1997:87(7):1207.

34. *FDA Consumer,* Sept. 1996.

Chapter 6: Sex Matters

1. H. S. Kaplan, *The New Sex Therapy* (New York: Brunner/Mazel, 1974).
2. R. Basson, The female sexual response: a different model, *J Sex & Marital Ther* 2000:26:51.
3. R. J. Levin, Sex and the human female reproductive tract—what really happens during and after coitus, *Int J Impotence Research* 1998:1(suppl):S14.
4. W. H. Masters, V. E. Johnson, *Heterosexuality* (New York: HarperCollins, 1994).
5. Ibid.
6. Ibid.
7. W. D. Petok, A practical approach to evaluating female sexual dysfunction, *ObG Management* 1999 Mar:68.
8. Basson, The female sexual response.
9. Masters, *Heterosexuality*.
10. Boston Women's Health Book Collective, *Our Bodies, Ourselves for the New Century* (New York: Touchstone, 1998).
11. E. Grafenberg, The role of the urethra in female orgasm, *Int J Sexol* 1950:3:145; H. Alzate, Vaginal eroticism: a replication study, *Arch Sex Behav* 1985:14:529; J. K. Davidson, C. A. Darling, C. Conway-Welch, The role of the Grafenberg spot and female ejaculation in female orgasmic response: an empirical analysis, *J Sex Marital Ther* 1989:15:102; M. Zaviacic, A. Zaviacicova, I. K. Holoman, J. Molcan, Female urethral expulsions evoked by local digital stimulation of the G spot: differences in the response patterns, *J Sex Res* 1988:24:311.
12. J. D. Perry, B. Whipple, Pelvic muscle strength of female ejaculators: evidence in support of a new theory of orgasm, *J Sex Res* 1981:17:22.
13. J. Berman, L. Berman, *For Women Only: A Revolutionary Guide to Overcoming Sexual Dysfunction and Reclaiming Your Sex Life* (New York: Henry Holt and Company, 2001).
14. Ibid.
15. Boston Women's Health Book Collective, *Our Bodies, Ourselves for the New Century*.
16. R. M. Moglia, J. Knowles, eds., *All About Sex: A Family Resource on Sex and Sexuality* (New York: Three Rivers Press, 1997).
17. B. R. Komisaruk, B. Whipple, The suppression of pain by genital stimulation in females, *Ann Rev Sex Research* 1995(6):151.
18. D. Symons, *The Evolution of Human Sexuality* (New York: Oxford University Press, 1979), 75; A. C. Kinsey, *Sexual Behavior in the Human Female* (Philadelphia: W. B. Saunders, 1953); S. Hite, *The Hite Report on Female Sexuality* (New York: Macmillan, 1976).
19. R. P. Maines, *The Technology of Orgasm* (Baltimore: The Johns Hopkins University Press, 1999), 1–8.
20. E. Bergler, W. S. Kroger, *Kinsey's Myth of Female Sexuality* (New York: Grune and Stratton, 1954), 7, 35, 70, 76.
21. S. D. Cochran, V. M. Mays, Sex, lies and HIV, *N Engl J Med* 1990:48:384.
22. Moglia and Knowles, *All About Sex*.
23. W. Leary, Female condom approved for market, *New York Times,* May 11, 1993, C5.
24. Moglia and Knowles, *All About Sex*.
25. J. D. Forrest, Timing of reproductive life stages, *Obstet Gynecol* 1993:82:105.
26. L. J. Piccinino, W. D. Mosher, Trends in contraception use in the United States: 1982–1995, *Fam Plann Perspect* 1998:30:24.
27. S. K. Henshaw, Unintended pregnancy in the United States, *Fam Plann Perspect* 1998:30:24.
28. L. M. Koonin, J. C. Smith, M. Ramick, et al., Abortion surveillance—United States, 1995, *MMWR* 1998:47:31.
29. S. Harlap, K. Kost, J. D. Forrest, *Preventing Pregnancy, Protecting Health: A New Look at Birth Control Choices in the United States* (New York: Alan Guttmacher Institute, 1991).

Chapter 7: The Most Bothersome Symptoms

1. W. Montagna, P. Parakkal, *Structure and Function of Skin* (New York: Academic Press, 1974).
2. K. Lidell, Smell as a diagnostic marker, *Postgrad Med J* 1976:52:136.
3. G. Ohloff, Recent developments in the field of naturally occurring aroma components, in W. Herz, H. Grisebach, and G. W. Kirby, eds., *Progress in the Chemistry of Organic Natural Products* (New York: Springer-Verlag, 1978), 431.
4. J. G. Kostelc, G. Preti, P. R. Zelson, et al., Salivary volatiles as indicators of periodontitis, *J Periodical Res* 1980:15:185; A. Zlatkis, H. M. Liebich, Profile of volatile metabolites in human urine, *Anal Chem* 1971:17:592.
5. R. F. Curtis, J. A. Ballantine, E. B. Keverne, et al., Identification of primate sexual pheromones and the properties of synthetic attractants, *Nature* 1971:232:396; G. Preti, G. R. Huggins, J. Bares, Analysis of human vaginal secretions by gas chromatography–mass spectrometry, *Isr Chem* 1978:17:215.
6. G. Preti, G. R. Huggins, Organic constituents of vaginal secretions, in E. S. E. Hafez, T. N. Evans, eds., *The Human Vagina* (New York: Elsevier/North Holland, 1978).
7. G. Preti, G. R. Huggins, H. J. Lawley, L. Schmidt, Monell Chemical Senses Center, unpublished results, 1980.
8. D. M. Mulherin, T. P. Sheeran, D. S. Kumararatne, et al., Sjögren's syndrome and other autoimmune diseases, *Arthritis Rheumatol* 1994:37:465.

Chapter 8: Now What?

1. J. T. Allen-Davis, Why we can't diagnose based on symptoms alone, *OBG Management*, 1998 November suppl:2–5.

Chapter 9: The Ideal V Exam

1. S. L. Hillier, Improving the diagnosis of vaginal complaints, *OBG Management*, 1998 November suppl:6–11.
2. C. Northrup, *Women's Bodies, Women's Wisdom* (New York: Bantam, 1998), 283.
3. J. N. Kreiger, M. R. Tam, C. E. Stevens, et al., Diagnosis of trichomoniasis: comparison of conventional wet-mount examination with cytologic studies, cultures and monoclonal antibody staining of direct specimens, *JAMA* 1988:259:1223–27.
4. D. S. Guzick, Efficacy of screening for cervical cancer: a review, *Am J Public Health* 1978:68:125.
5. H. J. Soost, H. J. Lange, W. Lehmacher, B. Ruffling-Kullmann, The validation of cervical cytology: sensitivity, specificity, and predictive values, *Acta Cytologica* 1991:35:8.
6. M. T. Fahey, L. Irwig, P. Macaskill, Meta-analysis of Pap test accuracy, *Am J Epidemiol* 1995:141:680; K. Nanda, D. C. McCrory, E. R. Myers, et al., Accuracy of the Papanicolaou test in screening for and follow-up of cervical cytologic abnormalities: a systematic review, *Ann Intern Med* 2000:132:810.
7. K. D. Hatch, N. F. Hacker, Intraepithelial disease of the cervix, vagina, and vulva, in *Novak's Gynecology*, J. S. Berek, E. Y. Adashi, P. A. Hillard, eds. (Baltimore: Williams & Wilkins, 1996), 447.
8. N. August, Cervicography for evaluating the "atypical" Papanicolaou smear, *J Reprod Med* 1991:36:89.
9. Northrup, *Women's Bodies, Women's Wisdom*.
10. D. E. D. Jones, W. T. Creasman, R. A. Dombroski, et al., Evaluation of the atypical Pap smear, *Am J Obstet Gynecol* 1987:157:544.
11. M. Borst, C. E. Butterworth, V. Baker, et al., Screening for women with atypical Pap smears, *J Reprod Med* 1991:36:95.
12. B. B. Bennett, K. Takezawa, E. J. Wilkinson, et al., Atypical glandular cells of undetermined significance and other glandular abnormalities in a high risk population, *J Lower Genit Tract Dis* 1998:2(3):132; G. Eddy, B. Strumpf, E. Wljtowycz, C. T. Pirano, M. T. Mazur, Biopsy findings in five hundred thirty-one patients with atypi-

cal glandular cells of uncertain significance as defined by the Bethesda system, *Am J Obstet Gynecol* 1997:177(5):1188.

13. J. S. Noumoff, Atypia in cervical cytology as a risk factor for intraepithelial neoplasia, *Am J Obstet Gynecol* 1987:156:628.

14. G. J. van Oortmarssen, J. D. F. Habbema, Epidemiologic evidence for age-dependent regression of preinvasive cervical cancer, *Br J Cancer* 1991:64:559.

15. Hatch, Intraepithelial disease of the cervix, vagina, and vulva.

16. K. Naisell, V. Roger, M. Nasiell, Behavior of mild cervical dysplasia during long-term follow-up, *Obstet Gynecol* 1986:5:665.

17. K. Syrjanen, V. Kataja, M. Yliskoski, et al., Natural history of cervical human papillomavirus lesions does not substantiate the biologic relevance of the Bethesda system, *Obstet Gynecol* 1992:79:675–821

18. Hatch, Intraepithelial disease of the cervix, vagina, and vulva.

Chapter 10: Yeast Infections

1. D. G. Ferris, J. Hendrich, P. M. Payne, et al., Office laboratory diagnosis of vaginitis: clinician-performed tests compared with a rapid nucleic acid hybridization test, *J Fam Pract* 1995:31(6):575–81.

2. R. Hurley, Recurrent *Candida* infection, *Clin Obstet Gynecol* 1981:8:209–13.

3. F. C. Odds, *Candida and Candidosis* (London: Balliere Tindall, 1988).

4. R. Skowronski, D. Feldman, Characterisaton of an estrogen binding protein in the yeast *Candida albicans, Endocrinology* 1989:124:1965–72; B. L. Powell, D. I. Druta, Estrogen receptor in *Candida albicans:* a possible explanation for hormonal influences in vaginal candidiasis, in *Program and Abstracts of the 23rd Annual Interscience Conference on Antimicrobial Agents and Chemotherapy* (Washington, D.C.: American Society for Microbiology, 1983), abstr. 751, 222.

5. O. S. Kinsman, K. Pitblado, C. J. Coulson, Effect of mammalian steroid hormones and luteinising hormone on the germination of *Candida albicans* and implications for vaginal candidiasis, *Mycoses* 1988:31:617–26.

6. J. D. Sobel, A comprehensive strategy for managing recurrent VVC, *ObG Management* 1998 Aug:suppl:14.

7. A. J. E. Barlow, T. Aldersley, F. W. Chattaway, Factors present in serum and seminal plasma which promote germ-tube formation and mycelial growth of *Candida albicans, J Gen Microbiol* 1974:82:261.

8. J. D. Sobel, G. Muller, H. R. Buckley, Critical role of germ tube formation in the pathogenesis of candidal vaginitis, *Infect Immun* 1984:576.

9. S. S. Witkin, Failure of sperm-induced immunosuppression: association with anti-sperm antibodies in women, *Am J Obstet Gynecol* 1989:68:696.

10. L. J. Douglas, Mannoprotein adhesions of *Candida albicans,* in *New Strategies in Fungal Diseases*, J. E. Bennett, R. J. Hay, P. K. Peterson, eds. (Edinburgh: Churchill Livingstone, 1992), 34–53.

11. N. Friedreich, Uber das constante vorkommen von plezen bei diabetischen, *Arch Pathol Anat Physiol Virchow* 1864:30:477.

12. J. D. Sobel, Recurrent candidiasis and "malcarbohydrate metabolism," *Am J Obstet Gynecol* 1998:179(2):557–58.

13. J. D. Sobel, P. G. Myers, D. Kaye, et al., Adherence of *Candida albicans* to human vaginal and buccal epithelial cells, *J Infect Dis* 1981:143:76.

14. B. J. Horowitz, S. W. Edelstein, L. Lippman, Sugar chromatography studies in recurrent *Candida* vulvovaginitis, *J Reprod Med* 1984:29(7):441–43.

15. W. G. Crook, *The Yeast Connection,* 3rd ed. (Jackson, Tenn.: Professional Books, 1986).

16. B. B. Jorgensen, Bakers yeast allergy in candidiasis patients, *J Adv Med* 1994:7(1):43.

17. J. D. Sobel, Epidemiology and pathogenesis of recurrent vulvovaginal candidiasis, *Am J Obstet Gynecol* 1985:152:924.

18. J. E. Edwards Jr., *Candida* species, in *Principles and Practices of Infectious Diseases,* 3rd ed., G. L. Mandell, R. G. Douglas, J. E. Bennett, eds. (New York: Churchill Livingstone, 1990), 1943–48.

19. A. Spinillo, E. Capuzzo, S. Acciano, et al., Effect of antibiotic use on the prevalence of symptomatic vulvovaginal candidiasis, *Am J Obstet Gynecol* 1999:180:14.

20. B. Foxman, The epidemiology of vulvovaginal candidiasis: risk factors, *AJPH* 1990:80(3):329–31.

21. H. C. Gugnani, F. K. Nzelibe, P. C. Gini, et al., Incidence of yeasts in pregnant and nonpregnant women in Nigeria, *Mycoses* 1987:32:131–34; C. J. Carroll, R. Hurley, V. D. Stanley, Criteria for diagnosis of *Candida* vulvovaginitis in pregnant women, *J Obstet Gynecol* 1973:80:258–61.

22. V. K. Hopsu-Havu, M. Gronroos, and R. Punnonen, Vaginal yeasts in parturients and infestation of the newborns, *Acta Obstet Gynecol Scand* 1980:59:73–77; B. D. Reed, W. Huck, and P. Zazove, Differentiation of *Gardnerella vaginalis, Candida albicans*, and *Trichomonas vaginalis* infections of the vagina, *J Fam Pract* 1989:28:304–7.

23. B. L. Powell, D. I. Druta, Estrogen receptor in *Candida albicans:* a possible explanation for hormonal influences in vaginal candidiasis, abstr. 751, 222. In: Program and abstracts of the 23rd Annual Interscience Conference on Antimicrobial Agents and Chemotherapy, Washington, D.C.: American Society for Microbiology, 1983; O. S. Kinsman, K. Pitblado, C. J. Coulson, Effect of mammalian steroid hormones and luteinizing hormone on the germination of *Candida albicans* and implication for vaginal candidiasis, *Mycoses* 1988:31:617–26.

24. F. Davidson, J. K. Oates, The pill does not cause "thrush," *Brit J Obstet Gynaecol* 1985:90:374–81; Foxman, The epidemiology of vulvovaginal candidiasis.

25. A. M. Geiger, B. Foxman, Risk factors for vulvovaginal candidiasis: a case-control study among university students, *Epidemiology* 1996:7(2):182–87; A. Spinillo, F. Capuzzo, S. Nicola, et al., The impact of oral contraception on vulvovaginal candidiasis, *Contraception* 1995:51:293–97.

26. B. D. Reed, Risk factors for candida vulvovaginitis, *Obstet Gynecol Survey* 1992:47(8):551–60.

27. J. D. Sobel, A comprehensive strategy for managing recurrent VVC, *ObG Management* 1998 Aug (suppl):15.

28. W. Chaim, B. Foxman, J. D. Sobel, Association of recurrent vaginal candidiasis and secretory Abo and Lewis phenotype, *J Infect Dis* 1997:76:828–36.

29. I. W. Fong, P. McCleary, Cellular immunity of patients with recurrent or refractory vulvovaginal moniliasis, *Am J Obstet Gynecol* 1992:166:887.

30. S. S. Witkin, J. Hirsch, W. J. Ledger, A macrophage defect in women with recurrent *Candida* vaginitis and its correction in vitro by prostaglandin inhibitors, *Am J Obstet Gynecol* 1983:155:790.

31. S. S. Witkin, A. Kalo-Kelin, L. Galland, et al., Effect of *Candida albicans* plus histamine on prostaglandin E2 production by peripheral blood mononuclear cells from healthy women and women with recurrent candidal vaginitis, *J Infect Dis* 1991:164:396.

32. M. Crandall, Allergic predisposition in recurrent vulvovaginal candidiasis, *J Adv Med* 1991:4(1):21.

33. N. Rosedale, K. Browne, Hyposensitisation in the management of recurring vaginal candidiasis, *Ann Allergy* 1979:43:250; D. Rigg, M. M. Miller, W. J. Metzger, Recurrent allergic vulvovaginitis: treatment with *Candida albicans* allergen immunotherapy, *Am J Obstet Gynecol* 1990:162:332.

34. S. L. Hillier, address sponsored by 3M Pharmaceuticals, April 24, 2001, Boston.

35. R. Chaponis, P. Bresnick, R. Weiss, et al., *Candida* vaginitis: signs and symptoms aid women's self-recognition, *J Clin Res Drug Dev* 1993:7:17–23.

36. P. Nyirjesy, M. V. Weitz, M. H. Grody, et al., Over-the-counter and alternative medicines in the treatment of chronic vaginal symptoms, *Obstet Gynecol* 1997:90(1):50–53.

37. D. G. Ferris, C. Dekle, M. S. Litaker, Women's use of over-the-counter antifungal medications for gynecologic symptoms, *J Fam Pract* 1996:42(6):595–600.

38. M. I. O'Conner, J. D. Sobel, Epidemiology of recurrent vulvovaginal candidiasis: identification and strain differentiation of *Candida albicans*, *J Infect Dis* 1986:154:358–63.

39. Sobel, A comprehensive strategy for managing recurrent VVC.

40. Ibid.

41. R. Javanovic, E. Congema, H. T. Nguyen, Antifungal agents vs. boric acid for treating chronic mycotic vulvovaginitis, *J Repro Med* 1991:36(8):593.

42. M. C. Maberry, Vulvovaginitis, in *Conn's Current Therapy*, R. E. Rakel, ed. (Philadelphia: W. B. Saunders, 1991).

43. K. K. Van Slyke, V. P. Michel, M. F. Rein, Treatment of vulvovaginal candidiasis with boric acid powder, *Am J Obstet Gynecol* 1981:141:145.

44. D. Rigg, M. M. Miller, W. J. Metzger, Recurrent allergic vulvovaginitis: treatment with *Candida albicans* allergen immunotherapy, *Am J Obstet Gynecol* 1990:162:332.

45. S. Vilupillai, R. N. Thin, Treatment of vulvovaginal yeast infection with Nystatin, *Practitioner* 1977:219:897–901.

Chapter 11: BV

1. D. J. Lash, A. G. Tagumpay, Diagnosis and treatment of vaginitis, *The Female Patient* 1998 May:23:73–93.

2. J. Sobel, Bacterial vaginosis: therapeutic dilemmas, *Infect in Med* 1990:5:24–30.

3. Ibid.

4. H. L. Gardner, C. D. Dukes, *Haemophilus vaginalis* vaginitis: a newly defined specific infection previously classified "nonspecific" vaginitis, *Am J Obstet Gynecol* 1955:69:962.

5. Sobel, Bacterial vaginosis.

6. S. J. Klebanoff, S. L. Hillier, D. A. Eschenbach, et al., Control of the microbial flora of the vagina by H_2O_2-generating lactobacilli, *J Infect Dis* 1991:164:94–100.

7. D. A. Eschenbach, Bacterial vaginosis: emphasis on upper genital tract complications, *Obstet Gynecol Clin North Am* 1989:16:593–610.

8. D. Avonts, M. Sercu, P. Heyerick, et al., Incidence of uncomplicated genital infections in women using oral contraception or an intrauterine device: a prospective study, *Sex Transm Dis* 1990:17:23.

9. L. V. H. Hill, J. A. Embil, Vaginitis: current microbiologic and clinical concepts, *Can Med Assoc J* 1986:134:321–31.

10. S. E. Hawes, S. L. Hillier, J. Benedetti, et al., Hydrogen peroxide–producing lactobacilli and acquisition of vaginal infection, *J Infect Dis* 1996:174:1058–63.

11. S. L. Hillier, The prevalence of bacterial vaginosis in sexually inexperienced women, sexually inactive women and women having one or more sexual partners, paper presented at the Infectious Diseases Society of Obstetrics and Gynecology Annual Scientific Meeting, August 5–8, 1998; R. C. Bump, W. J. Buesching, Bacterial vaginosis in virginal and sexually active females: evidence against exclusive sexual transmission, *Am J Obstet Gynecol* 1988:158:935–39.

12. M. Haukkamaa, P. Stranden, H. Jousimses-Somer, et al., Bacterial flora of the cervix in women using different methods of contraception, *Am J Obstet Gynecol* 1986:154:520–24.

13. J. L. Thomason, S. M. Gelbert, L. M. Wilcoski, et al., Proline aminopeptidase activity as a rapid diagnostic test to confirm bacterial vaginosis, *Obstet Gynecol* 1988:171:607–11.

14. P. Meis, R. Goldenberg, J. Iams, et al., Vaginal infections and spontaneous preterm birth, *Am J Obstet Gynecol* 1995:172:410.

15. C. Stevens-Simon, J. Jamison, J. A. McGregor, J. M. Douglas, Racial variation in vaginal pH among healthy sexually active adolescents, *Sex Trans Dis* 1994:21:168–72.

16. Hawes et al., Hydrogen peroxide–producing lactobacilli.

17. G. H. Eltabbakh, G. D. Eltabbakh, F. F. Broekhuizen, et al., Value of wet mount and cervical cultures at the time of cervical cytology in asymptomatic women, *Obstet Gynecol* 1995:85:499–503; M. A. Byrne, M. J. Turner, M. Griffiths, et al., Evidence that patients presenting with dyskaryotic cervical smears should be screened for genital-tract infections other than human papillomavirus infection, *Eur J Obstet Gynecol Reprod Biol* 1991:41:129–33.

18. J. Paavonen, K. Teisala, P. K. Heinonen, et al., Microbiological and histopathological findings in acute pelvic inflammatory disease, *Br J Obstet Gynaecol* 1987:94:454–60; S. Faro, M. Martens, M. Macato, et al., Vaginal flora and pelvic inflammatory disease, *Am J Obstet Gynecol* 1993:169(2S):470–74.

19. M. G. Gravett, D. Hammel, D. A. Eschenbach, et al., Preterm labor associated with subclinical amniotic fluid infection with bacterial vaginosis, *Obstet Gynecol* 1986:67:229–37; J. Martius, M. A. Krohn, S. L. Hillier, et al., Relationships of vaginal *Lactobacillus* species, cervical chlamydia trachomatis, and bacterial vaginosis to preterm birth, *Obstet Gynecol* 1988:76:89–95; T. Kurki, A. Sivonen, O. V. Renkonen, et al., Bacterial vaginosis in early pregnancy and pregnancy outcome, *Obstet Gynecol* 1992:80:173–77.

20. J. A. McGregor, D. Lawellin, A. Franco-Buff, et al., Protease production by microorganisms associated with reproductive tract infection, *Am J Obstet Gynecol* 1986:154:109–14.

21. W. J. Morales, S. Schorr, J. Albritton, Effect of metronidazole in patients with preterm birth in preceding pregnancy and bacterial vaginosis: a placebo-controlled, double-blind study, *Am J Obstet Gynecol* 1994:171(2):345–47; J. C. Hauth, R. L. Goldenberg, W. W. Andrews, M. B. Dubard, et al., Reduced incidence of preterm delivery with metronidazole and erythromycin in women with bacterial vaginosis, *N Engl J Med* 1995:333(26):1732–36.

22. H. M. McDonald, J. A. O'Loughlin, R. Vigeswaran, et al., Impact of metronidazole therapy on preterm birth in women with bacterial vaginosis flora *(Gardnerella vaginalis):* a randomised, placebo-controlled trial, *Br J Obstet Gynaecol* 1997:104(12):1338–40.

23. M. R. Joesoef, S. L. Hillier, G. Wiknjosastro, H. Sumampouw, et al., Intravaginal clindamycin treatment for bacterial vaginosis: effects on preterm delivery and low birth weight, *Am J Obstet Gynecol* 1995:173(5):1527–31; J. A. McGregor, J. I. French, W. Jones, et al., Bacterial vaginosis is associated with prematurity and vaginal fluid mucinase and sialidase: results of a controlled trial of topical clindamycin cream, *Am J Obstet Gynecol* 1994:170(4):1048–59.

24. J. Swedberg, J. F. Steiner, F. Deiss, et al., Comparison of single-dose vs. one-week course of metronidazole for symptomatic bacterial vaginosis, *JAMA* 1985:254:1046.

25. Sobel, Bacterial vaginosis.

26. S. L. Hillier, address sponsored by 3M Pharmaceuticals, February 1999, Boston.

27. Ibid.

28. Ibid.

29. P. Burtin, A. Taddio, O. Ariburnu, et al., Safety of metronidazole in pregnancy: a meta-analysis, *Am J Obstet Gynecol* 1995:172:525–29.

30. Joesoef et al., Intravaginal clindamycin cream.

31. Hillier, 1999 address.

Chapter 12: Trich

1. F. G. Bowden, G. P. Garnett, *Trichomonas vaginalis* epidemiology: parameterising and analysing a model of treatment interventions, *Sexually Transmitted Infections* 2000:76(4):248.

2. H. L. Kent, Epidemiology of vaginitis, *Am J Obstet Gynecol* 1991:165(4):1168–79.

3. A. Donne, Animacules observés dans les matières purulentes et le produit des secretions des organes genitaux de l'homme et de la femme, *C R Acad Sci* (III) 1836:3:385–86.

4. O. Hoehne, *Trichomonas vaginalis* als haufiger erregar einer typischen colpitis prurlenta, *Zentralbl Gynakol* 1916:40:4–14; G. Johnson, R. E. Trussell, Experimental basis for the chemotherapy of *Trichomonas vaginalis*, *Proc Soc Exp Biol Med* 1943:54:245–49.

5. C. Cosar, L. Julou, Activité de l'(hydroxy-2-ethyl)-1-methyl-2-nitro-5-imidazole (R.P. 8823) vis-à-vis des infections experimentales a *Trichomonas vaginalis*, *Ann Inst Pasteur Microbiol* 1959:96:238–41.

6. R. A. Underhill, J. Peck, Causes of therapy failure after treatment of *T. vaginalis*, *Br J Clin Pract* 1974:28:134.

7. M. F. Rein, M. Muller, *Trichomonas vaginalis*, in *Sexually Transmitted Diseases*, K. K. Holmes, P.-A. Mardh, P. F. Sparling, P. J. Weisner, eds. (New York: McGraw-Hill, 1984), 525–36.

8. D. A. Eschenbach, Vaginal infection, *Clin Obstet Gynecol* 1983:26:186–202.

9. L. G. Keith, J. Friberg, N. Fullan, G. S. Berger, The possible role of *Trichomonas vaginalis* as a vector for the spread of other pathogens, *Int J Fertil* 1986:31:272–77.

10. M. R. Spence, Trichomoniasis, *Contemp Ob/Gyn* 1992 Nov:132–41.

11. A. Fouts, S. Kraus, *Trichomonas vaginalis:* re-evaluation of its clinical presentation and laboratory diagnosis, *J Infect Dis* 1980:141:137–43.

12. J. G. Lossick, Treatment of *Trichomonas vaginalis* infections, *Rev Infect Dis* 1982:4(suppl):801–18.

13. C. H. Livengood, J. G. Lossick, Resolution of resistant vaginal trichomonas associated with the use of intravaginal nonoxynol-9, *Obstet Gynecol* 1991:78:954–56.

14. CDC, Sexually transmitted disease treatment guidelines, *MMWR* 1997:46:72–73.

15. B. D. Reed, A. Eyler, Vaginal infections: diagnosis and management, *Am Fam Phys* 1993:47(8):1805–16.

16. CDC, Sexually transmitted disease treatment guidelines.

Chapter 13: Vag Itch, Continued

1. M. K. Beard, Atrophic vaginitis: can it be prevented as well as treated? *Postgrad Med* 1992:91:257–60.

2. A. Miodrag, P. Ekelund, R. Burton, C. M. Castleden, Tamoxifen and partial oestrogen agonism in postmenopausal women, *Age and Ageing* 1991:20:52–54.

3. Ibid.

4. M. Taylor, Alternatives to conventional hormone replacement, *Menopausal Medicine* 1998:6:1–6.

5. S. R. Davis, A. L. Murkies, G. Wilcox, Phytoestrogens in clinical practice, *Int Med* 1998:1:27–34.

6. M. C. Roberts, S. L. Hillier, F. D. Schoenknecht, et al., Comparison of gram stain, DNA probe, and culture for the identification of species of *Mobiluncus* in female genital secretions, *J Infect Dis* 1985:152:74.

7. J. L. Thomason, P. C. Schreckenberger, W. N. Spellacy, et al., Clinical and microbiological characterization of patients with nonspecific vaginosis associated with mobile, curved anaerobic rods, *J Infect Dis* 1983:148:817.

8. Ibid.

9. J. K. Oates, D. Rowen, Desquamative inflammatory vaginitis: a review, *Genitourin Med* 1990:66:725–29; L. A. Gray, M. L. Barnes, Vaginitis in women: diagnosis and treatment, *Am J Obstet Gynecol* 1965:92:125–27; H. L. Gardner, Desquamative inflammatory vaginitis: a newly defined entity, *Am J Obstet Gynecol* 1968:102:1102–5.

10. P. Lynch, Desquamative inflammatory vaginitis with oral lichen planus, presented at Second International Congress of the International Society for the Study of Vulvar Disease (Key Biscayne, Florida), E. G. Friedrich, W. E. Josey, eds.; M. Pelisse, D. Leibowitch, D. Sedel, J. Hewitt, Un nouveau syndrome vulvo-vagino-gingival: lichen plan erosive pluriuqueux, *Acta Derm Venereol* (Paris) 1982:109:797–98; J. Hewitt, M. Pelisse, D. Lessan-Leibowitch, D. Sedel, et al., Le syndrome vulvo-vaginal-gingival, *Rev Stomatol Chir Maxillofac* 1985:86:57–65; L. Edwards, E. G. Friedrich Jr., Desquamative vaginitis: lichen planus in disguise, *Obstet Gynecol* 1988:71:832–36.

11. J. D. Sobel, Desquamative inflammatory vaginitis: a new subgroup of purulent vaginitis responsive to topical 2% clindamycin therapy, *Obstet Gynecol* 1994:171(5):1215–20.

12. L. J. Cibley, L. J. Cibley, Cytolytic vaginosis, *Am J Obstet Gynecol* 1991:165:1245–49.

13. C. Marty-Taysset, F. de la Torre, J. Garel, Increased production of hydrogen peroxide by lactobacillus delbruecki subspecies bulgaricus upon aeration: involvement of an NADH oxidase in oxidative stress, *Applied and Environmental Microbiology* 2000(Jan): 66(1):262.

Chapter 14: Could You Be Allergic?

1. J. V. Bosso, M. J. Aiken, R. A. Simon, Successful prevention of local and cutaneous hypersensitivity reactions to seminal fluid with intravaginal cromolyn, *Allergy Proc* 1991:12(2):113–16.

2. I. L. Bernstein, B. E. Englander, J. S. Gallagher, P. Nathan, et al., Localized and systemic hypersensitivity reactions to human seminal fluid, *Ann Int Med* 1981:94(1):459–65; S. A. Friedman, I. L. Bernstein, M. Enrione, Z. H. Marcus, Successful long-term immunotherapy for human seminal plasma anaphylaxis, *JAMA* 1984:251(20):2684–87.

3. W. R. Jones, Allergy to coitus, *Aust NZ J Obstet Gynaecol* 1991:31:137–41.

4. J. A. Bernstein, R. Sugumaran, D. I. Bernstein, I. L. Bernstein, Prevalence of human seminal plasma hypersensitivity among symptomatic women, *Ann Allergy* 1997:78:54–58.

5. Jones, Allergy to coitus.

6. Ibid.

7. Ibid.

8. M. H. Goldenhersh, A. Saxon, Seminal fluid hypersensitivity (SFH): a new approach (abstract), *Ann Allergy* 1989:6:256.

9. B. N. Halpern, T. Ky, B. Robert, Clinical and immunological study of exceptional case of reaginic type sensitization to human seminal fluid, *Immunology* 1967:12:247; S. M. Matloff, Local intravaginal desensitization to seminal fluid, *J Allergy Clin Immunol* 1993:91:1230–31; Bernstein et al., Prevalence of human seminal plasma hypersensitivity.

10. M. B. Sell, Sensitisation to thioridazine through sexual intercourse, *Am J Psych* 1985:142:271–72; W. J. Paladine, T. J. Cunningham, M. A. Donovan, Possible sen sitivity to vinblastine in prostatic or seminal fluid, *N Engl J Med* 1975:29:52; R. L. Green, M. H. Green, Postcoital urticaria in a penicillin sensitive patient, *JAMA Assoc* 1985:254:531; Z. H. Haddad, Food allergens, *Persp Allergy* 1978:1:2–3.

11. B. H. Berman, Seasonal allergic vulvovaginitis caused by pollen, *Ann Allergy* 1964:22:594–97.

12. S. S. Witkin, J. Jeremias, Q. J. Ledger, A localized vaginal allergic response in women with recurrent vaginitis, *J Allerg Clin Immunol* 1989:81:412–16.

13. A. Nel, C. Gujuluva, Latex antigens: identification and use in clinical and experimental studies, including crossreactivity with food and pollen allergens, *Ann Allergy* 1998:81:388–98.

14. C. Perniciaro, S. Alberto, J. Busamante, M. Gutierrez, Two cases of vulvodynia with unusual causes, *Acta Derm Venereol* (Stockholm) 1993:73:227–28.

Chapter 15: When Skin Gets Sick

1. P. J. Lynch, *Dermatology* (Baltimore: Williams & Wilkins, 1994), 305.

2. P. Marren, F. Wojnarowska, Allergic contact dermatitis and vulvar dermatoses, *Br J Dermatol* 1992:126:52.

3. Marren, *Br J Dermatol.*

4. Lynch, *Dermatology,* 46.

5. C. M. Ridley, Lichen sclerosus: a review, *Eur J Dermatol* 1994:4:99.

6. C. M. Ridley, S. M. Neill, Non-infective cutaneous conditions of the vulva, in *The Vulva,* C. M. Ridley, S. M. Neill, eds. (Oxford, England: Blackwell Science, 1999),157.

7. R. H. Meyrick-Thomas, C. M. Ridley, D. H. McGibbon, et al., Lichen sclerosus et atrophicus and autoimmunity—a study of 350 women, *Br J Dermatol* 1988:108:41.

8. Ridley, Lichen sclerosus: a review.

9. R. C. D. Staughton, E. B. Lane, et al., The cytokeratin profile of normal vulval epithelium and vulval lichen sclerosus, *Br J Dermatol* 1990:123(suppl 37):62; S. H. Tan, E. Derrick, P. H. McKee, et al., Altered p53 expression and epidermal proliferation is seen in vulval lichen sclerosus, *J Cutan Path* 1994:21:316; Y. Soini, P. Paako, K. Vahkangas, S. Vuopala, V. P. Lehto, Expression of p53 and proliferating cell nu-

clear antigen in lichen sclerosus et atrophicus with different histological features, *Int J Gyn Path* 1994:13:199.

10. P. Carli, A. Cattaneo, N. Pimpinelli, et al., Immunohistochemical evidence of skin immune system involvement in vulvar lichen sclerosus and atrophicus, *Dermatologica* 1991:182:18; P. M. Marren, P. R. Millard, F. Wojnarowska, Vulval lichen sclerosus: lack of correlation between duration of clinical symptoms and histological appearances, *J Eur Acad Dermatol Vener* 1997:8:212.

11 K. I. Dalziel, P. R. Millard, F. Wojnarowska, The treatment of vulvar lichen sclerosus with a very potent topical steroid, *Br J Derm* 1991:124:461.

12. K. I. Dalziel, F. Wojnarowska, Long term control of vulvar lichen sclerosus after treatment with a potent topical steroid cream, *J Repro Med* 1993:38:25.

13. G. L. Bracco, P. Carli, L. Sonni, et al., Clinical and histologic effects of topical treatments of vulvar lichen sclerosus, *J Repro Med* 1993:38:37.

14. J. J. Powell, F. Wojnarowska, Lichen sclerosus, *Lancet* 1999:22(353):9166.

15. Ridley, Neill, Non-infective cutaneous conditions of the vulva.

16. M. Sideri, M. Origoni, L. Spinaci, A. Ferrari, Topical testosterone in the treatment of vulvar lichen sclerosus, *Int J Gynecol Obstet* 1994:46:53.

17. M. T. Bousema, U. Romppanen, J. M. Geiger, et al., Acitretinin in the treatment of severe lichen sclerosus et atrophicus of the vulva: a double-blind placebo controlled study, *J Am Acad Dermatol* 1994:30:225.

18. A. Virgili, M. Corazzo, A. Bianchi, et al., Open study of topical 0.025% tretinoin in the treatment of vulvar lichen sclerosus, *J Reprod Med* 1995:40:614.

19. M. Kartamaa, S. Reitamo, Treatment of lichen sclerosus with carbon dioxide laser vaporization, *Br J Dermatol* 1997:135:356.

20. M. McKay, Vulvar dermatoses, *Clin Obstet Gynecol* 1991:34:614.

21. S. Zellis, S. H. Pincus, Treatment of vulvar dermatoses, *Sem Dermatol* 1996:15(1):71.

22. Ridley, Neill, Non-infective cutaneous conditions of the vulva.

23. E. M. De Jong, The course of psoriasis, *Clin Dermatol* 1997:15:687.

24. M. D. Zanolli, Psoriasis and Reiter's syndrome, in *Principles and Practice of Dermatology*, 2nd ed., W. W. Sams, P. J. Lynch, eds. (New York: Churchill Livingstone, 1996).

25. N. Han, P. Nowakowski, D. West, Common skin disorders: acne and psoriasis, in *Pharmacotherapy: A Pathophysiologic Approach*, J. DiPiro, R. L. Talbert, G. C. Yee, et al., eds. (Stamford, Conn.: Appleton & Lange, 1999), 1489.

26. E. Bardolph, R. Ashton, Psoriasis: a review of present and future management, *Nurs Stand* 1998:12:43.

27. H. Tagami, Triggering factors, *Clin Dermatol* 1997:15:677.

28. J. P. Ortonne, Aetiology and pathogenesis of psoriasis, *Br J Dermatol* 1996:135(suppl 49):1.

29. B. P. Peters, F. G. Weissman, M. A. Gill, Pathophysiology and treatment of psoriasis, *Am J Health-Syst Pharm* 2000:57(7):645.

30. Ibid.

31. J. P. Ortonne, Aetiology and pathogenesis of psoriasis, *Br J Dermatol* 1996:135(suppl 49):1.

32. B. J. Nickoloff, The immunologic and genetic basis of psoriasis, *Arch Dermatol* 1999:135:1104.

33. K. Kragballe, B. T. Gjertsen, D. D. Hoop, et al., Double-blind right/left comparison of calcipotriol and betamethasone 17-valerate in patients with psoriasis vulgaris, *Lancet* 1991:337:193.

34. G. S. Drew, Psoriasis, *Primary Care* 2000:27(2):385; European FK506 Multicenter Psoriasis Study Group, Systemic tacrolimus (FK506) is effective for treatment of psoriasis in a double-blind, placebo-controlled study, *Arch Dermatol* 1996:132:419.

35. C. Scully, M. el-Kom, Lichen planus: review and update on pathogenesis, *J Oral Pathol* 1985:14:431.

36. G. O. Fischer, The commonest causes of symptomatic vulvar disease: a dermatologist's perspective, *Australas J Dermatol* 1996:37:12.

37. F. M. Lewis, M. Shah, C. I. Harrington, Vulval involvement in lichen planus: a study of 37 women. *Br J Dermatol* 1996:135:89.

38. R. S.-H. Tan, P. D. Samman, Ulcerative colitis, myasthenia gravis, atypical lichen planus and vitiligo, *Proc Roy Soc Med* 1974:67:196; R. S.-H. Tan, P. D. Samman, Thymoma, acquired hypogammaglobulinaemia, lichen planus and alopecia areata, *Proc Roy Soc Med* 1974:67:196.

39. S. M. Neill, Erosive lichen planus: diagnosis and management (syllabus of the postgraduate course), International Society for the Study of Vulvovaginal Disease, October 1999.

40. C. M. Ridley, Chronic erosive vulval disease, *Clin Exp Dermatol* 1990:15:245.

41. F. M. Lewis, Vulval lichen planus, *Br J Dermatol* 1998:138:569.

42. M. Pelisse, Erosive vulvar lichen planus and desquamative vaginitis, *Semin Dermatol* 1996:15:47.

43. M. Pelisse, The vulvo-vaginal-gingival syndrome: a new form of erosive lichen planus, *Int J Dermatol* 1989:28:381.

44. H. J. Wallace, Lichen sclerosus et atrophicus, *Transactions St. John's Dermatol Soc* 1971:57:9; F. M. Lewis, C. L. Harrington, Squamous cell carcinoma arising in vulval lichen planus, *Br J Dermatol* 1994:131:703; C. M. Dweyer, R. E. I. Kerr, D. W. M. Millan, Squamous carcinoma following vulvar lichen planus, *Arch Dermatol* 1098:125:1677; I. Zaki, K. L. Dalziel, F. A. Solomonsz, A. Stevens, The underreporting of skin disease in association with squamous cell carcinoma of the vulva, *Clin Exper Dermatol* 1997:21:334.

45. O. Wiltz, D. J. Schoetz Jr., J. J. Murray, et al., Perianal hidradenitis suppurativa: the Lahey Clinic experience, *Dis Colon Rectum* 1990:33:731.

46. C. C. Yu, M. G. Cook, Hidradenitis suppurativa: a disease of follicular epithelium, rather than apocrine glands, *Br J Dermatol* 1990:122:763.

47. T. J. Brown, T Rosen, I. F. Orengo, Hidradenitis suppurativa, *South Med J* 1998:91:1107.

48. J. Lapins, C. Jarstrand, L. Emtestam, Coagulase-negative staphylococci are the most common bacteria found in cultures from the deep portions of hidradenitis suppurativa lesions, as obtained by carbon dioxide laser surgery, *Br J Dermatol* 1999:140:90.

49. A. J. Stellon, M. Wakeling, Hidradenitis suppurativa associated with use of oral contraceptives, *BMJ* 1989:298:28.

50. F. Lewis, A. G. Messenger, J. K. Wales, Hidradenitis suppurativa as a presenting feature of premature adrenarche, *Br J Dermatol* 1993:129:447.

51. J. H. Barth, A. M. Layton, W. J. Cunliffe, Endocrine factors in pre- and postmenopausal women with hidradenitis suppurativa, *Br J Dermatol* 1996:134:1057.

52. P. S. Mortimer, R. P. Dawber, M. A. Gales, R. A. Moore, Mediation of hidradenitis suppurativa by androgens, *Br Med J (Clin Res Ed)* 1986:292:245.

53. J. S. Fitzsimmons, P. R. Guilbert, E. M. Fitzsimmons, Evidence of genetic factors in hidradenitis suppurativa, *Br J Dermatol* 1985:113:1.

54. O. J. Clemmensen, Topical treatment of hidradenitis suppurativa with clindamycin, *Int J Dermatol* 1983:22:325; G. B. Jemec, P. Wendelboe, Topical clindamycin versus systemic tetracycline in the treatment of hidradenitis suppurativa, *J Am Acad Dermatol* 1998:39:971.

55. T. J. Brown, T. Rosen, I. F. Orengo, Hidradenitis suppurativa, *South Med J* 1998:91:1107.

56. M. L. Turner, oral presentation at the XIVth International Congress of the International Society for the Study of Vulvovaginal Disease, Baveno, Italy, September 14–18, 1997.

57. A. K. Banerjee, Surgical treatment of hidradenitis suppurativa, *Br J Surg* 1992:79:863.

58. P. S. Mortimer, R. P. Dawber, M. A. Gales, R. A. Moore, A double-blind controlled cross-over trial of cyproterone acetate in females with hidradenitis suppurativa, *Br J Dermatol* 1986:115:263.

59. J. Boer, M. J. P. van Gemert, Long-term results of isotretinoin in the treatment of 68 patients with hidradenitis suppurativa, *J Am Acad Dermatol* 1999:40:73; G. F. Webster, Acne vulgaris: state of the science [editorial: comment], *Arch Dermatol* 1999:135:1101.

60. Boer, van Gemert, Long-term results of isotretinoin.

61. M. Stegar, Acne inversa, in *Dermatology, Progress and Perspectives: The Proceedings of the 18th World Congress of Dermatology*, W. H. Burgdorf, S. I. Katz, eds. (New York: Parthenon Publishing Group, 1993), 366.

62. A. K. Gupta, C. N. Ellis, B. J. Nickoloff, et al., Oral cyclosporine in the treatment of inflammatory and noninflammatory dermatoses: a clinical and immunopathologic analysis, *Arch Dermatol* 1990:126:339; D. A. Buckley, S. Rogers, Cyclosporin-responsive hidradenitis suppurativa, *J R Soc Med* 1995:88:289P.

Chapter 16: V Bumps and Color Changes

1. E. G. Friedrich Jr., *Vulvar Disease* (Philadelphia: W. B. Saunders, 1983).

2. S. C. J. Van der Putte, Anogenital "sweat" glands: histology and pathology of a gland that may mimic mammary glands, *Am J Dermatopathol* 1991:13:557.

3. J. D. Oriel, Infective conditions of the vulva, in *The Vulva*, C. M. Ridley, S. M. Neill, eds. (Oxford: Blackwell Scientific, 1999).

4. C. M. Ridley, S. M. Neill, Non-infective cutaneous conditions of the vulva, in *The Vulva*, C. M. Ridley, S. M. Neill, eds. (Oxford: Blackwell Scientific, 1999).

Chapter 17: "It Hurts"

1. D. C. Foster, Treating vulvodynia, *NVA News* 1995 spring:1(2):1–9.

2. T. G. Thomas, ed., *Practical Treatise on the Diseases of Woman* (Philadelphia: Henry C. Lea's Son, 1880), 145–47; A. J. C. Skene, *Treatise on the Diseases of Women* (New York: Appleton and Company, 1889).

3. Burning vulva syndrome: report of the ISSVD task force, *J Reprod Med* 1984:29:457.

4. K .D. Jones, S. T. Lehr, Vulvodynia: diagnostic techniques and treatment modalities, *Nurse Pract* 1994:34–46.

5. J. Paavonen, Vulvodynia—a complex syndrome of vulvar pain, *Acta Obstet Gynecol Scand* 1994:74:243–47; A. W. Young, H. M. M. Tovell, O. Lermand, G. Rodke, The changing incidence of vulvar disease in clinical practice, *Cutaneous Vulvar Service St Luke's/Roosevelt Hospital* 1991:1:1.

6. M. F. Goetsch, Vulvar vestibulitis: prevalence and historic features in a general gynecologic practice population, *Am J Obstet Gynecol* 1991:164:1609–16.

7. J. T. Cox, Deconstructing vulval pain, *Lancet* 1995:345:53.

8. L. V. Westrom, R. Willen, Vestibular nerve fiber proliferation in vulvar vestibulitis syndrome, *Obstet Gynecol* 1998:91:572–76; N. Bohm-Starke, M. Hilliges, C. Falconer, E. Rylander, Increased intraepithelial innervation in women with vulvar vestibulitis syndrome, *Gynecol Obstet Invest* 1998:46(4):256.

9. D. C. Foster, J. D. Hasday, Elevated tissue levels of interleukin-1b and tumor necrosis factor-a in vulvar vestibulitis, *Obstet Gynecol* 1997:89:291–96.

10. T. F. Warner, S. Tomic, C. K. Chang, Neuroendocrine cell–axonal complexes in the minor vestibular gland, *J Reprod Med* 1996:41:397–402.

11. J. Jeremias, W. J. Ledger, S. S. Witkin, Interleukin-1 receptor antagonist gene polymorphism in women with vulvar vestibulitis, *Am J Obstet Gynecol* 2000:182:283.

12. S. C. Marinoff, M. L. Turner, R. P. Hirsch, R. Guylaine, Intralesional alpha interferon: cost-effective therapy for vulvar vestibulitis syndrome, *J Reprod Med* 1993:38:19–24.

13. D. Clauw, Disorders associated with vulvodynia, *NVA News* 1996:11(1):1–4.

14. M. McKay, Subsets of vulvodynia, *J Reprod Med* 1988:33:695–98; S. Bazin, C. Bouchard, J. Brisson, et al., Vulvar vestibulitis syndrome: an exploratory case-control study, *Obstet Gynecol* 1994:83:47–50.

15. W. Chaim, C. Meriwether, B. Gonik, et al., Vulvar vestibulitis subjects undergoing surgical intervention: a descriptive analysis and histopathological correlates, *Eur J Obstet Gynecol Reprod Biol* 1996:68:165–68.

16. P. Nyirjesy, J. D. Sobel, et al., Cromolyn cream for recalcitrant idiopathic vulvar vestibulitis: results of a placebo controlled study, *Sex Trans Infec* 2001:7(1):53.

17. G. Chiang, P. Patra, et al., Pentosanpolysulfate inhibits mast cell histamine secretion and intracellular calcium ion levels: an alternative explanation of its beneficial effect in interstitial cystitis, *J Urol* 2000:164(6):2119.

18. M. L. Turner, S. C. Marinoff, Association of the human papillomavirus with vulvodynia and the vulvar vestibulitis syndrome, *J Reprod Med* 1988:33:533–37; S. A. Umpierre, R. K. Kaufman, E. Adam, et al., Human papillomavirus DNA in tissue biopsy specimens of vulvar vestibulitis patients treated with interferon, *Obstet Gynecol* 1991:78:693; J. Bornstein, S. Shapiro, M. Rahat, et al., Polymerase chain reaction search for viral etiology of vulvar vestibulitis syndrome, *Am J Obstet Gynecol* 1996:175:139; E. J. Wilkinson, E. Guerrero, R. Daniel, et al., Vulvar vestibulitis is rarely associated with human papillomavirus infection types 6, 11, or 18, *Int J Gynecol Pathol* 1993:12:344–49; J. M. De Deus, J. Focchi, J. N. Stavale, G. R. DeLima, Histologic and biomolecular aspects of papillomatosis of the vulvar vestibule in relation to human papillomavirus, *Obstet Gynecol* 1995:86:758–63; C. Bergeron, M. Moyal-Barracco, M. Pelisse, et al., Vulvar vestibulitis: lack of evidence for a human papillomavirus etiology, *J Reprod Med* 1994:39:936–38; S. Bazin, C. Bouchard, J. Brisson, C. Morin, et al., Vulvar vestibulitis syndrome: an exploratory case-control study, *Obstet Gynecol* 1994:83:47; M. F. Goetsch, Vulvar vestibulitis: prevalence and historic features in a general gynecologic practice population, *Am J Obstet Gynecol* 1991:164:1609–16; C. Morin, C. Bouchard, J. Brisson, M. Fortier, et al., Human papillomaviruses and vulvar vestibulitis, *Obstet Gynecol* 2000:95:683.

19. H. H. Balfour, Acyclovir therapy for herpes zoster: advantages and adverse effects (editorial), *JAMA* 1986:255:387.

20. J. Bornstein, S. Shapiro, M. Rahat, et al., Polymerase chain reaction search for viral etiology of vulvar vestibulitis syndrome, *Am J Obstet Gynecol* 1996:175:139–44.

21. B. M. Peckham, D. G. Maki, J. J. Patterson et al., Focal vulvitis: a characteristic syndrome and cause of dyspareunia, *Am J Obstet Gynecol* 1986:154:855–64; M. S. Mann, R. H. Kaufman, D. Brown, et al., Vulvar vestibulitis: significant clinical variables and treatment outcome, *Obstet Gynecol* 1992:79:122–25.

22. M. Baggish, J. R. Miklos, Vulvar pain syndrome: a review, *Obstet Gynecol Survey* 1995:50 (8):618–27.

23. S. C. Marinoff, M. L. C. Turner, Vulvar vestibulitis syndrome: an overview, *Am J Obstet Gynecol* 1991:165:1228–31.

24. R. Reid, M. D. Greenberg, Y. Daoud, et al., Colposcopic findings in women with vulvar pain syndromes, *J Reprod Med* 1988:33:525; Goetsch, Vulvar vestibulitis; L. R. Shover, D. D. Youngs, R. Cannata, Psychosexual aspects of the management of vulvar vestibulitis, *Am J Obstet Gynecol* 1992:167:630–36.

25. H. I. Maibach, C. T. Mathias, Vulvar dermatitis and fissures: irritant dermatitis from methyl benzethonium chloride, *Contact Derm* 1985:5:340–45.

26. S. Bazin et al., Vulvar vestibulitis syndrome: an exploratory case-control study, *Obstet Gynecol* 1994:83(1):47–50.

27. J. Willems, New direction in medical management of vulvar vestibulitis, *Vulvar Pain Newsletter* 1994 fall:5–7; K. L. Noller, Diagnosis and treatment of chronic vulvar pain syndrome, *Women's Health Reports* 1995 Jul 24:1(8):65–72.

28. Noller, Diagnosis and treatment of chronic vulvar pain syndrome.

29. C. C. Solomon, M. H. Melmed, S. M. Heitler, Calcium citrate for vulvar vestibulitis, *J Reprod Med* 1991:36:879–82.

30. M. S. Baggish, E. H. Sze, R. Johnson, Urinary oxalate excretion and its role in vulvar pain syndrome, *Am J Obstet Gynecol* 1997:177:507–11.

31. W. Ledger, Observations on patients with vulvar vestibulitis, *NVA News* 2000:VI(1):1.

32. J. Bornstein, D. Zarfati, Z. Goldik, et al., Vulvar vestibulitis: physical or psychosexual problem? *Obstet Gynecol* 1999:93:876.

33. D. E. Stewart, A. E. Reicher, A. H. Gerulath, et al., Vulvodynia and psychological distress, *Obstet Gynecol* 1994:84:587–90.

34. E. G. Friedrich Jr., Vulvar vestibulitis syndrome, *J Reprod Med* 1987:32:110; Schover et al., Psychosexual aspects of the management of vulvar vestibulitis; L. Edwards, M. Mason, M. Phillip, et al., Childhood sexual and physical abuse: incidence in patients with vulvodynia, *J Reprod Med* 1997:42(3):135–39.

35. L. M. Klein, R. M. Lavker, W. L. Matis, et al., Degranulation of human mast cells induces an endothelial antigen central to leukocyte adhesion, *Proc Natl Acad Sci USA* 1989:86:8922–26.

36. M. McKay, Vulvodynia diagnostic patterns, *Derm Clin* 1992:10(2):423–32.

37. R. E. Pyka, E. J. Wilkinson, E. G. Friedrich Jr., B. P. Croker, The histopathology of vulvar vestibulitis syndrome, *Int J Gynecol Pathol* 1988:7:249–57.

38. Baggish, Miklos, Vulvar pain syndrome: a review.

39. R. D. France, The future for antidepressants: treatment of pain, *Psychopathology* 1987:20(suppl 1):99–113.

40. Ibid.

41. M. McKay, Dysesthetic ("essential") vulvodynia, *J Reprod Med* 1993:38(1):9–13.

42. S. C. Marinoff, Vulvodynia: a perplexing disorder, *NVA News* 1995:1(1):1–9; H. Emsellem, Chronic pain: a neurologist's perspective, *NVA News* 1995:1(3):1–8.

43. A. Eisen, Venlafaxine therapy for vulvodynia, *Pain Clinic* 1995:8:365–67.

44. B. Ben-David, M. Friedman, Gabapentin therapy for vulvodynia, *Anesth Anal* 1999:89:1459.

45. Ben-David, Gabapentin therapy for vulvodynia..

46. H. I. Glazer, G. Rodke, C. Swencionis, et al., Treatment of vulvar vestibulitis syndrome with electromyographic biofeedback of pelvic floor musculature, *J Reprod Med* 1995:40:283–90.

47. D. Hartmann, Managing vulvar pain with physical therapy, *NVA News* 1996:11(11):1–7.

48. Mann et al., Vulvar vestibulitis; H. L. Kent, P. M. Wisniewski, Interferon for vulvar vestibulitis, *J Reprod Med* 1990:35:1138–40; Umpierre et al., Human papillomavirus DNA in tissue biopsy specimens; S. C. Marinoff, M. L. Turner, R. P. Hirsch et al., Intralesional alpha-interferon: cost-effective therapy for vulvar vestibulitis syndrome, *J Reprod Med* 1993:38:19–24; J. Bornstein, B. Pascal, H. Abramovici, Intramuscular interferon treatment for severe vulvar vestibulitis, *J Reprod Med* 1993:38:117–20.

49. Mann et al., Vulvar vestibulitis.

50. S. M. Hurtado, L. D. Treene, S. C. Marinoff, Effectiveness of interferon therapy for the treatment of vulvar vestibulitis, International Society for the Study of Vulvovaginal Disease, XVth World Congress, September 26–30, 1999; S. K. Tyring, Interferon therapy of genital human papillomavirus infection, *Clin Pract Gynecol* 1989:2:233–44.

51. Emsellem, Chronic pain.

52. Marinoff, Vulvodynia: a perplexing disorder.

53. Ibid.

54. J. D. Woodruf, T. H. Parmley, Infection of the minor vestibular glands, *Obstet Gynecol* 1983:62:609–12.

55. Bornstein et al., Vulvar vestibulitis: physical or psychosexual problem?

56. J. Bornstein, Z. Goldik, Z. Alter, et al., Persistent vulvar vestibulitis: the continuing challenge, *Obstet Gynecol Survey* 1997:53(1):39–44.

57. J. Bornstein, R. H. Kaufman, Perineoplasty for vulvar vestibulitis, *Harefuah* 1989:116:90–92.

58. Baggish, Miklos, Vulvar pain syndrome: a review.

59. J. J. Yount, The vulvar pain newsletter, 1995:5:1–8.

60. J. Bornstein, H. Abramovici, Combination of subtotal perineoplasty and interferon for the treatment of vulvar vestibulitis, *Gynecol Obstet Invest* 1997:44:53–56.

61. J. Bornstein, D. Zarfati, Z. Goldik, et al., Treatment of intractable vulvar vestibulitis, *Isr J Obstet Gynecol* 1994:5:149–52.

62. M. McKay, Vulvodynia: a multifactorial problem, *Arch Dermatol* 1989:125:256–62.
63. T. G. Bohl, Vulvodynia and its differential diagnoses, *Semin Cutan Med Surg* 1998 Sept:17(3):189.
64. M. L. C. Turner, S. C. Marinoff, Pudendal neuralgia, *Am J Obstet Gynecol* 1991:165:1233–36.
65. Ibid.
66. J. Bonica, Pudendal neuralgia, in J. Bonica, ed., *The Management of Pain*, 2nd ed. (Philadelphia: Lea & Febiger, 1990), 190.
67. A. M. Verdeja, T. E. Elkins, A. Odol, et al., Transvaginal sacrospinous colpopexy: anatomic landmarks to be aware of to minimize complications, *Am J Obstet Gynecol* 1995:173(5):1468–69.
68. E. G. Friedrich Jr., *Vulvar Disease* (Philadelphia: W. B. Saunders, 1983).
69. W. Hunter et al., Abdominal pain from strain of intrapelvic muscles (letter), *Clin Orthop* 1970:279–80; P. M. King, Musculoskeletal origins of chronic pelvic pain, *Obstet Gynecol Clin North Am* 1993 (Philadelphia: W. B. Saunders), 719–41; P. M. King et al., Musculoskeletal factors in chronic pelvic pain, *J Psychosom Obstet Gynaecol* 1991:12:87–98; J. C. Slocumb, Neurological factors in chronic pelvic pain: trigger points in the abdominal pelvic pain syndrome, *Am J Obstet Gynecol* 1984:149:536–43; J. G. Travell, D. G. Simons, *Myofascial Pain and Dysfunction: The Trigger Point Manual* (Baltimore: Williams & Wilkins, 1983).
70. F. C. Greiss Jr., Equestrian dyspareunia, *Am J Obstet Gynecol* 1984:150:168.
71. R. B. Layzer, M. A. Connant, Neuralgia in recurrent herpes simplex, *Arch Neurol* 1974:31:233–37; E. J. Howard, Postherpetic neuralgia, *JAMA* 1985:253:2196.
72. F. Tognetti, M. Poppi, G. Gaist, et al., Pudendal neuralgia due to solitary neurofibroma, *J Neurosurg* 1982:56:732–33; Turner, Marinoff, Pudendal neuralgia.
73. F. M. Lewis, C. I. Harrington, Use of magnetic resonance imaging in vulvodynia, *J Reprod Med* 1997:42:169.
74. R. K. Portenoy, Opioid and adjuvant analgesics (syllabus for diagnosis and treatment of neuropathic pain), sponsored by Beth Israel Medical Center, Department of Pain Medicine, September 23, 2000.
75. B. A. Meyerson, Electrostimulation procedures: effects, presumed rationale, and possible mechanisms, in *Advances in Pain Research and Therapy*, vol. 5, J. J. Bonica et al., eds. (New York: Raven, 1983), 495–534.
76. D. C. Foster, C. Robinson, K. M. Davis, Urethral pressure variation in women with vulvar vestibulitis syndrome, *Am J Obstet Gynecol* 1993:169:107–12.
77. W. M. McCormack, Two urogenital sinus syndromes: interstitial cystitis and focal vulvitis, *J Reprod Med* 1990:35:873–75; C. C. Fitzpatrick, J. O. L. DeLancey, T. E. Elkins, et al., Vulvar vestibulitis and interstitial cystitis: a disorder of urogenital sinus-derived epithelium? *Obstet Gynecol* 1993:81:860–62.
78. J. Gunter, M. Clark, J. Weigel, Is there an association between vulvodynia and interstitial cystitis? paper presented to the annual meeting of the American College of Obstetricians and Gynecologists, San Francisco, May 2000.

Chapter 18: Sexual Healing

1. K. Hawton, *Sex Therapy: A Practical Guide* (New York: Oxford University Press, 1985).
2. C. Price, Psychologist addresses sexual, emotional aspects of vulvodynia, *NVA News* 1995:1(1):1.
3. J. M. Kessler, Sexual issues and vulvar pain, *The Vulvar Pain Newsletter* 1998:15:4.
4. B. Whipple, Research concerning sexual response in women, *Health Psychol* 1995:17(3):16.
5. R. L. Timmers et al., Treating goal-directed intimacy, *Social Work* 1976:401.
6. Kessler, Sexual issues and vulvar pain.
7. G. Rodke, Vulvar conditions, pregnancy and childbirth, *NVA News* 2000:VI (1):5.
8. S. Hutchison, Becoming pregnant with vulvodynia, *NVA News* 1999:V(1):6.
9. Rodke, Vulvar conditions, pregnancy and childbirth.

10. American Psychological Association, *Diagnostic and Statistical Manual of Mental Disorders*, 4th ed. (Washington, D.C.: APA, 1997).

11. J. Bengtson, The vagina, in *Kistner's Gynecology*, K. J. Ryan, R. S. Berkowitz, R. L. Barbieri, eds. (St. Louis: Mosby, 1995).

12. J. R. Berman, L. A. Berman, I. Goldstein, Female sexual dysfunction, *Medical Aspects of Human Sexuality* 1998:1(5):15.

13. B. Whipple, K. Brash McGreer, Management of female sexual dysfunction, in *Function in People with Disability and Chronic Illness: A Health Professional's Guide* (Gaithersburg, Md.: Aspen Publications, 1997), 511.

14. R. C. Rosen, S. R. Leiblum, Hypoactive sexual desire, *Psych Clin North Am* 1995:18(1):107.

15. D. A. Rivas, M. B. Chancellor, Management of erectile dysfunction, in *Sexual Function in People with Disability and Chronic Illness: A Health Professional's Guide*, M. L. Sipski, C. Alexander, eds. (Gaithersburg, Md.: Aspen Publications, 1997), 437.

16. D. Schardt, Peddling potency: do impotence-busters work? *Nutrition Action* 2000:27(6):9.

17. Ibid.

18. M. Loe, Female sexual dysfunction: for women or for sale, *The Network News* 2000 Jan–Feb:5.

Chapter 19: Bladder Pain

1. J. P. Patton, D. B. Nash, E. Abrutyn, Urinary tract infection: economic considerations, *Med Clin North Am* 1991:75:495.

2. J. P. Sanford, Urinary tract symptoms and infections, *Ann Rev Med* 1975:25:485.

3. S. D. Fihn, Behavioral aspects of urinary tract infection, *Urology* 1988:32(suppl):168.

4. R. Tuomala, Gynecologic infections, in *Kistner's Gynecology*, K. J. Ryan, R. S. Berkowitz, R. L. Barbieri, eds. (St. Louis: Mosby, 1996), 518.

5. S. D. Fihn et al., Association between diaphragm use and urinary tract infection, *JAMA* 1985:254:240; B. L. Strom et al., Sexual activity, contraceptive use, and other risk factors for symptomatic and asymptomatic bacteriuria, *Ann Int Med* 1987:107:816.

6. K. Gupta, A. E. Stapleton, T. M. Hooten, et al., Inverse association of H_2O_2-producing lactobacilli and vaginal Escherichia colonization in women with recurrent urinary tract infections, *J Infec Dis* 1998:178:446.

7. S. Smith, J. P. Hughes, T. M. Hooten, et al., Antecedent antimicrobial use increases the risk of uncomplicated cystitis in young women, *Clin Infect Dis* 1996:25:63.

8. L. E. Nicolle, A. R. Ronald, Recurrent urinary tract infection in adult women: diagnosis and treatment, *Infect Dis Clin North Am* 1987:1:793; R. Raz, W. E. Stamm, A controlled trial of intravaginal estriol in postmenopausal women with recurrent urinary tract infection, *N Engl J Med* 1993:329:753.

9. W. E. Stamm, T. M. Hooten, Management of urinary tract infections in adults, *N Engl J Med* 1993:329(18):1328.

10. Raz, Stamm, A controlled trial of intravaginal estriol.

11. Ibid.

12. L. Cardoza et al., Low dose oestrogen prophylaxis for recurrent urinary tract infections in elderly women, *Br J Obstet Gynaecol* 1998:105:403.

13. B. C. Eriksen, A randomized, open, parallel-group study on the preventive effect of an estradiol-releasing vaginal ring (Estring) on recurrent urinary tract infections in postmenopausal women, *Am J Obstet Gynecol* 1999:180:1072.

14. A. A. Hovelius, P.-A. Mardh, *Staphylococcus saprophyticus* as a common cause of urinary tract infection, *Rev Infect Dis* 1984:6:328.

15. Tuomala, Gynecologic infections.

16. Ibid.

17. Ibid.

18. A. J. Schaeffer, Infections of the urinary tract, in *Campbell's Urology*, P. C. Walsh,

A. B. Retik, E. D. Vaughan, A. J. Wein, eds. (Philadelphia: W. B. Saunders, 1998).

19. P. G. Pappas, Laboratory in the diagnosis and management of urinary tract infections, *Med Clin North Am* 1991:75:339.

20. W. E. Stamm, Protocol for diagnosis of urinary tract infection: reconsidering the criterion for significant bacteriuria, *Urology* 1988:32(suppl 2):6; W. E. Stamm et al., Diagnosis of coliform infection in acutely dysuric women, *N Engl J Med* 1984:307:463.

21. J. E. Fowler, E. T. Pulaski, Excretory urography, cystography, and cystoscopy in the evaluation of women with urinary tract infection: a prospective study, *N Engl J Med* 1981:3034:462; Stamm, Hooten, Management of urinary tract infections in adults.

22. Schaeffer, Infections of the urinary tract.

23. J. S. Elder, Congenital anomalies of the genitalia, in *Campbell's Urology,* P. C. Walsh, A. B. Retik, E. D. Vaughan, A. J. Wein, eds. (Philadelphia: W. B. Saunders, 1998).

24. G. E. Lemack, B. Foster, P. E. Zimmern, Urethral dilation in women: a questionnaire-based analysis of practice patterns, *Urology* 1999:54(1):37.

25. S. R. Norrby, Short-term treatment of uncomplicated lower urinary tract infections in women, *Rev Infect Dis* 1990:12:458; T. M. Hooten, C. Johnson, C. Winter, et al., Single-dose and three-day regimens of ofloxacin versus trimethoprim-sulfamethoxazole for acute cystitis in women, *Antimicrob Agents Chemother* 1991:35:1479; A. R. Ronald, L. E. Nicolle, G. K. Harding, Standards of therapy for urinary tract infections in adults, *Infection* 1992:3:S164.

26. C. D. Bacheller, J. M. Bernstein, Urinary tract infections, *Med Clin North Am* 1997:81(3):719.

27. Stamm, Hooten, Management of urinary tract infections in adults.

28. Ibid.

29. J. R. Johnson, W. E. Stamm, Urinary tract infections in women: diagnosis and treatment, *Ann Intern Med* 1989:111:906.

30. T. M. Hooten, W. E. Stamm, Management of acute uncomplicated urinary tract infection in adults, *Med Clin N Am* 1991:75:339.

31. A. R. Ronald, Optimal duration of treatment for kidney infection, *Ann Intern Med* 1987:106:467.

32. A. Stapleton, W. E. Stamm, Prevention of urinary tract infection, *Med Clin N Am* 1997:11:719.

33. A. Pfau, T. Sacks, D. Engelstein, Recurrent urinary tract infections in pre-menopausal women: prophylaxis based on an understanding of the pathogenesis, *J Urol* 1983:129:1153; A. Stapleton, R. H. Latham, C. Johnson, et al., Postcoital antimicrobial prophylaxis for recurrent urinary tract infection: a randomized, double-blind, placebo-controlled trial, *JAMA* 1990:264:703.

34. E. S. Wong, M. McKevitt, K. Running, et al., Management of recurrent urinary tract infections with patient-administered single-dose therapy, *Ann Intern Med* 1985:102:302.

35. N. Ho, J. A. Koziol, C. L. Parsons, Epidemiology of interstitial cystitis, in *Interstitial Cystitis,* G. R. Sant, ed. (Philadelphia: Lippincott-Raven, 1997); K. J. Propert, A. J. Schaeffer, C. M. Brensinger, et al., A prospective study of interstitial cystitis: results of longitudinal follow-up of the interstitial cystitis data base cohort, *J Urol* 2000:163:1434.

36. C. L. Parsons, Epithelial coating techniques in the treatment of interstitial cystitis, *Urol* 1997:49(suppl 5A):100.

37. A. Elbdawi, Interstitial cystitis: a critique of current concepts with a new proposal for pathologic diagnosis and pathogenesis, *Urol* 1997:49(suppl 5A):14.

38. C. L. Parsons, Interstitial cystitis: clinical manifestations and diagnostic criteria in over 200 cases, *Neurourol Urodyn* 1990:9:241.

39. Ho et al., Epidemiology of interstitial cystitis.

40. D. A. Nigro, A. J. Wein, Interstitial cystitis: clinical and endoscopic features, in *Interstitial Cystitis,* G. R. Sant, ed. (Philadelphia: Lippincott-Raven, 1997).

41. C. S. Bradley, G. S. Singh, Interstitial cystitis, in *The Female Patient* 2000:25:83.
42. M. Pontari, P. Hanno, A. Wein, Logical and systemic approach to the evaluation and management of patients suspected of having interstitial cystitis, *Urol* 1997:49(suppl 5A):114.
43. Ibid.
44. G. R. Sant, C. L. Parsons, R. J. Evans, et al., The diagnosis and treatment of interstitial cystitis (syllabus for continuing medical education telephone conference), sponsored by the Postgraduate Institute for Medicine and Medi-Topics, Inc, 2000.
45. C. L. Parsons, M. Greenberger, L. Gabal, et al., The role of urinary potassium in the pathogenesis of interstitial cystitis, *J Urol* 1998:159:1862.
46. D. Chaiken, J. Blaivas, S. Blaivas, Behavioral therapy for the treatment of refractory interstitial cystitis, *J Urol* 1993:149:1445.
47. J. Koziol, D. Clark, R. Gittes, E. Tan, The natural history of interstitial cystitis: a survey of 374 patients, *J Urol* 1993:149:465.
48. Bradley, Singh, Interstitial cystitis.
49. G. R. Sant, D. LaRock, Standard intravesical therapies for interstitial cystitis, *Urol Clin N Am* 1994:21:73.
50. Ibid.
51. G. A. Barbalias, E. N. Liatsikos, A. Athanasopoulos, G. Nikiforidis, Interstitial cystitis: bladder training with intravesical oxybutynin, *J Urol* 2000:163:1818.
52. T. C. Theoharides, G. R. Sant, Hydroxyzine therapy for interstitial cystitis, *Urology* 1997:49(suppl 5A):108.
53. P. Hanno, Amitriptyline in the treatment of interstitial cystitis, *Urol Clin N Am* 1994:21:89.
54. P. M. Hanno, Analysis of long-term Elmiron therapy for interstitial cystitis, *Urology* 1997:49(suppl 15A):93.
55. G. Chiang, P. Patra, et al., Pentosanpolysulfate inhibits mast cell histamine secretion and intracellular calcium ion levels: an alternative explanation of its beneficial effect in interstitial cystitis, *J Urol* 2000:164(6):2119.
56. P. Hwang, B. Auclair, D. Beechinor, et al., Efficacy of pentosan polysulfate in the treatment of interstitial cystitis: a meta-analysis, *Urology* 1997:50:39.
57. Hanno, Analysis of long-term Elmiron therapy.
58. P. M. Hanno, A. J. Wein, Medical treatment of interstitial cystitis other than Remso–50, Elmiron. *Urology* 1987:29(suppl 4):22.

Chapter 20: The Lifetime Virus

1. L. Corey, H. H. Handsfield, Genital herpes and public health: Addressing a global problem, *JAMA* 2000:283:791.
2. B. J. Sullivan, Neonatal herpes simplex virus infections in King County, Washington: increasing incidence and epidemiologic correlations, *JAMA* 1983:256:3059.
3. A. G. Nahmias, W. E. Josey, Epidemiology of herpes simplex viruses 1 and 2, in *Viral Infections of Humans, Epidemiology and Incidence*, A. S. Evans, ed. (New York: Plenum, 1982), 351.
4. B. Raab, A. L. Lorinez, Genital herpes simplex—concepts and treatment, *J Amer Acad Dermatol* 1981:5:249.
5. J. D. Oriel, Infective conditions of the vulva, in *The Vulva*, C. M. Ridley, S. M. Neill, eds. (London: Blackwell Science, 1999), 351.
6. L. Corey, K. K. Holmes, Clinical course of genital herpes simplex virus infection in men and women, *Ann Int Med* 1983:48:973.
7. L. Corey, W. C. Reeves, K. K. Holmes, Cellular immune responses in genital herpes simplex virus infections, *N Engl J Med* 1978:299:286.
8. L. Koutsky, R. Ashley, et al., The frequency of unrecognized type 2 herpes simplex virus infection among women, *Sexually Transmitted Dis* 1990:17:90; J. F. Rooney, J. M. Felser, J. Ostrave, et al., Acquisition of genital herpes from an asymptomatic sexual partner, *N Engl J Med* 1986:314:1561.

9. G. J. Mertz, O. Schmidt, R. Ashley, et al., Frequency of acquisition of first episode of genital infection with herpes simplex virus from symptomatic and asymptomatic contacts, *Sexually Transmitted Dis* 1985:12(1):83.

10. S. N. Nader, C. G. Prober, Herpesvirus infections of the vulva and vagina, in *Vulvovaginitis,* P. Elsner, J. Martius, eds. (New York: Dekker, 1993), 229.

11. B. Borck, S. Selk, J. Benedetti, et al., Frequency of asymptomatic shedding of herpes simplex virus in women with genital herpes, *JAMA* 1990:19:263; S. N. Nader, C. G. Prober, Herpesvirus infections of the vulva, *Sem Dermatol* 1996:15(1):8.

12. M. K. Breinig, L. A. Kingsley, Epidemiology of genital herpes in Pittsburgh: Serologic, sexual and racial correlations of apparent and inapparent herpes simplex infection, *J Infect Dis* 1990:162:299; R. Johnson, A. Nahmias, L. Magder, et al., A seroepidemiologic survey of the prevalence of herpes simplex virus type 2 infection in the United States, *N Engl J Med* 1989:321:7; F. Bonchet, I. Yasukawa, R. Bronzan, et al., A prospective evaluation of primary genital HSV-2 infection acquired during pregnancy, *Ped Inf Dis* 1990:9:499.

13. Corey, Holmes, Clinical course of genital herpes simplex virus infection.

14. L. Corey, Genital herpes, in *Sexually Transmitted Diseases,* 2nd ed., K. K. Holmes, P.-A. Mardh, P. F. Sparling, P. J. Weisner, eds. (New York: McGraw-Hill, 1989), 391.

15. Corey, Genital herpes.

16. L. Corey, H. G. Adams, Z. A. Brown, et al., Genital herpes simplex virus infections: clinical manifestations, course and complications, *Ann Int Med* 1983:98:958.

17. Nader, Prober, Herpesvirus infections of the vulva.

18. W. E. Lafferty, R. W. Coombs, J. Benedetti, et al., Recurrences after oral and genital herpes simplex virus infection. Influence of site of infection and viral type, *N Engl J Med* 1987:316:1444.

19. W. C. Reeves, L. Corey, H. G. Adams, et al., Risk of recurrence after first episode of genital herpes: relation to HSV type and antibody response, *N Engl J Med* 1981:305:315.

20. A. Mindel, D. Coker, et al., Recurrent genital herpes: clinical and virological features in men and women, *Genitourin Med* 1988:164:103.

21. L. Corey, Genital herpes.

22. Nader, Prober, Herpesvirus infections of the vulva.

23. R. C. Moseley, L. Corey, D. Benjamin, et al., Comparison of viral isolation, direct immunofluorescence, and indirect immunoperoxidase techniques for detection of genital herpes simplex virus infection, *J Clin Microbiol* 1981:13:918.

24. R. Ashley, A. Cent, V. Maggs, L. Corey, Inability of enzyme immunoassays to discriminate between infections with herpes simplex virus type 1 and 2, *Ann Int Med* 1991:115:520.

25. A. Wald, New therapies and prevention strategies for genital herpes, *Clin Infec Dis* 1999:28(suppl 1):S4.

26. Corey, Genital herpes.

27. Wald, New therapies and prevention strategies.

28. A. Wald, J. Benedetti, G. Davis, et al., A randomized, double-blind, comparative trial comparing high and standard dose oral acyclovir for first episode genital herpes infections, *Antimicrob Agents Chemother* 1994:38:174.

29. Wald, New therapies and prevention strategies.

30. G. R. Kinghorn, I. Abeywickreme, M. Jeavons, et al., Efficacy of combined treatment with oral and topical acyclovir in first episode genital herpes, *Genitourin Med* 1986:62:186.

31. R. C. Reichman, C. J. Badger, G. J. Mertz, et al., Treatment of recurrent genital herpes simplex infections with oral acyclovir: a controlled trial, *JAMA* 1984:251:2103.

32. Nader, Prober, Herpesvirus infections of the vulva and vagina.

33. Wald, New therapies and prevention strategies.

34. J. M. Douglas, C. Critchlow, J. Benedetti, et al., Prevention of recurrent genital herpes simplex virus infection with daily oral acyclovir: a double-blind trial, *N Engl J Med* 1984:310:1551.

35. K. H. Fife, C. S. Crumpacker, G. J. Mertz, et al., Recurrence and resistance patterns of herpes simplex virus following cessation of >6 years of chronic suppression with acyclovir, *J Infect Dis* 1994:169:1338; L. G. Kaplowitz, D. Baker, L. Gelb, et al., Prolonged continuous acyclovir treatment of normal adults with frequently recurring genital herpes simplex virus infection: the Acyclovir Study Group, *JAMA* 1991:265:747; L. H. Goldberg, R. Kaufman, T. O. Kurtz, et al., Long-term suppression of recurrent genital herpes with acyclovir, *Arch Dermatol* 1993:129:582.

36. L. Corey, R. Ashley, R. Sekulovich, et al., Lack of efficacy of a vaccine containing recombinant gD2 and gB2 antigens in MF59 adjuvant for the prevention of genital HSV-2 acquisition, in *Program and Abstracts of the 37th Interscience Conference on Antimicrobial Agents and Chemotherapy (Toronto)* (Washington, D.C.: American Society for Microbiology, 1997).

37. American Academy of Pediatrics, *Herpes simplex*, in G. Peter, ed., *1994 Red Book: Report of the Committee on Infectious Diseases*, 23rd ed. (Elk Grove Village, Ill.: American Academy of Pediatrics, 1994), 242.

38. K. M. Stone, C. A. Brooks, M. E. Guinan, et al., National surveillance for neonatal herpes simplex virus infections, *Sex Transm Dis* 1989:16:152.

39. J. Sullivan Bolyai, H. F. Jull, C. Wilson, et al., Neonatal herpes simplex virus infection in King County, Washington: increasing incidence and epidemiologic correlates, *JAMA* 1983:250:3059.

40. Z. A. Brown, S. A. Selke, J. Zeh, et al., Acquisition of herpes simplex virus during pregnancy, *N Engl J Med* 1997:337:509.

41. L. L. Scott, P. J. Sanchez, G. L. Jackson, et al., Acyclovir suppression to prevent cesarean delivery after first-episode genital herpes, *Obstet Gynecol* 1996:87:69.

42. L. A. Vontver, D. E. Hickok, Z. A. Brown, et al., Recurrent genital herpes simplex virus infection in pregnancy: infant outcome and frequency of asymptomatic recurrences, *Am J Obstet Gynecol* 1982:143:75.

43. Z. A. Brown, L. A. Vontver, J. Benedetti, et al., Genital herpes in pregnancy: risk factors associated with recurrences and asymptomatic shedding, *Am J Obstet Gynecol* 1985:153:24.

44. T. Lissauer, D. Jeffries, Preventing neonatal herpes infection, *Br J Obstet Gynaecol* 1989:96:1015.

45. L. L. Scott, P. B. Sanchez, G. L. Jackson, et al., Acyclovir suppression to prevent cesarean delivery after first-episode genital herpes, *Obstet Gynecol* 1996:87:69.

46. B. Stray-Pedersen, Acyclovir in late pregnancy to prevent neonatal herpes simplex, *Lancet* 1990:336:756.

47. Centers for Disease Control and Prevention, Pregnancy outcomes following systemic prenatal acyclovir exposure—June 1, 1984–June 30, 1993, *MMWR* 1993:42:806.

48. A. S. Yaeger, Use of acyclovir in premature and term neonates, *Am J Med* 1982:73:205.

Chapter 21: The Crafty Virus

1. T. V. Sedlacek, Advances in the diagnosis and treatment of human papillomavirus infections, *Clin Obstet Gynecol* 1999:42(2):206.

2. American College of Obstetrics and Gynecology, Sexually transmitted diseases, in *Precis V: An Update in Obstetrics and Gynecology* (Washington, D.C.: ACOG, 1994), 87.

3. G. Y. Ho, R. Bierman, L. Beardsley, C. H. Chang, R. D. Burk, Natural history of cervicovaginal papillomavirus infection in young women, *N Engl J Med* 1998:338:423.

4. C. Volter, Y. He, H. Delius, et al., Novel HPV types present in oral papillomavirus lesions from patients with HIV infection, *Int J Cancer* 1996:66:453.

5. K. R. Beutner, D. J. Wiley, J. M. Douglas, et al., Genital warts and their treatment, *Clinical Infectious Diseases* 1999:28(suppl 1):537.

6. Beutner, Genital warts and their treatment.

7. C. Sonnek, Human papillomavirus infection with particular reference to genital disease, *J Clin Path* 1998:51(9):643.

8. Ibid.
9. B. J. Monk, R. A. Burger, New therapies for genital condyloma in women, *Contemporary ObGyn* 1998 February:81.
10. H. W. Buck and the Task Force on Human Papillomavirus Disease, *Genital Human Papillomavirus (HPV) Disease: Diagnosis, Management, and Prevention* (Rockville, Md.: American College Health Association, 1989).
11. W. C. Phelps, K. A. Alexander, Antiviral therapy for human papillomavirus: rational and prospects, *Ann Int Med* 1995; 123(5):368.
12. E. G. Friedrich Jr., *Vulvar Disease* (Philadelphia: W. B. Saunders Company, 1983), 194.
13. L. Kjellberg, G. Wadell, F. Bergman, et al., Regular disappearance of the human papillomavirus genome after conization of cervical dysplasia by carbon dioxide laser, *Am J Obstet Gynecol* 2000:183:1238.
14. L. A. Koutsky, K. K. Holmes, C. W. Critchlow, et al., A cohort study of the risk of cervical intraepithelial neoplasia grade 2 or 3 in relation to papillomavirus infection, *N Engl J Med* 1992:327:1272.
15. C. Ley, H. M. Bauer, A. Reingold, et al., Determinants of genital papillomavirus infection in young women, *J Natl Cancer Inst* 1991:83:997.
16. K. Nasiell, V. Roger, M. Nasiell, Behavior of mild cervical dysplasia during long-term follow-up, *Obstet Gynecol* 1986:5:665.
17. A. L. Herbst, Intraepithelial neoplasia of the cervix, in *Comprehensive Gynecology*, A. L. Herbst, D. R. Mishell, M. S. Stenchever, W. Droegemueller, eds. (St. Louis: Mosby–Year Book, 1992), 835.
18. K. Nasiell, M. Nasiell, V. Vaclavinkova, Behavior of moderate cervical dysplasia during long-term follow-up, *Obstet Gynecol* 1983:61:609; Nasiell et al., Behavior of mild cervical dysplasia.
19. Herbst, Intraepithelial neoplasia of the cervix.
20. M. F. Mitchell, G. Tortolero-Luna, E. Cook, et al., A randomized clinical trial of cryotherapy, laser vaporization, and loop electrosurgical excision for treatment of squamous intraepithelial lesions of the cervix, *Obstet Gynecol* 1998:92:737.
21. K. D. Hatch, N. F. Hacker, Intraepithelial disease of the cervix, vagina, and vulva, in *Novak's Gynecology*, J. S. Berek, E. Y. Adashi, P. A. Hillard, eds. (Baltimore: Williams & Wilkins, 1996), 447.
22. D. E. Townsend, Cryosurgery for CIN, *Obstet Gynecol Surv* 1979:34:828.
23. V. C. Wright, Carbon dioxide laser surgery for the cervix and vagina: indications, complications and results, *Comprehensive Ther* 1988:14:54.
24. Hatch, Hacker, Intraepithelial disease of the cervix, vagina, and vulva.
25. M. S. Baggish, Laser management of cervical intraepithelial neoplasia, *Clin Obstet Gynecol* 1983:26:968.
26. T. C. Wright, S. Gagnon, R. M. Richart, A. Ferenczy, Treatment of cervical intraepithelial neoplasia using the loop electrosurgical excision procedure, *Obstet Gynecol* 1991:79:173.
27. P. C. Gunasekera, J. H. Phipps, B. V. Lewis, Large loop excision of the transformation zone (LLETZ) compared to carbon dioxide laser in the treatment of CIN: a superior mode of treatment, *Br J Obstet Gynaecol* 1990:97:995.
28. W. Prendiville, J. Cullimore, S. Norman, Large loop excision of the transformation zone (LLETZ): a new method of management for women with cervical intraepithelial neoplasia, *Br J Obstet Gynaecol* 1989:96:1989; P. F. Whiteley, K. S. Olah, Treatment of cervical intraepithelial neoplasia: experience with the low-voltage diathermy loop, *Am J Obstet Gynecol* 1990:162:1272.
29. H. W. Jones, R. E. Butler, The treatment of cervical intraepithelial neoplasia by cone biopsy, *Am J Obstet Gynecol* 1980:137:882.

Chapter 22: V Cancer and Precancer

1. J. S. Park, R. W. Jones, M. R. McLean, et al., Possible aetiological heterogeneity of vulvar intraepithelial neoplasia: a correlation of pathologic characteristics with human papillomavirus detection by in-situ hybridization and polymerase chain

reaction, *Cancer* 1991:67(6):1599; E. J. Wilkinson, I. K. Stone, *Atlas of Vulvar Disease* (Baltimore: Williams & Wilkins, 1995).

2. A. Singer, J. M. Monaghan, *Lower Genital Tract Precancer* (Boston: Blackwell Scientific Publications, 1994).

3. E. G. Friedrich, E. J. Wilkinson, Y. S. Fu, Carcinoma in situ of the vulva: a continuing challenge, *Am J Obstet Gynecol* 1980:136:830.

4. Ibid.

5. C. Bergeron, Z. Naghashfar, C. Canaan, et al., Human papillomavirus type 16 in intraepithelial neoplasia (Bowenoid papulosis) and co-existent invasive carcinoma of the vulva, *Int J Gynecol Pathol* 1987:6:1.

6. R. Li Vigni, A. Turans, M. Colombi, et al., Histological human papillomavirus-induced lesions: trypitzation by molecular hybridization techniques, *Eur J Gynecol Oncol* 1992:13(3):236.

7. J. H. Dorsey, Understanding CO_2 laser surgery of the vulva, *Colposcopy & Gynecol Laser Surgery* 1984:1(3):205–13; A. L. Kaplan, et al., Intraepithelial carcinoma of the vulva with extension to the anal canal, *Obstet Gynecol* 1981:58:368–71.

8. Park et al., Possible aetiological heterogeneity of vulvar intraepithelial neoplasia; T. Toki, R. J. Kurman, J. S. Park, et al., Probable non-papillomavirus aetiology of squamous cell carcinoma of the vulva in older women: a clinico-pathological study using in-situ hybridization and polymerase chain reaction, *Int J Gynecol Pathol* 1991:10:107.

9. R. W. Jones, M. R. McLean, Carcinoma in situ of the vulva: a review of 31 treated and 5 untreated cases, *Obstet Gynecol* 1986:68:499.

10. J. D. Thompson, J. A. Rock, *Te Linde's Operative Gynecology* (Philadelphia: J. B. Lippincott, 1992).

11. A. Singer, J. M. Monaghan, *Lower Genital Tract Precancer* (Boston: Blackwell Scientific Publications, 1994).

12. Ibid.

13. M. J. Campion, N. F. Hacker, Vulvar intraepithelial neoplasia and carcinoma, *Semin Cutan Med Surg* 1998 September:17(3):205; V. Kuppers, M. Stiller, T. Somville, H. G. Bender, Risk factors for recurrent VIN: role of multifocality and grade of disease, *J Reprod Med* 1997:42(3):140.

14. Thompson, Rock, *Te Linde's Operative Gynecology*.

15. R. W. Jones, D. M. Rowan, Vulvar intraepithelial neoplasia: III. A clinical study of the outcome in 113 cases with relation to the later development of invasive vulvar carcinoma, *Obstet Gynecol* 1994:84:741.

16. J. Fanning, L. Lambert, T. M. Hale, et al., Paget's disease of the vulva: prevalence of associated vulvar adenocarcinoma, invasive Paget's disease, and recurrence after surgical excision, *Am J Obstet Gynecol* 1999:180:24.

17. P. J. DiSaia, W. T. Creasman, *Clinical Gynecologic Oncology* (St. Louis: Mosby Year Book, 1993), 263.

18. Fanning et al., Paget's disease of the vulva.

19. M. Sugase, T. Matsukara, Distinct manifestations of HPV in the vagina, *Int J Cancer* 1997 Jul 29:72(3):412.

Index

Note: Page numbers in *italic* refer to illustrations

acid-base balance (pH) test, 170
acidity, vaginal, 48–49, 56, 170
acidophilus, 53, 201–202
acrochordons (skin tags), 281, *281*
acyclovir, 373–375, 376–377
A fibers, 299–300
AGUS (atypical glandular cells of undeter-
    mined significance), 185
AIDS, 124, 295
albinism, 290
Aldara (imiquimod), 282, 384, 386, 401, 406
allergic seminal vulvovaginitis, 248–250
allergies, 247–253
  definition, 247–248
  dryness and, 147
  hives, 253
  latex, 251–253
  leading allergens, 259
  semen, 248–250
  yeast, 206–207
allodynia, 299
amitriptyline (Elavil), 275, 309, 311, 312,
    363
anaphylaxis, 248
Angier, Natalie, 31
angiokeratomas, 282
antiandrogens, 277
antibiotics, yeast and, 198, 202–204
antidepressants, tricyclic, 309–312
antihistamines, 261
aphthous ulcers, 294
art, female genitalia in, 5–6, 14, 18, 22, 125
ASCUS (atypical squamous cells of undeter-
    mined significance), 185–186
Astroglide, 112
asymptomatic shedders, 368–369
atrichia, 23
atrophic vaginitis, 237–239
atypical glandular cells of undetermined sig-
    nificance (AGUS), 185
atypical squamous cells of undetermined sig-
    nificance (ASCUS), 185–186
AutoPap, 181

babies, vulvovaginal development, 61–63
bacterial vaginosis (BV), 219–228
  diagnosis, 223–224
  odor, 134
  organism, 221
  pregnancy and childbirth and, 69, 222–223
  recurrence, 226
  risk factors, 221–222
  symptoms, 220
  treatments, 225–226
  yeast *vs.*, 220

bacteria, vaginal, 52–57. *See also* lactobacilli
Bartholin's duct cysts and abscesses,
    285–286, *286*
Bartholin's glands, 32, *32*
bathing practices, 83, 140, 147
Behcet disease, 296
Berman, Laura, 335
biopsies
  cone, *394*, 395–396
  vulvar, 173–174
birth control
  and bacterial vaginosis, 222
  device maintenance, 83
  diaphragms and urinary tract infections,
    350
  douching and, 101
  importance of, 128–129
  vaginal dryness and, 148
  yeast infections and, 198, 204–205
bladder infections. *See* urinary tract infec-
    tions
bladder pain. *See* interstitial cystitis; urinary
    tract infections
boric acid, 217–218, 227
branding, labial, 107
Bright, Susie, 66
Brown, Helen Gurley, 76
bubble bath, 64, 83
bumps, 279–288
  acrochordons (skin tags), 281, *281*
  angiokeratomas, 282
  Bartholin's duct cysts and abscesses,
    285–286, *286*
  endometriosis, 284
  fibroids, 287–288
  fibromas, 286
  Fox-Fordyce disease, 285
  Gartner's duct cysts, 283
  hemangiomas, 281–282
  hematomas, 286–287
  hernias, 287
  herpes simplex virus, 370–373
  hidradenoma, 283, *284*
  inclusion cysts, *280*, 280–281
  lipomas, 286
  lymphogranuloma venereum (LGV), 287
  molluscum, 282
  neurofibromas, 281
  pilonidal cysts, 283–284
  pyogenic granulomas, 282
  syringomas, 283
  vestibular cysts, 283
  vulvar cancer and precancer, 399, 403–404
  warts (human papillomavirus), 380–386
BV. *See* bacterial vaginosis (BV)

Camphausen, Christina, 22
cancer. *See also* precancer
  cervical, 379–380, 386–389
  definition, 388
  vulvar, 403–404
Candida albicans. See yeast infections
canker sores, 294
Carlson, Mary, 4
cell-mediated immunity, 368
cervical cancer, 379–380, 386–389. *See also*
  Pap test
cervical ectropion, 145
cervical precancer (cervical intraepithelial
    neoplasia, CIN)
  definition, 182, 387–388
  etiology, 390–392
  grades of, 182, 391–392
  HPV testing and, 389
  risk factors, 390
  treatment, 392–396
cervicography, 183
cervix, 50–52. *See also* Pap test
C fibers, 299–300
chancroid, 124, 295
chastity belts, 127
childbirth. *See* pregnancy and childbirth
childhood, vulvovaginal development,
    62–64, 63–65
chlamydia, 124, 174
chronic inflammation, 299–300, 303, 403
CIN. *See* cervical precancer
CIN 1, 185–186, 187, 391–392
CIN 2, 187, 392
CIN 3, 392
circumcision, female, 77
Claire, Ruth, 68
clindamycin, 225–226, 277
clinicians, vulvovaginal, 155–158
clitoris, 29–31, *30*
  clitorodynia, 328
  and orgasm, 116–117
  during sexual excitement, 113–114
clitorodynia, 328
clobetasol, 266–267
clothing, 83, 98–100, 139–140, 204, 262
clue cells, 223, *224*
color changes, 279–280, 288–296
  erythrasma, 289
  folliculitis, 288
  intertrigo, 290
  lentigo, 291
  melanomas, 293
  nevus (mole), *291*, 291–292
  partial albinism (piebaldism), 290
  postinflammatory hypopigmentation
    (leukoderma), 290
  pubic lice (crabs), 292
  radiation damage, 290
  reactive hyperpigmentation, 292
  ringworm of the groin, 289
  seborrheic keratosis, 292–293
  vitiligo, 289–290
colposcopy, 183
columnar epithelium, 390
condoms
  latex allergy and, 252, 253
  sexually transmitted diseases and, 127–128,
    376, 381

conization, *394*, 395–396
contraception. *See* birth control
cortisone, 244, 256–257, 270, 273–274
crabs (pubic lice), 292
cranberry juice, 348, 356
Crohn's disease, 295
cryotherapy, 393
cyclical vulvovaginitis. *See* yeast infections
cyclosporine, 277
cystitis. *See* urinary tract infections
cysts. *See under* bumps
cytolytic vaginosis, 245

dehydroepiandrosterone (DHEA), 76–77
Denman, Thomas, 10
depilatories, 104
dermatitis, 258–262
dermographism, 253
DES (diethylstilbestrol), 406
desensitization, 250
desquamative inflammatory vaginitis (DIV),
    242–245
detergents and soaps, 262
DHEA (dehydroepiandrosterone), 76–77
diaphragms, 350
diethylstilbestrol (DES), 406
Diflucan (fluconazole), 208, 211, 216–217,
    218, 225
dilators, 274, 315
discharge (secretions), 47–59
  amounts, 48, 51–52, 57–59, 144
  bacteria and, 52–57
  as birth control, 58
  cervix and, 50–52
  douching and, 101
  menstrual cycle and, 48–50
  normal, 47, 57–59
  postmenopausal, 59
  during pregnancy, 68, 69, 70
  problem finder, 192
  sexual lubrication, 112–113
  sources of, 47
  unusual, 144–146, 154
DIV. *See* desquamative inflammatory
    vaginitis
Dodson, Betty, 121
douching, 82, 100–102, 103, 222
dryness
  artificial lubricants, 112
  causes, 147–149
  menopause and, 73, 78, 149
  painful intercourse and, 148, 331
  problem finder, 192
dysesthetic vulvodynia. *See* vulvodynia
dyspareunia. *See* painful intercourse
dysplasia, 398

ectopic pregnancy, 102
eczema, 258–262
ejaculation, by women, 119
Elavil. *See* amitriptyline
electrolysis, 105–106
Elmiron (pentosan), 363
EMLA, 173–174
endometriosis, 88–90, 284
Ensler, Eve, 42
episiotomy, 34–35, 69
epithelium, 390

Eros, 344
erythrasma, 289
Escherichia coli, 53–54, 351, 355
escutcheons, *22*, 22–23
estrogen
  babies and children, levels of, 62, 63
  itching and, 143
  menopause and, 72–74, 237–239
  at puberty, 66
  urinary tract infections and, 351
  vaginal bacteria and, 55–56
  vaginal secretions and, 48–50
  vestibulodynia and, 304
  yeast infections and, 195–196
estrogen creams, 238–239
euphemisms and slang, 4, 13, 55, 64, 65

Fallopio, Gabriele, 9
female circumcision, 77, 79
FemExam, 171–172
feminine hygiene sprays, 82, 262, 304
fibroids, 287–288
fibromas, 286
fistulas, 146
Flagyl, 223, 225–226, 233–234
fluconazole. *See* Diflucan
folliculitis, 288
fourchette, 27
Fox-Fordyce disease, 285
Frank, Anne, 65
frenulum, *26*, 27
Freud, Sigmund, 120
Friedrich, Edward, 306
fumigation, 7, *7*

gabapentin (Neurontin), 312–313
Galen, Claudius, 7–8
Gartner's duct cysts, 283
glans clitoris, *26*, 29, *29*, 31. *See also* clitoris
Glazer, Howard, 314
Goetsch, Martha, 298
gonorrhea, 124, 174
Goodell, William, 10
Graaf, Regnier de, 9–10
granuloma inguinale (GI), 294–295
group B strep (GBS), 69, 240
G spot, 46, 117–118
gynecological examinations
  acid-base balance (pH) test, 169–170
  appointments, timing of, 160–161
  cervicography, 183
  colposcopy, 183
  diagnosis by telephone, 155–156
  evaluating symptoms, 151–155
  FemExam, 171–172
  finding and choosing a clinician, 155–158
  first, 187
  health history, 161–164
  Pap test (*See* Pap test)
  pelvic exams, 165–169
  skin scrapings, 173
  trichomonas cultures, 173
  vaginal cultures, 172
  vulvar biopsy, 173–174
  wet prep (wet mount, vaginal smear), 171
  whiff test, 170–171
  yeast cultures, 172–173

gynecologists, 155–158, 161, 171
gynecology, history of, 6–14

Haas, Earle, 81
hair follicles, blockage of, 275–277
hair removal, 102–106
hemangiomas, 281–282
hematomas, 286–287
hepatitis, 124
hernias, 287
herpes simplex virus (HSV), 365–378
  diagnosis, 372–373
  etiology, 366–367
  pregnancy and, 375–378
  prevention, 376
  risk factors, 368
  symptoms, 369–372
  transmission, 367–369, 375
  treatment, 373–375
  vestibulodynia and, 303
  vulvodynia and, 324, 326
herpes zoster (shingles), 324
heterochromia, 24
hidradenitis suppurativa (HS), 275–277
hidradenoma, 283, *284*
history of gynecology, 5–14
hives, 253
HIV, yeast infections and, 205
hormone replacement therapy (HRT), 73–74,
  239
hormones. *See specific hormones*
hot flashes, 78
HPV. *See* human papillomavirus
HRT. *See* hormone replacement therapy
HS. *See* hidradenitis suppurativa
HSIL (high-grade dysplasia, CIN2, CIN3),
  187
human papillomavirus (HPV), 379–396
  cervical cancer, 386–388, 395
  cervical precancer and, 388–394
  diagnosis, 382–383
  risk factors, 380, 381
  symptoms, 379–381
  transmission, 381
  treatment, 383–386
  types, 380, 395
  vestibulodynia and, 303, 304
  vulvar precancer, 397–403
hymen
  anatomy of, *32*, 32–34, *33*
  imperforate, 68
  virginity, 66–68, 90, 91, 93
hyperalgesia, 299
hypertrophy of the labia minora, 35
hypotrichosis, 22
hysterectomy, 396
hysteria, 119, 120

IgE, 247
imiquimod. *See* Aldara
immunosuppression and yeast infections, 205
imperforate hymen, 33–34, 68
inclusion cysts, *280*, 280–281
incontinence, 44, 136–137
inflammatory bowel disease (Crohn's
  disease), 295
intercourse, painful. *See* painful intercourse
interferon, 315–316

interstitial cystitis (IC), 358–364
  causes, 359
  diagnosis, 360–361
  symptoms, 359–360
  treatment, 361–364
  vulvodynia and, 327–328
intertrigo, 290
intraepithelial neoplasm, 388. *See also* cervical precancer; Paget's disease; vaginal precancer; vulvar precancer
intralabial folds, 25, *25*
intralabial sulcus, *25*
introitus, *28*, 29
irritants
  dryness and, 147
  eczema and, 258–259
  itching and, 140–142
  leading vulvar, 259
  vestibulodynia and, 304
  vulvar cancer and, 403
itching
  causes, 138–144
  evaluating, 154
  problem finder, 192

James, D. W., 249
Johnson, Virginia, 110, 114

Kegel exercises, 44
kidney infections, 353
K-Y jelly, 112

labia décor, 107
labial adhesion, 63–65
labial reduction, 35
labia majora, *19*, *20*, *21*, *23*, 23–25, *25*
labia minora, *25*, 25–27, *26*, 35
laboratory standards, 177–178
lactobacilli, 52–55
  bacterial vaginosis and, 221
  menopause and, 72
  overgrowth of, 245
  during pregnancy, 68
Lane, Dorrie, 125
laser hair removal, 106
laser treatment, 393–394
latex allergy, 251–253
LSC. *See* lichen simplex chronicus
LEEP (loop electrosurgical excision procedure), 394–395
lentigo, 291
leukoderm (postinflammatory hypopigmentation), 290
LGV. *See* lymphogranuloma venereum
lichen planus (LP), 243, 271–275
lichen sclerosus (LS), 262–269
  cancer and, 267
  cause, 264–265
  diagnosis, 265–266
  symptoms, 263–264, *264*
  treatment, 266–269
lichen simplex chronicus (LSC), 258–262
life cycle changes. *See* vulvovaginal life cycle changes
lipomas, 286
loop electrosurgical excision procedure (LEEP), 394–395

LP. *See* lichen planus
LS. *See* lichen sclerosus
LSC. *See* lichen simplex chronicus
LSIL (low-grade dysplasia, CIN1), 187
lubricants, artificial, 112
lymphogranuloma venereum (LGV), 287
Lynch, Peter, 242

mammarylike glands (MLG), 284
Margesson, Lynette, 326
Masters, William, 110, 114
masturbation, 121, 122–123
melanomas, 293
Melmed, M. Herzl, 305
menopause
  atrophic vaginitis, 237–239
  DHEA and, 76–77
  estrogen loss, 72–73
  hormone replacement therapy (HRT), 73–74
  painful intercourse, 331
  testosterone replacement, 74–76
  urinary tract infections, 351
  vaginal discharge after, 58–59
  vaginal dryness, 149
menstruation
  menstrual cups, 96–97
  pads, 93–95, 97–98
  panty liners, 95–96
  sea sponges, 98
  tampons (*See* tampons)
  vaginal bacteria, 55–56
  vaginal dryness and, 148
  vaginal secretions and, 48–50
merkins, 104
mobiluncus vaginitis, 226, 241–242
moles (nevi), *291*, 291–292
molluscum, 282
mons, *21*, 21–22
Morris, Desmond, 114

neoplasm, 387–388
nerve blocks, 316–317
nerve fibers, 299–300
neurofibromas, 281
Neurontin (gabapentin), 312–313
nevi (nevus), *291*, 291–292
Nin, Anaïs, 18
nitric oxide, 111, 112

odor, 132–138
  bacterial vaginosis (BV), 134
  as communication tool, 135
  douching and, 101
  individual differences, 132–133, 137–138
  problem finder, 192
  sweat, 135–136
  trichomonas and, 135
  from urine, 136–137
  yeast infections and, 134
orgasm, 116–121
orgasmic platform, 115
orthopedic injuries, vulvodynia and, 323–324
oxalate, 304–305, 308–309

pads, menstrual, 93–95, 97–98
Paget's disease, 404–407

painful intercourse (dyspareunia), 298. *See also* vestibulodynia; vulvodynia
  causes, 330–332
  clitorodynia, 328
  coping with, 336, 337–339
  desquamative inflammatory vaginitis (DIV), 242–245
  effects of, 332–334
  partner's reactions, 334–335
  problem finder, 192
  vaginismus, 341–343
pain theory, 298–301
panties, 98–100
panty hose, 99
panty liners, 82, 95–96
PAPNET, 181
Pap test, 174–187. *See also* cervical precancer
  abnormal, 182–187
  accuracy of, 181–182
  guidelines for good samples, 176–177
  interpretation of, 177–178, 180
  questions about, 179–180
  trichomonas and, 233
paraurethral glands, 29
PC (pubococcygeus) muscle, 44, 313–314
PDR (*Physicians' Desk Reference*), 310
pelvic exams, 6–7, 10, 10–11, 11, 165–167. *See also* gynecological examinations
pelvic inflammatory disease (PID), 101–102
pemphigoid, 295–296
pemphigus, 295–296
pentosan (Elmiron), 363
perimenopause, 71–72, 149, 238, 331
perineum, 18, 34
pheromones, 135
pH, vaginal, 48–49, 56, 170
Physicians' Desk Reference (PDR), 310
piercing, labial, 107
pigmentation changes. *See* color changes
pilonidal cysts, 283–284
pinworms, 143–144
plaque psoriasis, 269–271
polymer chain reaction (PCR), 389
postinflammatory hypopigmentation (leukoderma), 290
precancer
  cervical (*See* cervical precancer)
  vaginal, 407
  vulvar, 397–403
pregnancy and childbirth
  atrophic vaginitis and, 238
  bacterial vaginosis and, 69, 222–223
  douching and ectopic pregnancy, 102
  group B strep, 69
  herpes and, 375–378
  Pap tests, 180
  trichomonas, 69, 234
  urinary tract infections, 350
  vaginal bacteria during, 56
  vulvar precancer and, 402
  vulvodynia and, 324, 336, 339–341
  vulvovaginal changes during, 68–71
  yeast infections, 198, 204
prepuce, *26*
problem finder, 192
psoriasis, 269–271
puberty, 65–68, 187

pubic hair, *21, 22, 22–23, 24*
  dyeing, 106–107
  puberty and, *66*
  removal, 102–106
pubic lice (crabs), 292
pubikini, 104
pubococcygeus (PC) muscle, 44, 313–314
pudendal nerve, 321, 322–324, *323*
pyogenic granulomas, 282

Q-tip test, 307

radiation damage, 290
radioallergosorbent test (RAST), 249
reactive hyperpigmentation, 292
Replens, 228
retinoids, 277
ringworm of the groin, 289
rugae, 46

sea sponges, 98
seborrheic keratosis, 292–293
sebum, 24
secretions. *See* discharge
self-examination, 35–39, 409–410
semen allergy, 248–250
sexual activity
  bacterial vaginosis and, 221–222
  urinary tract infections and, 349–350, 351
  yeast infections and, 197–200
sexual desire, 75–76, 110, 343–344
sexual intercourse, painful. *See* painful intercourse
sexually transmitted diseases (STDs). *See also* herpes simplex virus; human papillomavirus
  AIDS, 295
  chancroid, 295
  chart, 124
  discharge, 145
  douching and, 101
  granuloma inguinale (GI), 294–295
  lymphogranuloma venereum (LGV), 287
  molluscum, 282
  routine testing for, 174
  safer sex guide, 82, 123–128
  syphilis, 294
  trichomonas (*See* trichomonas)
sexual response, stages of, 110–122
  excitement, *111*, 111–114
  orgasm, 116–121
  plateau, 114–115, *115*
  resolution, 122, *122*
Shakespearean euphemisms, 55
shaving, 104
shingles, 324
Skenes ducts, 29
skin conditions, 255–278
  eczema/dermatitis, 258–262
  hygiene rules, 262
  irritants, 259
  itching and, 142
  lichen planus (LP), 271–275
  lichen sclerosus (LS), 262–269
  lichen simplex chronicus (LSC), 260, 261
  psoriasis, 269–271
skin tags (acrochordons), 281, *281*

slang. *See* euphemisms and slang
Sobel, Jack, 242–243
Solomons, Clive, 304–305
speculums, 166–167, 169, *175, 177*
squamo-columnar junction (SCJ), 390–391
squamous epithelium, 46, 390
STDs. *See* sexually transmitted diseases
    (STDs)
steroids, 256–258
Stevens-Johnson syndrome, 295
strep vaginitis, 69, 240–241
striae, 256
sugar-yeast link, 200–201
superinfections, 240
sweat, odor from, 24–25, 135–136
symbolism, 4–5, 8, 19
syphilis, 124, 294
syringomas, 283

talcum powder, 82
tamoxifen, 239
tampons, 81–93, 94
    absorbency ratings, 86
    asbestos and dioxin in, 87
    deodorant, 82, 92
    endometriosis and, 88–90
    fit and comfort, 94
    history of, 81, 83–84
    lost or forgotten, 92, 137
    teens and, 67
    tips for use, 91–93
    toxic shock and, 84–86
    vaginal ulcers and, 87–88
    virginity and, 67, 90, 91, 93
tattoos, labial, 107
Taussig, Frederick, 10
testosterone, 65–66, 74–76
tests, gynecological. *See* gynecological exami-
    nations
Theroux, Alexander, 118
ThinPrep Pap test, 181
thongs, 100
Tinea cruris (ringworm of the groin), 289
toxic shock syndrome (TSS), 84–86
trichomonas, 124, 229–235
    cultures, 173
    diagnosis, 232–233
    odor, 135
    organism, 229–230
    premature delivery and, 69
    symptoms, 230–231
    transmission, 231
    treatment, 233–235
tricyclic antidepressants, 309–312

ulcers, 293–296. *See also* herpes simplex virus
    AIDS, 295
    Behcet disease, 296
    canker sores, 294
    chancroid, 295
    granuloma inguinale (GI), 294–295
    hidradenitis suppurativa (HS), 275–277
    inflammatory bowel disease (Crohn's dis-
        ease), 295
    pemphigus and pemphigoid, 295–296
    Stevens-Johnson syndrome, 295
    syphilis, 294
    tampons and, 87–88

underwear, 98–100
urethral opening, *28, 29*
urethral syndrome, 359
urinary tract, *28, 29, 349*
urinary tract infections (UTI), 347–358
    causative bacteria, 351
    cranberry juice and, 348, 356
    diagnosis, 353–355
    kidney infection and, 353
    prevention, 357–358
    recurrence and relapse, 351–352
    risk factors, 349–351
    self-treatment, 348
    symptoms, 348
    treatment, 355–357

vagina, 41–59
    absence of, 63
    bacteria of, 52–57
    description, 42–43, 45–47
    function of, 41–42
    medical knowledge of, 7–10
    size of, 45
vaginal cancer, 407
vaginal discharge. *See* discharge
vaginal precancer (vaginal intraepithelial
    neoplasia, VAIN), 407
vaginal smear. *See* wet prep
vaginismus, 298, 331, 341–343
vaginitis, 237–245. *See also* allergies; bacterial
    vaginosis; yeast infections
    atrophic (estrogen loss), 237–239
    desquamative inflammatory (DIV), 242–245
    lactobacillus overgrowth, 245
    little girls and, 64
    mobiluncus, 241–242
    premature delivery and, 69
    strep, 240–241
vaginosis. *See* bacterial vaginosis
VAIN, 407
varts, 115
Vaseline, 112
VBD. *See* vestibulodynia
VENIS (very erotic noninsertive sex), 335
Vesalius, Andreas, 8
vestibular cysts, 283
vestibule, 20–21, *21, 27,* 27–29
vestibulectomy, *316,* 317–320
vestibulitis. *See* vestibulodynia
vestibulodynia (VBD), 301–320
    antiseizure medications, 312–313
    causes, 302–306
    counseling, 316
    diagnosis, 306–307
    discomfort levels, 302
    inflammatory pain theory, 299–300
    interferon, 315–316
    interstitial cystitis and, 327–328
    oxalate and, 308–309
    physical therapy and biofeedback, 313–315
    primary *vs.* secondary, 302
    surgery, *316,* 316–320
    symptoms, 301–302
    tricyclic antidepressants, 309–312
    vaginismus and, 331, 342
Viagra, 111, 343–344
vibrators, 118, 121, 123
VIN. *See* vulvar precancer

Virapap, 389
virginity, 33, 67, 90, 91
vitiligo, 289–290
vulva, anatomy of, 17–39
  Bartholin's glands, 31–32, 32
  clitoris, 29–31, 30
  defined, 18–20, 19, 20, 21
  hymen, 32, 33, 33–34
  labia majora, 19, 20, 21, 23, 23–25, 25
  labia minora, 25, 25–27, 26, 35
  mons, 21, 21–22
  perineum, 34
  pubic hair, 21, 22, 22–23, 24
  purpose of, 18
  self-examination, 35–39
  urethral opening, 28, 29
  vestibule, 20, 21, 27, 27–29
vulva puppets, 125
vulvar biopsy, 173–174
vulvar cancer, 403–404
vulvar precancer (vulvar intraepithelial neo-
    plasia, VIN), 397–403
  categories, 398, 400
  diagnosis, 399–400
  pregnancy and, 402
  recurrence, 402
  treatment, 400–403
  in women over fifty, 399, 403
  in young women, 398
vulvodynia (VVD), 321–328. See also vestibu-
    lodynia
  causes, 300–301, 322–324
  definition, 297–298
  diagnosis, 324–325
  dryness and, 148
  interstitial cystitis and, 327–328
  pregnancy and, 336
  prevalence of, 298
  sex and, 337–338
  symptoms, 321–322
  treatment, 324–327
  Viagra and, 343–344
vulvo-vaginal-gingival syndrome (VVG), 273
vulvovaginal health care
  education and research, 411–413
  individual responsibility, 409–410

vulvovaginal life cycle changes
  childhood, 62–64
  menopause, 72–79
  pregnancy and childbirth, 68–71
  prenatal and newborn, 61–63
VVD. See vulvodynia

warts, 380–386
waxing, 105
West, Mae, 333
wet prep (wet mount, vaginal smear), 55,
    171
whiff test, 170–171
Woodruff, Donald, 318

yeast cultures, 172–173, 207–208
yeast infections, 190–218
  as allergy, 206–207, 218
  alternative/herbal remedies, 213
  antibiotics and, 202–204
  causative organism, 193–195, 194
  clothing and, 204
  complicated vs. uncomplicated,
    214
  contraceptives and, 204–205
  diagnosis, 190–192, 207–210
  diet and, 200
  estrogen and, 195–196
  as factor in other diseases, 203
  genetics and, 205–206
  immunosuppression and, 205
  odor, 134
  painful intercourse, 330
  recurrent, 212–214
  reservoir of infection theory, 218
  risk factors, 197–207
  self-diagnosis and treatment,
    208–212
  sex and, 197–200
  symptoms, 196–197
  systemic, 203
  treatment, 216–218
  vestibulodynia and, 303–304
  vs. bacterial vaginosis, 220
yogurt and yeast infections, 201–202
yoni, 5, 5–6

About the Authors

Elizabeth Gunther Stewart, M.D., FACOG, a Boston-based gynecologist, is director of the Stewart-Forbes Vulvovaginal Specialty Service at Harvard Vanguard Medical Associates. Dr. Stewart is also Assistant Professor of Obstetrics and Gynecology at Harvard Medical School and a member of Brigham and Women's Hospital staff. She speaks extensively about vulvovaginal disease to medical professionals. Her perspectives as a full-time vulvovaginal practitioner, a researcher, and a teacher shape her prominence as one of the leading voices advocating the emerging importance of her specialty. This book is an extension of her lectures, her clinical experience with patients, and patient-education materials she has prepared for them.

Paula Spencer specializes in health and family subjects for *Woman's Day, Glamour, Parenting, Baby Talk, USA Weekend,* and other publications. She is the author of four books on pregnancy and parenting, including *Everything ELSE You Need to Know When You're Expecting* (St. Martin's Press).